MANUAL OF OSTEOPATHIC PRACTICE

By the same author

MANUAL OF OSTEOPATHIC TECHNIQUE

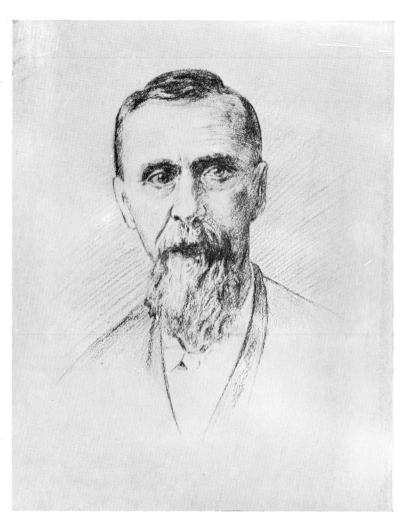

Dr. Andrew Taylor Still

MANUAL OF OSTEOPATHIC PRACTICE

ALAN STODDARD

M.B. B.S. D.O. D.Phys.Med

Consultant in Physical Medicine, Brook Hospital, London

HUTCHINSON

London Melbourne Sydney Auckland Johannesburg

Hutchinson & Co. (Publishers) Ltd

An imprint of the Hutchinson Publishing Group

17–21 Conway Street, London WIP 6JD

Hutchinson Group (Australia) Pty Ltd
30–32 Cremorne Street, Richmond South, Victoria 3121
PO Box 151, Broadway, New South Wales 2007

Hutchinson Group (NZ) Ltd
32–34 View Road, PO Box 40–086, Glenfield, Auckland 10

Hutchinson Group (SA) (Pty) Ltd
PO Box 337, Bergvlei 2012, South Africa

First published 1969
Reprinted 1974, 1977, 1980 and 1982

Printed in Great Britain by The Anchor Press Ltd
and bound by Wm Brendon & Son Ltd
both of Tiptree, Essex

ISBN 0 09 089790 0

This manual of osteopathic practice and its companion volume on osteopathic technique are dedicated to all those practitioners of whatever persuasion who wish to excel in the art of manipulation.

CONTENTS

Preface   xiii

1 THE PRINCIPLES OF OSTEOPATHY   1

Definition   1
Structure governs function   4
Mechanical effects on:
  1 Nerves   6
  2 Blood-vessels   19
  3 Viscera   23
  4 Bone   23
  5 Joints   24
  6 Muscle   32
  7 Skin   33
Compensatory mechanisms   33
The osteopathic spinal lesion   36
  Features   39
  Mobility   43
  Position   44
  Pain and tenderness   50
  Reflex muscular contraction   53
  Reflex changes   55

2 MECHANICAL DIAGNOSIS   56

General considerations   57
  Body types   57
  Occupational and outdoor activities   62
  Trauma   63
  Gross mechanical disorders   64
Detailed considerations in the differential diagnosis of
mechanical lesions   65
  Pain   66
  Tenderness   72

Paraesthesiae (hyperaesthesia and anaesthesia)   73
Mobility   74
Locking   81
Displacement   83
Muscle tone   87
Soft-tissue changes   89
Skin changes   91
Clinical examination and procedure   92
Radiological examination   99
Interpretation of symptoms and signs relative to the spine 100
Local anaesthesia   106

3 CLINICAL SPINAL SYNDROMES AND THEIR MANAGEMENT 108

List of causes of spinal pain   110
List of clinical spinal syndromes   112
   1   Adhesion   114
   2   Ligamentous strain   119
   3   Acute episodic   136
   4   Chronic degenerative   150
   5   Lordosis   156
   6   Nerve-root   168
   7   Peripheral nerve lesions of the lower extremity   183
   8   Sacro-iliac   184
   9   Ankylosing spondylitis   190
  10   Coccygeal   193
  11   Thoracic and rib   194
  12   Brachial   203
  13   Occipital and upper cervical   219
  14   Cervical myelopathy and amyotrophic neuropathy   234
  15   Soft tissue   236
  16   Osteochondritis   240
  17   Kyphosis   244
  18   Scoliosis   252
  19   Spinal gout   255
  20   Spinal osteitis   260
  21   Neoplastic bone and nerve   261
  22   Miscellaneous and rare spinal diseases   264
  23   Visceral backache   265
  24   Psychogenic   267

4 THE ART OF OSTEOPATHY   270

Appendix   1   Contra-indications to manipulation   279
           2   Osteopathic research   281

References   291

Index   297

ACKNOWLEDGMENTS

I am much indebted to Dr. John Barrett and Dr. Doreen Handel, who during the preparation of this book helped me so much with constructive criticisms. To my secretaries my thanks for their patient typing and retyping of my illegible script. I am also most grateful to all those who have made contributions to osteopathy and to all the knowledge which I have tried to amalgamate into a presentable manual of osteopathic practice. The idea of this book emanated from readers of my *Manual of Osteopathic Technique* who sent appreciative comments, implying, however, that it was not sufficient merely to know techniques, but one must know how to apply them under the right conditions at the correct time on the correct patient and in a correct sequence. These ideas were constantly in my mind as I wrote the following pages in the hope that the book would be helpful to those who, having acquired good techniques already, would like to apply them to maximum advantage.

Zeal without knowledge is
Fire without light

OLD ENGLISH PROVERB

PREFACE

The practice of osteopathy has changed radically since its inception in 1874 when Dr. Andrew Taylor Still first promulgated his ideas on health and disease and their relationship to the physical structures of the body. His knowledge, and indeed the world's knowledge, of medical subjects in those days was very limited compared with that of the present day. With this increase of knowledge medicine has changed completely, and the practice of osteopathy has inevitably been modified; yet the basic ideas enunciated by Still remain sound.

His basic concept was that the body is a vital machine—an anatomical structure with physiological functions—that would remain healthy so long as it remained structurally normal; and if structurally disturbed this would have an adverse effect on its function. He contended that one of the main reasons for illness was structural abnormality. He maintained that structure governed function, and, although we cannot agree nowadays that this is entirely true, there is sufficient truth in the rule that structure controls function to make it invaluable in its practical application.

We know that structure and function are reciprocal and complementary. During growth physiological processes have a dominant influence, but once the body has achieved its final structural form it remains almost static. Alteration of structure, as for example by injury, then adversely affects the function of the injured part, and, when serious enough, the functioning of the body as a whole suffers. Similarly, the alteration of structure by faulty posture or occupational stress influences bodily function adversely.

Osteopathy is concerned with the study of structural and mechanical faults in the body, and with the manner in which these faults influence physiological processes. In practice it is concerned with the diagnosis of mechanical derangements together with the methods by which these faults can be corrected mechanically. Some of the techniques for correction of mechanical faults in the spine are described in detail in the companion volume—a *Manual of Osteopathic Technique*. It is not the purpose of this book to reiterate those methods in detail. Here is explained not how to manipulate, but why, when, and where to manipulate.

Although manipulation is the keystone of osteopathic management, it is not the only mechanical procedure. Some mechanical problems require mechanical aids, supportive exercises, correction of posture, or even surgical procedures to restore proper mechanics. With other mechanical problems manipulations may be contraindicated. In Chapter 3 on 'Clinical Spinal Syndromes and their Management' treatment other than and in addition to manipulation is discussed.

In this book mechanical diagnosis (as distinct from the diagnosis of the osteopathic spinal lesion) is elaborated; and I shall describe the treatment immediately after consideration of the diagnosis of the individual syndromes, so that the reader can grasp the significance of the recommended management.

Osteopathy does not ignore the significance of the many other factors in health and disease, but its standpoint is the *emphasis* on mechanical factors. There was a stage in the history of osteopathy when mechanical faults were the be all and end all of its philosophy, and in the latter part of the nineteenth century this seemed reasonable because orthodox medicine had very little to offer. For example, on January 2nd, 1875, a writer in the *British Medical Journal* advised treating diabetes with mineral acids, bark, and opium. In the same issue Dr. Conrad said that vinegar had some power to modify the eruption of smallpox; cancer of the skin was treated with arsenical paste; and enuresis was treated with strychnine. In the light of modern therapeutics these were foolish and dangerous practices. A. T. Still recognised the uselessness of the drugs of those days, and started the first American School of Osteopathy in Kirksville, Missouri, in 1892. Still offered a practical alternative to blood-letting, leeches, and poisons, and he fostered the natural regenerative powers of the body. He was one of the vanguard in supporting drugless systems of healing. At that time, even within the ranks of the medical profession, doctors were beginning to question the efficacy of drugs. In 1894 William Osler first published his *Principles of Practice of Medicine*, in which he denigrated the use of drugs and extolled the value of diet, good nursing, and hydrotherapy. He stated: 'Medical antipyretics are not of much service in comparison with cold water. . . . The profession has long learned that typhoid fever is not a disease to be treated by medicines. . . . Many specifics have been vaunted in scarlet fever but they are all useless.'

In 1864 three of Still's children developed meningitis and died despite all the medical care he could get, and this shattered his faith in drugs. Quoting from his autobiography:[1]

It was when I stood gazing upon three members of my family, all dead from spinal meningitis, that I propounded to myself the serious question 'In, sickness, has God left man in a world of guessing? Guess what is the matter? What to give and guess the result? And when dead, guess where he goes?' I decided then, that God was not a guessing God but a God of truth. All His works spiritual and material are harmonious. His law of animal life is absolute. So wise a God had certainly placed the remedy within the material house in which the spirit of life dwells.

This tragedy in A. T. Still's life coloured all his thoughts appertaining to medicine, and he turned to religion and God to find an answer. Making the assumption that God had provided the gift of life, He must therefore provide the means of keeping the body healthy. To what should A. T. Still turn? Drugs were useless. What else was there? How did animals keep healthy? When disease affected them how did they recover? There must be some inherent healing force. How did this break down? What prevented the healing forces from working successfully in restoring health? These were the thoughts which plagued him. He had a mechanical turn of mind and had invented several mechanical devices for use on the farm where he lived. He began to think of the body as a machine. What went wrong with the machine to produce disease? Could it be that the mechanical components of the machine actually became displaced, so interfering with the mechanisms of circulation and of nerve-supply?

For ten years he studied the anatomy of the body; he dug up bodies from their graves and dissected them, and he carried bones with him in his pockets in order to dwell upon their structure and function. Then in 1874 he formulated his conception of health and disease and called it osteopathy. Quoting again from his autobiography (p. 343), he stated: 'I took the position in 1874 that the living blood swarmed with health corpuscles which were carried to all parts of the body. Interfere with that current of blood and you steam down the river of life and land in the ocean of death.' This picturesque style of writing did not endear him to medical readers. They rejected his ideas also, and in the light of modern knowledge we now know that much of what he said was wrong. Osteopathic theory has been severely criticised, but *no one in the osteopathic profession now maintains that lesions in the spinal column are the sole cause of disease.*

Still claimed that osteopathy was a complete system of healing, and he held the view that—apart from surgery and midwifery—there was no need to rely on any form of treatment other than the correction of the structural faults in the body. Basing his treatment on the theme that a structurally sound body should function healthily, he treated everything from typhoid fever to croup and from dislocated hips to dysentery by manipulating the spine and peripheral joints. He stopped using drugs, and he relied on natural immunity. In his own sphere of influence he put a stop to iatrogenic disease. His patients got better not merely because he manipulated their spines but because he inspired confidence and allowed the natural immunity of the body full play. Clearly Dr. Still misinterpreted the reason for his patients' recovery and attributed it to his manipulation of the spinal lesion.

So began to grow the excessive claims of the early osteopaths that osteopathy was a complete system in its own right. Over the past eighty years osteopaths have been slow to relinquish these claims, but a better perspective has been achieved by the majority. They realise that the scope of osteopathy is more limited than before, though there is difficulty in delineating its efficacy in any one patient. It is also impossible to say whether osteopathy is effective or not in any one disorder. So much depends in each case on the structural factors, the type of patient, and the competence of the practitioner, but it is still as true as ever, whatever the patient's disease, that he will have a better chance of full recovery if he is mechanically sound.

Early in its history the American Osteopathic Association adopted the definition (attributed to Dr. C. B. Atzen[2]): 'Osteopathy is the name of that system of the healing art which places chief emphasis on the structural integrity of the body mechanism as being the most important single factor in the maintenance of the well-being of the organism in health or disease.' The first part of this definition—that the system lays chief emphasis on structural integrity—still holds good; but the second part certainly cannot be maintained, and modern osteopathic teachers do not make any such claim.

The *Osteopathic Blue Book*, which was compiled in Britain by the Register of Osteopaths in 1956, states that 'osteopathy is a system of therapeutics which lays chief emphasis upon the diagnosis and treatment of structural and mechanical derangements of the body'. Here there is no claim to treat general disorders and diseases of the body, and the scope of osteopathy is vastly reduced. By limiting themselves to this sphere of action, osteopaths have become more acceptable to the medical profession, and in this lesser sphere their methods are already largely accepted even though much of the theory is still debatable.

As the reader peruses these chapters I hope he or she will glean some idea of the scope of osteopathic practice, realising that while the principle that structure governs function has no theoretical limit there are often very definite practical limits to its application.

It is my intention to present a realistic view of osteopathic theory and practice in this manual, and in this way I hope that the system will gain a further measure of recognition.

As medicine has advanced, the scope of osteopathy has diminished. This is not to decry the value of osteopathy, for we know its limitations, but it is more important that we know what it encompasses, and this is greater than our medical colleagues will admit.

While osteopathic teaching and ideas have been moulded by medical views, the converse is also true. In the past century and well into this one, medical men believed that brachial neuritis was caused by infection and rheumatism. Now the neuritis is recognised as essentially mechanical in origin from disc lesions, intervertebral foraminal compression, costoclavicular compression, carpal-tunnel compression, and cervical ribs. All these are mechanical faults which disturb the nerve-supply to the arm.

The influence of mechanical pressure on peripheral nerves has now been well documented. The study of the effect of mechanical faults on the central nervous system and the spinal cord is proceeding, but that related to the autonomic nervous system has hardly started. It is now well recognised that vasomotor disturbances occur in limbs secondarily to prolapsed discs, yet the wider implications of these observations are largely ignored.

The osteopathic profession has laid emphasis on the influence of mechanical lesions on nerve roots, on the autonomic nerves, and on the spinal cord. The research workers at Kirksville, Missouri, have made observations both in animals and humans on the effects of mechanical lesions on central and peripheral nerves, the effects of mechanical stress on the body framework, and the subsequent responses in the muscular, sudomotor and vasomotor systems. They have studied viscero-somatic reflexes, somatico-visceral reflexes, and viscero-visceral reflexes; but Cole,[3] who is one of the leading research workers in osteopathy, came to the conclusion that 'no basic study has ever completely substantiated the theories of osteopathic medicine'. Yet Korr,[4] another leading research worker at Kirksville, stated that

the osteopathic profession has earned its place in history and society, through having developed and effectively and skilfully applied a system of diagnosis and therapeutics based on the role of the somatic structures in disease. It has demonstrated, although it is not yet recognised by the other schools, that the somatic component can be most directly and effectively influenced and controlled by adjustment of the vertebral and paravertebral structures.

Much osteopathic research has been done and more is in preparation, and reference will be made to the results of this work as well as to the applications and implications of the new knowledge throughout the book as well as in the Appendix; but because research is such a complex study and the influence of mechanical faults on body function still remains incompletely understood, there must be room for conjecture. The substance of this book is therefore *based on clinical observations*, rationalised from existing knowledge and confirmed by favourable responses to treatment, rather than on theoretical considerations.

My objective in this *Manual of Osteopathic Practice* is to set down those aspects of osteopathic medicine which I personally think are significant. They are the culmination of some thirty years of careful study during which I have recorded my clinical observations, and I present those osteopathic procedures which in my experience are the most valuable. I have already set down in my *Manual of Osteopathic Technique* detailed descriptions of how to manipulate the spine. Now I want to explain in detail why, when, and where to use these techniques; to say something of the art of manipulation; to discuss the conduct of an osteopathic practice; and to describe the handling of patients as a whole and not merely their lesions.

In my technical manual there is no reference, except in the broadest sense, to the application of different techniques in the conditions which we are called upon to treat. Here I attempt to convey the osteopathic approach to mechanical problems—namely, how much treatment to give, when to give it and when to withhold it, the estimated duration of treatment, the progression, and what to expect from following technical procedures. This is the art of the application of techniques, not the description of the techniques themselves.

Osteopathic treatment is not something one can prescribe like a drug with a specific dosage three times a day, three times a week, or once a fortnight. Any attempt to prescribe in detail the exact amount of force or the exact sequence of each manœuvre is difficult, if not impossible. To learn osteopathy by a rigid set of rules is useless, and this is why it is not easy for a medical graduate to re-orientate himself into the osteo-pathic mode of thinking. He is schooled into thinking in terms of prescriptions—of drugs, of surgical procedures, or of a series of electro-convulsive therapy treatments. With this outlook he approaches mani-pulation in a similar way: he thinks, 'Here we have a disorder—a syn-drome if not a disease—in which manipulation is helpful. We must therefore prescribe a manipulation or a series of manipulations to tally exactly. This series should be set down step by step so that some auxiliary can do it'. This is the basis of medical thinking, as when a physiothe-rapist is given a series of, say, six set techniques to be performed on all disc lesions. If one does not work, proceed to the next.

This system, while it might be the best that can devised under some circumstances, is a poor second to the system whereby the physician himself, having a comprehensive grasp of his subject, makes the diagnosis as he goes along, and adapts his technique and programme accordingly—if necessary at every visit of his patient. In other words, the practice of osteopathy is not just manipulation: it calls for understanding of the mechanical problem and of the patient, the recognition of other contributory factors, and the adaption of the technique at the very moment when the patient is being treated: it is the *art of medicine applied in a particular sphere.*

A few techniques can be acquired by a physiotherapist or a general practitioner—or by a farmer, for that matter (and who can deny that lay bone-setters are sometimes successful!)—and applying them will give a measure of success; but this is not osteopathy. Osteopathy is infinitely wider: it is the application of healing using not merely the hands but the whole being of the doctor. His hands are his instruments, and what more delicate or refined instrument is there on this earth? The hands communicate. They are the liaison between physician and patient. They impart a manipulation, yes, but they should impart vastly more than this—namely, confidence, experience, healing, and the power of suggestion. The doctor who administers the remedy with his own hands is in a far stronger position to influence his patient than is the one who administers the remedy remotely—i.e. through a third person— however good is the technique or however good the technician. If the patient is treated by a third person the patient has to transfer his allegiance and his confidence to that third person before he can respond.

A good doctor inspires confidence in his patient because he relies on his knowledge and experience. He examines his patient manually and instantly transmits a feeling of assurance. The good osteopath not only does this at the first visit, but he does it repeatedly and all the time. In the mere handling of the patient the influence for good is tremendous without even going on to specific and skilled manipulations. Unless a rapport is established between doctor and patient, a good response is unlikely however skilled the doctor might be. Incidentally, a patient can tell almost at once whether the doctor has confidence in himself or not. A doctor who is unsure of himself as to his knowledge or experience or skill transmits this uncertainty directly to the patient as soon as manual contact is made. It is possible sometimes by words and demeanour for the doctor to give the impression of knowledge, but as soon as physical contact is made with the patient the sham of uncertainty is expressed and no disguise is possible.

In writing this book I assume that the reader has a good knowledge of the basic sciences of anatomy and physiology, and of clinical medicine.

I do not intend to describe the whole range of the application of osteopathy. It is not my purpose to write a textbook of medicine adding an osteopathic footnote disease by disease. I have left out the osteopathic treatment of pneumonia, for example, because it is irrelevant in these days of antibiotics. I have omitted the diagnostic features of tuberculosis because these are far better described in other textbooks. What I have tried to set down are the aspects of osteopathic practice which are different—i.e. those which I think are better than the ones in current orthodox practice. Therefore by omission I infer agreement, and by commission I infer an alternative and perhaps better approach. This may help to bring what is good in osteopathy into medicine, and therefore improve the medical management of mechanical problems; and I hope it will encourage a deeper recognition of the inherent powers of healing within the body so that reliance on extraneous agencies such as drugs will diminish.

My intention is to write in as practical a way as I know how, so that the reader will obtain as much first-hand information as I can offer. But without grasping the basic tenets of the theme—i.e. the principles of osteopathy—the practice will not follow smoothly or intelligently. Several whole books have been written on the principles of osteopathy, but it should be possible to state these briefly and succinctly; therefore I have devoted a relatively short chapter to 'principles' and the rest of the manual to 'practice'. I have not attempted to deal with individual diseases as such, except where some special practical technique appertains, because this would spoil the basic idea that whatever the disorder, the principle behind treatment is to restore proper and harmonious mechanics.

Any valid observations from any source, whether osteopathic or medical or purely scientific, concerning the structure and function of the body are gathered into the compass of osteopathy. A. T. Still originally stated a principle, that 'Structure governs function', and he attempted to apply this theme in diagnosis and treatment. Subsequent osteopathic physicians and societies have elaborated this idea. The osteopathic contributions are to be described here, but I make no excuse for using information relative to this theme from any source. Medical researches in this field have added materially to our knowledge of osteopathy and helped to confirm the osteopathic concept, and although the medical profession has been slow to accept the view that structural faults adversely influence function, osteopaths have been quick to absorb into their philosophy any medical knowledge which has been forthcoming and which is supportive to the main theme.

Undoubtedly the study of intervertebral disc degeneration and its clinical manifestations has focussed medical attention on to mechanical

disorders of the spine, and a more acceptable basis has been discovered
for some spinal syndromes; yet there is more to the spine than the discs.
The discs are just one component of a complex spinal segment consisting
of bones, cartilages, ligaments, nerves, and blood-vessels. All of these
have to be considered, and this is what osteopathy has emphasised over
the years. Intervertebral disc prolapse is a relatively terminal and
relatively pathological state of the osteopathic spinal lesion; and the
osteopathic lesion might have been present for years before the incapacitating clinical manifestations of disc protrusions ensue. If gastritis is
recognised and properly treated, ulceration and neoplastic changes ought
not to follow. If osteopathic spinal lesions are recognised and properly
treated, disc herniations and prolapses should not develop later.

The emphasis on mechanical disorders of the body does not or should
not blind the osteopath to other factors in health and disease, just as
the emphasis on mental stresses should not blind the psychotherapist
to the influences of bacteria or vitamin deficiencies. But the vast range of
human knowledge and endeavour precludes the study in detail of all
branches of medicine by any one man. The detailed study of mechanical
problems is the specialised contribution of osteopathy, and to that
extent we recognise the limitations of osteopathy both in diagnosis and
treatment. This is the limitation of specialisation; but one hopes that
the specialist in one field will not keep his mind and studies in water-
tight compartments. Let there be more co-ordination of all the branches
of medicine, and let osteopathy be a part of the whole. But until the
medical profession recognises and accepts the contribution which
osteopathy has made and can continue to make, the need for separate
schools will exist.

THE PRINCIPLES OF OSTEOPATHY

DEFINITION

Osteopathy is a system of healing in which chief emphasis is placed on the structural and mechanical problems of the body. The practice of osteopathy, while recognising that human beings are complex entities influenced by a wide range of environmental and inherent factors, is concerned primarily with the mechanics of the body—how far the body is structurally normal or where it is abnormal, how that abnormality influences its health, and how to restore normal mechanics or when that is not possible how best to help the body adapt itself to its structural weakness.

In this broad sense osteopathy is far from being a complete system of medicine, but it is in this context that this book is written. Our chief interest lies in the diagnosis and treatment of mechanical problems in spite of the fact that the effects of these problems impinge upon every branch of medicine. Any structure of the body in the head, the neck, the limbs, the torso, the viscera, and the spine can be affected by mechanical faults but the compass of such a vast subject is not attempted here. Only the spinal column and its faults are described in detail.

In Chapter 3 the reader will find my own attempt to classify, analyse, and treat the most common of the syndromes which involve the spinal column. The subject of spinal syndromes is dealt with in as practical a manner as possible without the introduction of too many theoretical considerations, so that those readers who wish to learn of the practical contributions of osteopathy to spinal problems should now turn to p. 108 for this purpose. In that chapter I have tried to draw spinal problems in balanced perspective, not to overemphasise the intervertebral disc or the defects of the partes interarticulares or the displacements of bones, but to list the causes of back problems and then to collate these into syndromes, and to try and bring some semblance of order into the confusion which is current in medical thought.

Although I hope that the description of syndromes and their treatment will be useful even to those who do not wish to go too deeply into the subject, the reader will be well advised to read on to obtain a broad grasp of the principles of osteopathic theory which underlie osteopathic practice. He will then be able to apply the treatment more effectively and more intelligently, rather than by rule of thumb.

The basic theme of osteopathy is that mechanical and structural abnormalities adversely affect the harmony and efficiency of the body. These faults can sometimes persist long enough for disease to ensue, though the body is constantly attempting to restore itself to health. Spontaneous restoration of well-being after accident or illness is the rule: how else would the human race survive? Even serious mechanical disruption caused by accidents can be restored by spontaneous healing. Most fractures unite whether we help Nature or not; but the result is functionally better if, during the repair, we splint the bones in correct alignment. Even if the alignment is faulty, the body tries to adapt itself and its structure to function as efficiently as possible. It should be our aim to help Nature as much as we can by removing any mechanical hindrance to the restoration of efficient function. Functional efficiency and harmonious physiology is what we and our patients desire rather than perfection in shape. Because of this the restoration of structural integrity is not the be all and end all of treatment, though in most cases the restoration of proper shape and alignment does result in the restoration of normal function. It is quite feasible, by surgery for example, to replace two broken bony fragments perfectly and yet to ignore the functional efficiency of adjacent joints—i.e. it is possible to restore normal alignment and yet not to restore good function. Ideally we should attempt to restore both perfection in structure and harmonious function, but of the two the function is the more important.

When we manipulate the spine, therefore, we are not so much concerned with putting a bone back into place as with removing any mechanical hindrance to the restoration of normal movements in the affected joints. Our concept embraces not merely that of static structural problems but also that of *dynamic mechanics*. The positional concept of osteopathy is incomplete: it may be essential in some cases to deal with the position of, say, the sacrum, because the base of the spine must be level, but in other spinal areas the mobility of the intervertebral joint is far more significant than is its positional relationship with the vertebrae below.

To use the analogy of fractures further, if a fracture involving a joint leads to irregularity of the joint surfaces, then the joint will be adversely affected and in time it will become diseased: osteo-arthritis will set in, the patient will suffer pain and stiffness, his body will have to adapt itself to that disease, and his general well-being will deteriorate.

If the joint is dislocated the bones must be replaced, otherwise it will never function efficiently again. Similarly if a joint is subluxated the joint must be realigned and the ligaments must be restored before it can function normally again: a subluxated joint *may* move fairly well, and the repair processes may be sufficient to restore it to functional efficiency, but often the joint remains only partially effective and recovery is imperfect. In some circumstances this matters a great deal, because an imperfectly functioning structure predisposes to disease. Imperfect function in joints matters most in the spinal column because of the proximity of the spinal cord and spinal nerves. If these vital structures are adversely affected by faulty mechanics, as will be shown later, then health is impaired and disease may ensue.

Local structural faults impair function locally, but adaptation may be so good that no generalised effect is apparent. For example, a chronic sprain of the ankle may merely slightly impede walking and never affect the body generally, but it can have a wider influence because the whole limb is slightly limited by the reduction in ankle movements; the gait and posture may be altered and so disturb the mechanics of the spine. In due course this may lead to ligamentous and muscular strains, and eventually to degenerative changes in the spine.

If a peripheral bone is fractured and the injury involves an adjacent nerve, then the function of that nerve is impaired. For example, a Colles fracture may alter the mechanics of the carpal tunnel so that the median nerve is irritated or compressed. The mechanical irritation can cause peripheral and central effects—pain in the thumb, index, and middle fingers, and also pain extending back to the forearm and arm. Similar changes can result from irritation of nerve-roots from mechanical injuries in the spine.

A fracture may involve blood-vessels and their vasomotor nerves to set up vascular spasm and sometimes trophic changes. A prolasped disc may not only press on peripheral nerves to produce paralysis, numbness, and loss of reflexes but also disturb vasomotor tone, leading to vascular changes at the periphery. Because vasomotor and viscero-motor nerves follow similar pathways, it is logical to assume that pressure and irritation of nerve-roots in the spinal column can impair viscero-motion as well as vasomotion. The best known example of this is in cauda equina lesions, when bladder and bowel control are lost. The peripheral effects of vasomotor irritation or paralysis are vasconstric-tion or vasodilatation, or an alternation of both; sudomotor activity is impaired, the skin becomes shiny and atrophic, and oedema and stiffness ensue. If severe enough or prolonged enough, ulceration or even gangrene can set in purely as the result of a mechanical effect on a peripheral nerve.

These are examples where altered structure affects function. At first the physiological disturbance is likely to cause an excess of activity. Later, owing to fatigue of the nerves, the activity tends to be reduced. In either case, if underactivity or overactivity of any function is protracted, pathological changes can ensue.

The effects of disturbed vasomotion are easy to observe in the extremities. It is less easy to see the effects of disturbed vasomotion and visceromotion in the thoracic and abdominal cavities, yet assuredly these disturbances do occur. The evidence for this will be discussed later in this chapter.

STRUCTURE GOVERNS FUNCTION

If the reader agrees with these premises so far, the theme can be developed still further. Physical and mechanical factors which influence the body are gravity, pressure, weight, inertia, compression, elasticity, leverage, movement, stretch, expansion, and contraction.

The mechanical effects of heat, light, sound, magnetism, and electricity do not concern us here, neither do the secondary mechanical effects of bacterial, chemical, and pathological changes. For example, the mechanical blockage of an artery by thrombosis or the mechanical pressure from an expanding neoplasm are not dealt with because the pathological processes themselves are not of mechanical origin.

The physical forces mentioned above work constantly and continuously: life could not go on without them. The normal contraction of muscle counteracts gravity; the elasticity of ligaments permits joints to move; movements like those of respiration affect the circulation of blood in the abdominal and thoracic cavities. Countless physical and mechanical forces act and interact with each other. This is the realm of applied mechanics in the human body, and there is much research both inside and outside medicine on these subjects.

Although the study of applied mechanics to the body is not the sole prerogative of osteopathy, it holds a special place because the erect posture of man places undue strains on the spine and peripheral joints; because the spine is vulnerable even to normal mechanical stresses; because the central nervous system depends upon the integrity of the spinal column; because all the afferent and efferent pathways between the brain, the spinal cord, and the peripheral nerves have to traverse the vulnerable intervertebral foramina; and because all these factors have a direct bearing on health and disease.

In the practical work of osteopathy we are concerned with abnormal mechanical forces: in *posture* we are concerned with the effects of gravity causing abnormal pressures on joints, viscera, blood-vessels, and nerves; in *occupational disease* we are concerned with the abnormal effects of stretching, weight-bearing, lifting, etc., on the locomotor system; and in *injuries* we are concerned with the effects of displacements of structures, tearing of tissues, contraction of scars, etc.

Goldthwait and others[5] in their book on body mechanics state, as their first paragraph:

> An individual is in the best health only when the body is so used that there is no strain on any of its parts. This means that when standing the body is held fully erect, with no strain on the joints, bones, ligaments, muscles, or any other structures. There should be adequate room for all the viscera, so that their functions can be performed normally, unless there is some congenital defect.

Goldthwait was one of the earliest medical writers to recognise a causal link between faulty mechanics and disease. His book presents evidence of the effects of faulty posture, and stress is laid on the correlation between certain body types and certain diseases.

Let us now consider in greater detail how faulty structure can lead to faulty function. Mechanical disturbances can adversely affect the body in the following ways:

1 Irritation or compression of *nerves* leads to increase or decrease of conduction, and later to trophic changes (p. 6).
2 Irritation or blocking of *blood-vessels* leads to ischaemia or congestion (p. 19).
3 Abnormal pressure or stretching of *viscera* leads to disturbed visceral function (p. 23).
4 Abnormal compression on *bone* leads to sclerosis or alteration of its shape and its internal architecture (p. 23).
5 Abnormal leverage at *joints* leads to weakness or tearing of ligaments; damage to cartilage, both articular and intra-articular; and irritation of synovial membranes (p. 24).
6 Abnormal forces on *muscles* lead to hypertrophy or atrophy (p. 32).
7 Abnormal pressure on *skin* and *connective tissues* leads to thickening or thinning (p. 33).

In addition to these local effects on each type of tissue, there are general effects on the whole body because each abnormal stress results in abnormal discharges of afferent impulses to the central nervous system. The cumulative effect of these abnormal sensory discharges leads to altered reflexes within the spinal cord (p. 11).

The treatment of the above mechanical disturbances consists in principle of removing the mechanical causes, where this is possible, and by encouraging repair processes; but if the effects of the mechanical

faults are irreversible, treatment must be directed towards assisting the
body to compensate mechanically for them. The practical methods of
achieving these mechanical objectives comprise the therapeutic contribution of osteopathy to medicine.

The mechanical stresses detailed above first adversely affect the
tissues directly but soon remote effects ensue, especially when the
primary tissue is a nerve or an artery. The mechanical stress may result
in severance of the tissue or merely the stretching of it. It may lead to
compression, intermittent compression, or irritation of the tissue. The
effects will also depend upon the degree of the stressed force. The remote
effects may be localised or generalised according to which tissue is
involved and to the degree of involvement.

Furthermore we must consider abnormal mechanical effects on areas
and systems of the body, not merely on isolated structures like bone,
ligament, artery, etc. For example, we study and treat abnormal
mechanical forces in the thorax as a whole, the abdomen as a whole, the
spinal column as a whole, or the whole nervous system. Mechanical
stresses lead to compensatory mechanisms and these have to be borne
in mind in management because we do not want to alter the compensation too much lest by so doing we make the condition worse.

Another factor relevant here is the vulnerability of certain tissues and
sites to mechanical stresses. The lower cervical and lower lumbar areas
of the spine are more likely to be strained than are other levels of the
spine. Nerves are more easily compressed in the intervertebral foramina
than in the rest of their course to the periphery. Some intervertebral
foramina are smaller than others and some have larger nerves passing
through them.

Consideration must also be given to the secondary effects which
persist after the primary causes have been removed. Reflexes which at
first may be protective and beneficial may hinder the return to normal.
Protective muscle action and abnormal posture or abnormal gait may
persist after the original source of pain has ceased to exist. These
abnormal reflex habits may need further attention for their correction.

I MECHANICAL EFFECTS ON NERVES

Nerves may be severed, compressed, intermittently compressed, or
stretched.

I *Severance* This leads to loss of conduction of the nerve. Wallerian
degeneration of the axon takes place distal to the cut and proximally as
far as the next node of Ranvier. Sometimes chromatolytic changes
develop in the neurone itself, especially if the damage is close to the

neurone. Later, regeneration takes place along the endoneurial tube if this persists and if the ends of the severed nerves have not been too widely separated. Loss of conduction leads to paralysis, numbness, absent reflexes, or altered autonomic balance according to which type of nerve-fibres is involved.

Persistent interruption of nerve conduction leads to trophic changes in the tissues supplied by those nerves. This has been recognised for many years, but only recently has the modus operandi been established. The research team at Kirksville under the leadership of I. M. Korr[6] has done some pioneer work in this field: they found that chemical substances not yet identified but traced by radioactive isotopes actually proceed from the cell body along the axon and into the muscle fibre, and that these substances advance at the rate of 5 mm a day (see Appendix 2, p. 285).

2 *Compression* If severe enough, the compression blocks the blood-supply to the nerve, which then loses its power of conduction. Wallerian degeneration will take place if the nerve-fibre dies. If compression is only temporary, conduction may only be impaired for a matter of minutes, hours, or days. The duration of the compression is significant: anything over thirty minutes leads to delay in recovery.

3 *Intermittent compression* is tantamount to mechanical irritation, and if long-continued it will lead to swelling of the nerve—that is, to neuritis—with pain and paraesthesiae, and sometimes to loss of power in the muscles supplied by the nerve. The swelling is both distal and proximal to the site of intermittent pressure, and the effects of this neuritis are directed centrally as well as distally.

4 *Traction* Severe traction may tear a nerve, and the effects then are those of severance. Less severe traction will cause irritation of the nerve and consequent neuritis. If the nerve-fibres are torn by traction the chances of regeneration are better as compared with a cleanly divided nerve, because some of the neurilemmal fibres persist so that an endo-neurial tube can form to facilitate regeneration.

The effects of severe injuries to nerves belong to the sphere of neuro-surgery and physical medicine, but the *effects of intermittent compression and traction of nerves are vitally important to the osteopathic concept.* These effects are:

(*a*) On the nerve trunk itself, inflammation—i.e. local swelling of the nerve, causing local pain and tenderness.
(*b*) On the nerve fibres, remote effects, both distal and central. The effect on motor fibres is to produce fibrillation, with loss of power or wasting of

muscle. The effect on sensory fibres is to produce paraesthesiae and pain felt peripherally. In addition increased afferent impulses are directed centrally to the spinal cord. These centripetal effects of increased afferent discharge to the spinal cord contribute to the facilitated segment at the same level (p. 11). Centrifugal effects on autonomic fibres lead to changes in vasomotor, visceromotor, and sudomotor tone.

Denny-Brown and Brenner[7] made a significant contribution in their study of the effects of compression on peripheral nerves and their conclusions were:

Compression of a nerve by a metal clip exerting a tension of 170 to 430 Gm for two hours induced transient paralysis lasting five to eighteen days. This paralysis was not associated with gross defect in sensation, and the distal portion of the nerve fibres did not degenerate. It was accompanied by intermittent loss of myelin at the nodes of Ranvier in the compressed area. The lesion was identical with the intermediate degree of pressure lesion induced by compression with a tourniquet. Though recovery of motor conduction was early, the restitution of the myelin defect was only slightly advanced after six to eight weeks and was still defective after six months.

Continuous compression of a nerve by a metal clip exerting a tension of 5 to 7 Gm did not interfere with conduction. The compressed segment was greatly narrowed, and the nerve was edematous on either side of the region of constriction. Striking histologic changes in myelin and axis-cylinder occurred in the edematous region. These changes appeared to be due to simple swelling of the myelin. They were associated with mobilisation of the large pale endoneural cells.

Continuous compression by a 44 Gm clip induced pressure necrosis of myelin and axis-cylinders under the clip, with edema and degeneration above and below the area of compression. The proximal degeneration was of the type due to excessive ischaemia.

Continuous compression by clips exerting a tension of 9 or 10 Gm induced delayed onset of motor paralysis on the fifth to the eighth day, which lasted up to twenty-five days, with rapid recovery and without necessarily any Wallerian degeneration or change in nerve endings or muscle. The lesion was associated with segmental loss of myelin, as well as the changes recognised as related to edema. Restitution of myelin was gradually taking place six weeks after the beginning of the experiment. The demyelinated axis-cylinder stained poorly, if at all, with silver impregnation.

The effect of pressure on nerve is considered to be due entirely to ischaemia, and the characteristic histologic lesion and dissociated paralysis form a distinctive type of neuro-pathologic reaction.

The histologic evidence indicates that the dissociation between sensory and motor function is due to a functional property of the disorder of the axoplasm, and not to selective effect related to the size of the fibre.

Continuing this study in a slightly different direction Barlow and Pochin[8] noticed that if ischaemia is repeated there is a reduction in the degree of recovery of the nerve. They summarised their findings by saying:

> After occlusion of the circulation to the human arm with a cuff for twenty-five minutes, movements and sensation return rapidly to normal. For a period of many hours, however, full recovery of the nerves can be shown to be incomplete, since in a second occlusion, motor and sensory changes develop earlier than in the first.
>
> Recovery is only complete in this sense after about ten hours, while at twenty-four hours after the first occlusion the nerves consistently have a slightly increased resistance to ischaemia, paralysis of thumb apposition occurring at a time greater by 10 per cent than in controlled occlusions.
>
> The slow recovery from occlusion appears to be an effect of ischaemia on the nerve below the cuff. The effect is not cumulant in a sequence of occlusions unless the periods of free circulation are small compared with those of circulatory occlusion.

The implications here are that pressure on a nerve which is sufficient to occlude the vasa nervorum will cause varying degrees of loss of conduction, and that repeated pressure will render the nerve more vulnerable.

Pressure affects conduction and it leads to oedema of the nerve-trunk. Clinically, however, nerves do not behave exactly as in experiments and a single nerve-fibre, although important for study purposes, is not a clinical entity because peripheral nerves normally carry the whole range of functional nerve-fibres. Consequently the effects of nerve irritation differ not only according to the severity of the neuritis but also according to which type of nerve-fibres are affected. (For example Frykholm[9] found that mechanical irritation of the posterior nerve-roots produced sharp pain, while mechanical irritation of the anterior nerve-roots produced dull poorly localised pain. He was able to do this by operating on the cervical spine under local anaesthesia.)

At the site of pressure there is secondary swelling both of the nerve and the connective tissues. If the nerve traverses a confined space or tunnel, this oedema can magnify the mechanical pressure and lead to venous obstruction. The venous congestion thus produced can impair the local supply of oxygen so that carbon dioxide and pH values are changed. These further influence nerve conduction. Because the mechanical pressure causes swelling of the nerve there is a further increase of pressure, and a vicious cycle is established, which may be sufficiently vicious to stop conduction altogether by blocking the arterial supply to the nerve, as in facial paralysis when the seventh cranial nerve is compressed by inflammatory oedema.

Some nerve sites in the body are more vulnerable than others to mechanical irritation and traction—e.g. the anterior and posterior nerve-roots are affected by abnormal tensions in the ligamentum denticulatum. The posterior nerve-root ganglia in the cervical intervertebral foramina and the combined nerve-roots in the intervertebral foramina can be irritated by pressure from osteophytes, disc displacements, arthritis and synovitis of the apophyseal joints, fibrosis, and oedema. More distally the nerves can be affected by abnormal muscle tensions—e.g. the scalene muscles and piriformis. The first rib may be elevated by anomaly or lesions of the first costo-vertebral joint, causing traction on the lower cord of the brachial plexus. The ulnar nerve at the medial epicondyle, the median nerve in the carpal tunnel, and the radial nerve in the spiral canal posterior to the humerus are all vulnerable to mechanical pressure. The lumbar nerves as they traverse the psoas muscle, the lateral cutaneous nerve of the thigh as it passes under the inguinal ligament, the peroneal nerve as it courses round the head of the fibula, the plantar nerve medial to the os calcis, and the digital nerves between the metatarsal heads are also mechanically vulnerable.

The track of a peripheral nerve will withstand a great deal of mechanical irritation without protest as, for example, an ulnar nerve slipping over the medial epicondyle due to either an anomalous shape or an old supracondylar fracture of the humerus. This is because nerves are elastic, and in this instance the nerve is not traversing a confined space so that it can swell without increasing the pressure upon itself; but even in this situation pain, paraesthesiae, and muscle weakness can ensue.

The initial effects of nerve irritation are exaggeration of the nerve conduction with abnormal stimulation of sensory, motor, and autonomic nerves, leading to pain, paraesthesiae, fibrillation of muscle, and vasoconstriction. Later, when neurological fatigue sets in or conduction fails, this hyperfunction is replaced by hypofunction and the symptoms change to numbness, loss of power, and vasodilatation. The response is centrifugal or centripetal, or both—for example, the carpal-tunnel compression syndrome evokes pain and paraesthesiae in the thumb and index and middle fingers, and loss of power in the thenar muscles; but also it can cause retrograde pain from the forearm to the arm. The effects may be temporary or permanent.

When an axon is compressed close to its neurone, there is a greater risk of the neurone being damaged than when the pressure is remote. For example, carpal-tunnel compression can lead to permanent loss of power in the thenar muscles, but it is unlikely to lead to permanent damage of posterior-root ganglion cells, whereas compression at the intervertebral foramen may well cause permanent damage in the posterior-root ganglion cells. Another consideration is that peripheral nerves carry only a few autonomic nerve-fibres because these have already separated off to pass down the limb in the coats of the arteries, whereas at the intervertebral foramen nerve-roots carry the white and grey rami communicantes of the autonomic nervous system along with the motor and sensory fibres of the central nervous system. Proximal mechanical pressure on nerves has a greater effect therefore on the autonomic nervous system than does distal pressure.

The *central effects*, as distinct from the peripheral effects, of nerve pressure and irritation are less well defined and they are open to some speculation, but osteopathic research has shed light on the problems and it has modified some of the older osteopathic theory.[10] The present view is that intermittent pressure on a peripheral nerve-trunk sets up abnormal afferent impulses. These impulses bombard the cord and create a 'summation effect' within the cord, leading to an increased central excitatory state. Then abnormal efferent impulses discharge from the excitable anterior horn cells along peripheral nerves to muscles, and from the excitable lateral horn cells along the autonomic nerves to blood-vessels, sweat-glands, and viscera. The increased central excitatory state creates what is called a *facilitated segment* because the threshold for the efferent discharge is lowered, and the transmission of impulses is thereby facilitated. But it must be remembered, however, that all afferent impulses are not necessarily excitatory; some are inhibitory and these may in fact reduce the excitability of the motor neurones, and reduce the central excitatory state, thereby reducing the adverse effects of mechanical lesions on the spinal cord.

The abnormal afferent impulses not only arise from mechanical irritation of nerve-trunks and nerve-roots, but from mechanical effects on sensory nerve-endings in muscle, tendon, ligament, periosteum, etc. These all have a cumulative effect and any persistence of the sensory bombardment of the cord leads to facilitation of reflexes.

The researches referred to above have demonstrated that the majority of adults—even those in good health—have one or more facilitated segments in their spinal column. The segment is characterised by a reduction in the thresholds of pain and touch in the dermatomes of the same segment. Vasomotor and sudomotor changes are also demonstrated in that dermatome, together with increased motor activity in the

related paravertebral muscles. Many of the facilitated segments become
chronic and persist for months or even years. The patterns of vasomotor
and sudomotor changes in dermatomes can be modified, at least
temporarily, by experimentally induced postural stresses and myofascial irritation—for example, by creating temporary curvatures in the
spine with heel lifts, or by injecting hypertonic saline into the spinal
ligaments.

Glover[11] made a study of hyperaesthesia in 100 cases of back pain,
which he termed a syndrome in preference to giving an exact diagnosis.
He described the areas of hyperaesthesia and stated that if the syndrome
was not treated or did not recover spontaneously, the hyperaesthesia
remained constant for up to two or more years. In this syndrome he
located a tender spot to palpation a half to two inches lateral to the mid-
line. The syndrome of back pain, hyperaesthesia, and paravertebral
tenderness was also accompanied by limitation of spinal movements.
There is no doubt that Glover is describing the hypomobile type of
spinal lesion (see p. 114), and his observations tally with those of the
osteopathic research team in Kirksville who have taken the study much
further.

In addition to the sensory changes which accompany the lesion and its
facilitated segment, there is a facilitated motor response. This has been
shown by applying pressure to the spinous processes and measuring the
force required to evoke a motor response:[12]

> Segmental motor reflex thresholds were determined by measuring
> in kilograms the amount of pressure applied to the spinous process of
> each segment which just evokes contraction of the paravertebral
> muscles at that segmental level. Muscular contractions were detected
> and evaluated by electromyographic recordings. Lesioned segments
> invariably required weaker stimuli than did non-lesioned segments.

Eble[13] demonstrated that stimulation of a viscus produced contraction of spinal muscles in two or three segments on the same side of the
spine and at the levels of the cord corresponding to its innervation. If
the stimulus is intense more segments show motor irritability. Sometimes
this irritability spreads to the contralateral side. When bilaterally
innervated viscera, like the intestine, were stimulated there was a
bilateral motor response.

Eble[14] demonstrated that a similar increase of paravertebral muscle
contractions occurred when the skin was stimulated. When the dorsal
aspect of the torso was stimulated the multifidus muscles showed increased motor action potentials, whereas when the ventral aspect of
the torso was stimulated it was the intertransversalis muscles which
showed increased motor action potentials. It is also well known that

chilling of the skin in the thoracic area can give rise to respiratory infection through some reflex effect on the mucous membrane in the bronchial tubes. Cold feet can reduce the circulation in the trachea. Nose-bleeding can be checked by applying cold to the neck. In reverse, too, heating the skin can increase the circulation in deep structures.

In these various ways the spine and the spinal segment react to abnormal afferent impulses whether from the skin, the ligaments, the bone or the segmentally related viscus. The cord segment becomes irritable and reflexes are facilitated. The anterior and lateral horn cells are the focal point through which the reflexes express themselves. Korr called them the 'neurologic lens' through which abnormal afferent impulses were magnified into abnormal efferent discharges. These discharges lead to abnormal function—in the first place to hyperfunction and later to hypofunction, and then if the abnormal stimuli persist long enough, pathological changes can ensue.

Somewhere along this sequence of events, however, other factors creep in to modify the central excitatory state. A compensating balancing process steps in to reduce the deleterious effects, and the adverse influence of mechanical faults is thereby minimised.

What constitutes this balancing force has not so far been investigated; but if there were no such mechanism, then the worst mechanical stresses would produce the worst effects. This is not so: many patients with serious scolioses and those who have had serious spinal injuries become otherwise quite healthy. In these subjects, therefore, whatever abnormal afferent impulses reach the cord to disturb the central excitatory state there is some compensatory mechanism to modify, mollify, and restore the resultant efferent impulses towards the normal.

The efferent discharges of the anterior horn cells are the result of the sum total of the afferent barrage, and if the afferent impulses from one source are in excess then other sources must be reduced by inhibition in some way or other. No one has yet worked out what this self-regulating mechanism is, and the very idea of such a mechanism is rarely considered.

The disturbed reflex mechanism and the altered central excitatory state which mechanical stresses evoke in the spinal cord must therefore usually be temporary and only rarely permanent. For example, in about 10 per cent of cases of lumbar disc prolapse there is a history (if suitable questions are put to the patient) of coldness or oedema in the affected limb, but this passes in a few days and is often forgotten or hardly noticed. Only about 1 per cent of such patients continue to have coldness or oedema or vasomotor instability. In the remainder either the autonomic nerves cease to be irritated or the self-regulating mechanism here postulated comes in to restore the balance.

Spanos and Andrew[15] studied the link between intermittent claudication and disc lesions: 'Many physicians will be familiar with cases of intermittent claudication in which the vascular insufficiency in the legs seems insufficient to account for the symptoms.' Spanos and Andrew maintained that such cases were usually neurological, and that the commonest cause was a prolapsed intervertebral disc. Root signs were not always present. They cited cases at operations when they found disc protrusion and the affected nerve-root was under tension, yet the disc was reducible by finger pressure.

Joffe[16] described two cases of pain, numbness, and weakness of the legs with exertion, never coming on at rest and being relieved by rest. Both the patients' leg arteries were normal to palpation, and both patients responded well to laminectomy. These are examples of disturbed vasomotion to the lower extremities due to pressure within the spinal canal, and they are examples of persisting autonomic disturbance from mechanical cause; but in my experience many of these cases are transient. Even surgical division of autonomic nerves only leads to temporary imbalance—for example:

> After a successful sympathectomy operation vasodilation immediately sets in, as is shown by a rise in skin temperature, flushing of the skin and increased loss of heat; the superficial veins are also relaxed. This occurs in subjects with normal blood-vessels (e.g. patients with hyperhidrosis) and in appropriately selected cases of vascular disorder. Reflex sweating and pilomotor reactions are abolished. Within the first day or two, blood through the hand may be increased eightfold, but the hyperaemia subsides quickly and after a week the blood is only double the initial value. . . . The rapid return of vascular tone after sympathectomy is not satisfactorily explained.[17]

Similarly after interruption of parasympathetic nerves—for example, in the treatment of peptic ulceration by dividing the vagus nerve—there is altered autonomic balance in the gastro-intestinal system, and diarrhoea is a frequent sequel to vagotomy; but in the majority of cases the diarrhoea is transient and the tendency is towards a return of normal bowel habit. When this happens some self-regulating mechanism must be operating to restore the balance in the autonomic nerve supply to the bowel.[18] Another example is that of cauda equina pressure effects on the sacral outflow of parasympathetic nerves, which are often only transient.

There is a self-regulating mechanism for the blood-supply of the kidneys. This was demonstrated in 1934 by van Slyke et al.,[19] who found that autoregulation of the blood-flow in the kidney is not dependent upon extrinsic nerves, because anaesthetisation of the renal pedicle of an exteriorised kidney did not abolish the autoregulation.

Hix, at Kirksville, has worked on this autoregulation mechanism.[20] He pointed out that there is a rich internal nerve-supply irrespective of the autonomic supply to the kidney. He showed that the kidney was capable of maintaining a renal blood-flow at 100 mm Hg irrespective of the general blood-pressure, and that this is possible even in a transplanted kidney which has had all its nerve-supply severed.

There may well be other self-regulating mechanisms within the autonomic nervous system which minimise the adverse influence of altered mechanics of the spine on visceral function. *However, the self-regulation is often incomplete and insufficient to restore balance,* and during the stage of increased central excitatory state the outflow of abnormal efferent impulses may be provoked by any other stimulus which reaches the anterior and lateral horn cells from anywhere in the rest of the nervous system. In other words, the irritable spinal segment—owing to mechanical causes—is vulnerable to other noxious influences; and, even if the mechanical fault in itself is not sufficient to evoke abnormal responses, the combination of it with other factors is sufficient to produce abnormal symptoms. Consequently *the mechanical fault can sometimes be aetiological or predisposing or exacerbating or susstaining in its adverse effects on the central nervous system.*

So many visceral symptoms are of a transient nature that they tend to be disregarded and their correlation with mechanical lesions is discounted. In any case it can be argued that if the recovery is spontaneous, the mechanically produced hyperactivity does not matter. This is so, except in those cases in which the disturbed visceromotion persists. Then the structural fault must be corrected not only for its own sake but for its visceral effects. When the structural fault persists other aetiological factors can then precipitate malfunction more easily. Most diseases have multiple aetiologies. The pneumococcus attacks the lungs of the smoker more readily than those of the non-smoker, and we say that the patient's resistance is weakened by the chemical irritant of the tobacco; the bacteria and the tobacco are both aetiological factors, and there may be others. Mechanical lesions are aetiological in many diseases, because the lesions weaken those viscera which are reflexly and segmentally linked with them.

To claim that mechanical lesions are the only aetiological factors in disease is, of course, ludicrous. They are rarely if ever totally responsible, but they cannot *or should not be discounted in any disease.* The degree of significance of mechanical factors varies from disease to disease and from patient to patient. The mechanical component in the aetiology of syphilis is negligible (if we ignore the mechanism of transmission !) but in the aetiology of sciatica it is all important; and in some cases of constipation, dysmenorrhoea, or asthma the mechanical factor may be so important that until the mechanics are put right the symptoms will persist.

When all medical investigations are negative in patients in whom symptoms persist, there is frequently a mechanical or structural basis for those symptoms even though the linkage seems tenuous. It is unwise to label such patients as neurotic until the mechanics of the spine have been properly assessed.

The abnormal afferent impulses from mechanical faults arising in muscles, ligaments, capsules, tendons, and periosteum are sometimes very persistent partly because the mechanical fault may be self-perpetuating. The pain causes an increase of muscle tension which in turn causes more pain to perpetuate the tension. In this way is established a vicious cycle to maintain the flow of abnormal afferent impulses, and this may be sufficient to overcome the self-regulating mechanism referred to above, creating chronicity of the symptoms.

The vicious cycle needs breaking. This may be achieved by manipulation in the appropriate case, but another effective way to break it is to force the muscle to relax by infiltrating the painful sites with local anaesthesia. Certainly this method is often successful clinically, and the relief of symptoms lasts considerably longer than the mere period of anaesthesia. Further examples will now be given of observed visceral disturbances secondary to mechanical faults. Lennart Herlin,[21] for example, when studying the effects of nerve-root compression in the lumbar spine, noticed how frequently the pain was accompanied by urogenital dysfunction:

> In painful chronic infections of the urogenital organs the author has found that one or several of the lower sacral nerve-roots (especially 2 and 3S) have been compressed or stretched by degenerated disc tissue. They may account for symptoms and signs previously attributed to local pelvic disorders—e.g. painful irregular menstruation, bladder dysfunction, or chronic infections such as prostatovesciculitis.

He also lists twenty-nine cases in which cauda equina symptoms were not present and yet disturbances of micturition, potency, liability to urogenital infection, and vaginal discharge occurred. He followed these cases after surgical removal of their disc protrusions, and noticed that these visceral symptoms subsided after the operation.

Roberts,[22] in his book on chronic structural low backache, described sixty-four cases in great detail and noticed the frequency of visceral disturbances which he considered could not have been merely coincidental: 2 patients noticed heavy bleeding of their haemorrhoids when the backache was at its worst; 8 cases were under treatment for their haemorrhoids at the same time as their backache, and dysuria occurred in 17 cases, haematuria in 6, dribbling in 7, congestion of the bladder in 2, and red and white blood cells were found in the urine in 12. These symptoms were accentuated by mechanical strain or relieved by rest. He poses the question (p. 69):

> Why cannot we go further and say that in march haematuria and orthostatic albuminuria there is over action of the muscles and soft tissues of the low back skeletal system with their consequent edematous swelling which disturbs the sympathetic or autonomic nervous system and its neurovascular control, so that blood, blood cells or albumin appear in the urine as a result of congestion of the urinary tract?

Love and Emmett[23] reported three cases of lumbar disc protrusions in women in which urinary retention was the presenting symptom without significant back or neurological symptoms. Removal of the disc protrusion cured the retention and they concluded that many transient retentions may be due to similar causes.

Lewis and Kellgren[24] state as a result of their own experimental studies with injections of hypertonic saline into the spinal ligaments:

> In man it has been shown that all the essential parts of the condition known as renal colic, pain diffused from loin to scrotum, iliac and testicular tenderness and cremasteric retraction, can be provoked by a stimulus confined to somatic structures such as muscle or ligament of the spine.

Freude and Ruhmann,[25] observing the stomach on a radiographic screen, noticed that its tone and peristalsis could be modified within two seconds by applying cold wooden discs to the epigastrium. Hansen and von Staa[26] observed that in left-sided renal lithiasis there was dilation of the left pupil, increased dermographia on the left side, hyperalgesia in the skin and muscles in the normal cutaneous zones of 10–12T, increased tone in the muscles in the same segmental area, and a secondary scoliosis in the lumbar area.

Dittmar[27] demonstrated that the application of cold or painful stimuli to the dermatomes 5–9T anteriorly on the left immediately inhibited the gastric motility of the rabbit or dog; peristalsis ceased at once and tonus diminished markedly. If, however, the posterior roots of the spinal cord segments 5–9T were cut this inhibitory effect was absent. A similar cutaneo-visceral effect can also be obtained with a human subject by pinching a fold of skin at 7T on the left. It can also be evoked by stimulating the contralateral dermatome. The effect of heat on a hyper-peristaltic stomach is diminution of peristalsis.

In like manner, by infiltrating the dermatome with procaine, it is possible to interrupt the cutaneo-visceral pathways and to exert a soothing effect on viscera.

Dittmar came to the conclusion that surgical and pharmacological measures which aim at cure of organic disease by interruption of the autonomic neural pathways are justified.

So, too, do we contend that by restoring normal mechanics we are achieving in a natural way the restoration of autonomic balance by calming the stimulated and over-excitable segment.

The central effects of mechanical faults upon the cord so far discussed concern the increased afferent bombardment, the facilitated segment and increased central excitatory state, the increased or modified discharges of the anterior and lateral horn cells and how these impulses alter the skin, the muscle, and the vascular and visceral activities of the involved segment. But this is not all, a further central effect could result from disturbed vasomotion to the blood-vessels of the spinal cord itself. There is, of course, a rich blood-supply to the spinal cord, and there is wide anastomosis between adjacent spinal arteries and adjacent veins. There are five longitudinal arteries to connect adjacent segments, and there are both internal and external venous plexuses with longitudinal channels and veins running right through the vertebral bodies, so that it seems unlikely that any mechanical lesion of the intervertebral joints (short of a massive disc prolapse or a fracture-dislocation) could block the arterial supply to the cord or cause so much venous congestion as to lead to symptoms from this source alone, but reflex vasomotor changes from disturbed central excitatory states could well lead to vasodilatation or vasoconstriction of the vasa nervorum of the cord and nerve-roots.

Any effects on the spinal cord from reflex vasomotor disturbances of its blood-supply would probably have to be sustained for a long time before symptoms could ensue, but once degenerative changes are established in the spinal cord the symptoms become permanent because of the innate inability of the cord to regenerate. This explains some of the disappointing results from the osteopathic treatment of diseases of the central nervous system. Once cervical myelopathy has been diagnosed with certainty, it is already too late to reverse the existing pathological changes.

Cervical myelopathy is so often associated with cervical spondylosis that a causal relationship must exist, with the myelopathy being secondary to the spondylosis, but there is no fixed relationship. Severe spondylosis often does not cause any central nervous system changes, and even the nerve-roots may escape. On the other hand, in serious myelopathy the degenerative changes may be only minor. Therefore factors other than purely mechanical ones must be invoked in the aetiology of myelopathy, and circulatory impairment is a highly probable explanation.

2 MECHANICAL EFFECTS ON BLOOD-VESSELS

The circulation of blood in the body is constantly adapting itself to innumerable local and general factors. If the need for blood is greater in one tissue or organ than in another, the arteries to it dilate, and if the need diminishes the arteries constrict. If the response is excessive, we call it hyperaemia or if it is not enough, ischaemia. Similarly, though less actively, the venous drainage is increased or decreased. If the drainage is inadequate it leads to congestion, stasis, and oedema.

The circulation depends upon the complex interrelationship between the heart, the arteries, the capillaries, and the veins. Many influences extraneous to the vessels themselves—mechanical factors, environmental temperature, the emotions, muscular activity, digestion, and so on—affect the flow of blood to and from the local tissues. All these influences are co-ordinated by the autonomic nervous system, which has its headquarters in the floor of the fourth ventricle and the major peripheral control in the spinal cord at the 2T to 2L levels. The lumen of normal arteries and veins is controlled by vasoconstrictor and vasodilator nerves which pass along the walls of the vessels.

There are several ways in which local circulation can be affected mechanically:

1 Through pressure on vasomotor nerves in the spinal canal. It has already been shown (p. 14) that a disc protrusion can cause coldness (from vasoconstriction) in one limb. Oedema in one limb (from vasodilation or congestion) can also result, though less frequently, from the same cause.

2 Through reflex mechanical disturbances of a spinal segment (see p. 13) it is postulated that the facilitated spinal segment emits abnormal efferent discharges along vasomotor nerves to alter the local blood-supply in the head, the thorax, the abdomen, or the spinal cord. There are considerable research difficulties in proving this, however, and there is much speculation within orthodox medicine as well as within osteopathic spheres about circulatory factors in disease. Medical thought is orientated round the pathological changes in the vessel walls, whereas osteopathic thought is orientated round the disturbed vasomotor control which is secondary to mechanical influences on the sympathetic nervous system. The difficulties in establishing causes for local abnormalities are increased, because many of the manifestations are transient and are easily modified by other factors. Examples of transient vaso-

motor disturbances are vaso-vagal attacks, drop attacks, angina, and postural hypertension; migraine, vertigo, and probably tinnitus have vascular disturbances as part of their aetiology.

3 Through direct mechanical pressure on blood-vessel walls. Pressure on an artery can, if hard enough, lead to ischaemia or even to necrosis of the tissues supplied by it. Pressure on veins leads to venous congestion and later to oedema. Both ischaemia and congestion, if prolonged, can lead to necrosis. Temporary ischaemia does no harm provided it is brief enough and not repeated too frequently.

4 Through postural defects. Faulty posture and gravity factors can impede the return of blood to the heart. The faulty posture has, of course, to be sustained for a considerable time before symptoms of venous congestion develop. Postural defects, inactivity, and poor respiratory function can all impede the return of venous blood to the heart.

The adverse effects of impaired circulation from whatever cause are due to lack of oxygen, the slowing up of local metabolism, and the accumulation of katabolites. These adverse effects are only temporary if the circulation is restored. In Raynaud's disease, for example, the temporary ischaemia in the limbs usually has no serious effects. Numbness and pallor are followed by tingling, redness, and oedema. During the ischaemic phase histamine and other metabolites are liberated, including pain-producing vasodilator kinins, but they are soon dispersed when blood flows freely again.

Hyperaemia is rarely if ever produced by mechanical factors except as a reaction to trauma. It is a process used by the body in the presence of inflammation to assist in healing and repair when there has been tissue damage of mechanical, chemical, or bacterial origin. Prolonged hyperaemia may have a damaging effect, as in bone when this leads to decalcification.

Hyperaemia develops in a limb during exercise and it lasts longer than the active phase. Similarly, an increase of circulation results from passive movements of limbs. The alternating stretching and squeezing of soft tissue during articulatory treatment has a pumping action on the veins, decongesting the part to allow more arterial blood to reach the area unimpeded by venous stasis.

Improvement in circulation is one of the objectives of osteopathic treatment, and one spends much time on articulatory types of manipulation with this objective in mind. Not only is the circulation of the body as a whole improved by general treatment, but treatment can be directed to any area of the body to improve its circulation locally.

Manual treatment can improve local circulation in three ways:

1 By local friction on the skin. This leads to the liberation of histamine which in turn causes hyperaemia of the skin. There is evidence to suggest that, through an axon reflex, the skin hyperaemia leads to hyperaemia in subjacent tissues also.
2 By the effleurage type of massage from the periphery towards the heart. This helps in the drainage of venous blood and decreases oedema.
3 By articulatory manipulations. These alternately squeeze and stretch the soft tissues in the area, and this acts like a pump on the local blood-flow.

In clinical practice the mechanical blockage of an artery from its outer walls does not exist, and mechanical blockage of a single vein is insignificant because of the wide anastomosis of superficial and deep veins. Generalised venous congestion—as in cardiac failure and portal obstruction—are not considered here; but postural faults when long sustained can lead to venous obstruction—e.g. prolonged sitting in a low chair and prolonged standing can lead to oedema of the ankles. Long-continued visceroptosis leads to haemorrhoids with anal thrombosis and fissures: it also impairs visceral function if the viscus is itself congested. Tight clothing is enough to cause venous congestion in the limbs and the abdomen. The effects of poor posture will increase as the individual grows older, when his vessels become less elastic.

Persistent venous congestion leads to the exudation of plasma into the tissue spaces. This oedema is at first soft and pits on pressure, but in time the exudates clot, leading to fibrosis of the connective tissues so that they become permanently hard and unyielding to finger pressure. Possibly this is also because the lymphatic drainage is impaired at this stage of venous congestion. The blocking of *lymphatic vessels* alone does not occur from mechanical causes because of their wide anastomosis: only certain diseases and surgical excision of lymphatic glands lead to blocking of lymphatic drainage, and then all the tissues distal to the affected glands become swollen and hard. The tissues do not pit on pressure. Mechanically produced oedema or, for that matter, oedema from any cause can have secondary mechanical effects if the oedema occurs in confined spaces—e.g. in the facial nerve canal, the intervertebral foramen, or the carpal tunnel—because it then increases the mechanical pressure, and a vicious cycle is established.

Venous congestion in the spinal column is important. Despite the advantages of widespread venous anastomoses and venous plexuses in the spinal canal, there is the disadvantage that the spinal veins have no valves within their lumen so that venous congestion probably occurs in some conditions and postures. Venous congestion in the spinal cord and canal may account for the exacerbation of symptoms in those patients who have more pain in bed than when upright. Many brachial neuritis syndromes are worse on lying down, when venous congestion in the cord is accentuated, whereas on sitting and standing venous drainage in the neck is helped by gravity, so that the area becomes decongested, swelling diminishes, pressure decreases, and pain subsides.

Conversely, many patients with sciatic neuritis find that their symptoms are relieved by lying down and aggravated by standing and sitting. This could be explained on a similar basis: venous congestion is increased in the lumbar spine in the erect position and relieved on lying down. Farkas[28] maintains that many symptoms in the spine are due to venous congestion: coughing, sneezing, and defaecation all accentuate the venous pressure in the spine and in turn accentuate the pain. He advocates raising the foot of the bed to help venous drainage, and claims improved results with this method of rest. This may not be the precise explanation because gravity has effects other than that on venous drainage—e.g. compression in the standing position may well cause a disc to herniate more, it may produce greater pressure from alteration of the shape of the intervertebral foramina, it may cause over-lap of articular facets as in lumbar lordosis, and it may produce more muscular tension and pain in the process of maintaining balance.

Roberts[22] contends that oedema is responsible for some of the symptoms in chronic structural low backache. He points out that when muscles and ligaments are overstrained they become swollen and oedematous. If these tissues are injected with a local anaesthetic there is a temporary increase of pain because the existing tension is thereby increased, and he says it is clinically noteworthy that pain and stiffness are often relieved by movements (active and passive) only to return again within minutes, presumably because oedema has re-collected.

Oedema is the result of and part of the slowing up of local circulation; but this has secondary effects on the chemistry of the blood in the area, and, because the oxygen content in the vessels diminishes, there is an accumulation of metabolites and the pH values change. Conduction in nerves is very sensitive to such an environment, and the larger fibres suffer from a lack of oxygen before the smaller fibres. There is therefore an interplay between the circulation and nerves in any area: impair the function of either and the other will suffer.

One other point relative to vessels and mechanical stimulation is that during surgical manipulation of vessels they often go into local spasm. Anaesthetists commonly find that the vein they are trying to penetrate with a needle has gone into spasm so that its lumen cannot be found. Similarly the introduction of a needle into an artery leads to its con-striction. But there is an element of trauma to the vessel walls under these circumstances, and a direct analogy cannot be made with mechanical pressure from the outside through intact skin.

3 MECHANICAL EFFECTS ON VISCERA

Abnormal mechanics in the spine and in the thoracic and abdominal cavities can adversely affect visceral function in the following ways:

1 By abnormal efferent visceral stimuli reaching the organ from the facilitated segment. This has been discussed at length (p. 15).
2 By abnormal vasomotor impulses to the blood-vessels which supply the organs.
3 By abnormal tensions and stretchings of the supports of the viscera.
4 By venous congestion through inactivity, faulty breathing, and sustained faulty posture.

Provided the physiological control of circulation and respiration is normal, their efficiency depends upon mechanical considerations. The mechanical pumping action of the heart relies on efficient valves, and the return of venous blood depends on negative pressure in the thorax during expiration, and on proper tone in the abdominal muscles and diaphragm. The activity of muscles in the limbs aids venous drainage through pressure on veins with efficient valves. Shallow respiration from a rigid chest wall, poor abdominal tone from a sagging belly, and lack of exercise all add to the strain on venous return to the heart. Venous congestion ensues, stasis develops, oedema and lack of oxygen add to the visceral embarrassment, and abnormal physiological responses are inevitable.

These considerations show the value of good posture and proper exercise for efficient cardiac and respiratory function. The same applies to the abdominal viscera. The mechanical inefficiency of a transverse colon which is sagging into the pelvis is obvious, and although a floating kidney may remain efficient enough for most needs it will suffer if ptosis persists, especially if the renal vessels become mechanically blocked.

4 MECHANICAL EFFECTS ON BONE

Abnormal pressure on bone leads to sclerosis and alteration in its shape. Conversely, a decrease of normal pressure leads to osteomalacia. Far from being a solid static structure, bone is adaptive and relatively pliable, and it is influenced by both calcium metabolism and marrow physiology. Its internal architecture becomes modified by the stresses placed upon it. It readily remodels itself after fracture by processes of absorption and reformation. A relatively soft structure like an aortic aneurysm, however, can press on the thoracic vertebrae and erode them away. Increased pressure within the intervertebral discs can cause expansion at the expense of bone, as seen in the Cupid's bow effect on the lower surfaces of the lower lumbar vertebrae. A Schmorl's node illustrates the malleable and reactive nature of bone: firstly the nuclear material of the disc protrudes into the vertebral body and then, to prevent further damage, the body lays down more calcium to limit the incursion. Lordosis in the lumbar spine provokes increased density in the posterior vertebral arches, and abnormal stresses in the form of chronic pulling strains on bone lead to osteophyte formation. Bed rest results in considerable outpouring of calcium as the unused skeleton is broken down. It involves loss of the bone parenchyma rather than just its calcium content, yet the bones can increase in response to mechanical demand—e.g. after the tibia has been divided the fibula hypertrophies, and bone grafts which are subjected to mechanical stress often increase in bulk and density.

All these points are succinctly covered in *Wolff's law*, which states: 'The form of the bone being given, the bone elements place or displace themselves in the direction of the functional pressures.'

5 MECHANICAL EFFECTS ON JOINTS

Mechanical stresses and strains affect joints in different ways according to which component of the joint is involved—ligament, cartilage or synovial membrane. In addition there are remote effects through the central nervous system due to the abnormal afferent discharge of nervous impulses from the joints. These effects are reflex muscle guarding and alteration of the central excitatory state of the spinal cord (p. 11).

1 Ligaments

The mechanical function of ligaments is to hold bones together and yet allow some measure of freedom. They are elastic structures, yet there is an elastic limit to the amount of stretch that they will take. They remain healthy in response to intermittent stretching. They keep strong and may even increase in strength in response to the normal demands of intermittent moderate stretching.

A separational stress beyond the ligament's elastic limit will tear it. This can occur in two ways—by a sudden sharp force, or by a prolonged uninterrupted stretch.

Tearing of fibres leads to haemorrhage, oedema, fibrin formation, and eventual repair, with the laying down of new fibres. If the ligament is given sufficient time and rest it will repair fully and grow as strong as before, but if the new fibres are stretched too soon the repair will be weak and incomplete, and elongation of the ligament will ensue.

Similarly if the separational force is sustained long enough without let-up, the ligament will elongate. There are some sites where ligaments are especially strong—e.g. the ilio-femoral ligament at the hip joint, and the plantar ligaments of the foot. These ligaments have to take the strain of body weight when standing, but even they will elongate if standing is prolonged. It is, of course, unusual for an individual to remain standing absolutely stationary for more than a few moments at a time, so that these ligaments only have to bear the stretch effect of the whole body weight intermittently. Pes planus is an example of the effects of prolonged stretching of ligaments; genu recurvatum occurs in poliomyelitis if the knee remains unsupported during the paralysis; but the commonest example of all is stretching in the ligaments of the lower lumbar spine due to sitting in slumped positions in low easy chairs or to lying on sagging mattresses in bed or to half sitting in bed reading for hours at a time, when the supraspinous and interspinous ligaments elongate and intervertebral joints become unstable at least in flexion (p. 131).

Traction treatment of the spine has become popular, and in some cases the use of sustained traction is justifiable; but on physiological grounds sustained traction has an adverse effect on the supportive ligaments, especially if excessive weights are used. Intermittent sustained traction, if it will achieve the benefits of sustained traction, is a more physiological method (p. 154).

Hypertrophy of ligaments sometimes occurs in response to continuing intermittent stretching of the ligaments, as in unstable joints. Nature attempts to stabilise the joints in this way. For example, surgeons exploring for disc protrusions have sometimes found the ligaments thickened (especially the ligamentum flavum) by even two or three times the normal thickness. The thick ligamentum flavum may also contribute to the mechanical pressure on nerve-roots at the intervertebral foramina.

2 Cartilage

The chief mechanical function of cartilage is to buffer the effects of compression upon bone. It is the chief shock absorber of the body, and it constitutes a quarter of the whole length of the spine. In some peripheral joints there are interarticular cartilages as well as hyaline cartilage to help absorb the effects of compression. The shock absorption is achieved more on the principle of the hydraulic system than by the elastic properties of a substance like rubber.

Charnley[29] reported the observation that under pressure articular cartilage behaves like a sponge and exudes a liquid which appeared identical with synovial fluid. Ekholm and Norbäch[30] make the point that 'Cartilage is bathed in and saturated by synovial fluid. If not, any compressive load would immediately induce elastic stress in the cartilaginous matrix. Cartilage is porous and external pressure causes excess fluid pressure in the pores. This fluid pressure will carry initially the most substantial load, leaving only a relatively small part of it to be supported by the solid material.'

Cartilage is nourished by synovial fluid, and if a piece flakes off it remains alive inside the joint cavity. But cartilage is also nourished from the subchondral bone by tissue-fluid diffusion: it has no direct blood-supply and no nerve-supply, so that it is a relatively passive structure. It is therefore slow to react to trauma, and it is slow and often incomplete in repair. These two facts have a considerable bearing on clinical practice because after trauma there is no immediate pain if cartilage alone is damaged. It is only when adjacent sensitive structures, like bones and ligaments, are damaged at the same time that pain follows immediately after injury.

The fact that cartilaginous damage occurs at times without the patient being aware of it has several consequences. One is that the same activity which caused the damage may be continued and further unnecessary damage may follow. Another consequence may be that adequate rest to allow for repair is not given to the joint. Repair is therefore often incomplete, and as a sequel to this degenerative changes occur earlier than need be.

Following trauma to any tissue there is swelling owing to the liberation of histamine and plasma kinins. This applies equally to cartilage. Cartilage even swells as a result of forced activity,[30] but because of the absence of blood-supply the oedema only develops slowly. Following injury two or more days may pass before cartilage swells, compared say with damaged ligaments which swell two or more hours after equivalent trauma.

The clinical significance of this lies in the delay in the onset of symptoms after injury. The swelling may stretch adjacent ligament or periosteum to cause pain, or the swelling may block the full range of movements in the joint.

These physiological facts apply equally well to the fibro-cartilage of the intervertebral disc as to the cartilage of peripheral joints. The discs are not bathed in synovial fluid, however, and they have to be nourished entirely by tissue-fluid diffusion from the vertebral body blood-supply. Between the nucleus pulposus and the cancellous bone of the vertebral body is a layer of hyaline cartilage (the end-plate) which is perforated by thousands of small holes through which the tissue fluid diffuses. The fluid diffuses both into and out of the discs. A disc has the quality of a sponge and is able to absorb fluid as well as dispel fluid from itself. There is in fact a diurnal variation in the turgidity of discs. Evidence for this is that the total height of an individual decreases at the end of the day and increases after a night's sleep. The difference may be anything from $\frac{1}{4}$ to $\frac{3}{4}$ in. This change in height cannot be accounted for by mere straightening of the curves of the spine, because the alteration is gradual. De Puky[31] maintained that there was diurnal dehydration and nocturnal hydration.

The proper interchange of tissue fluid between the vertebral bodies and the discs and the proper balance of pressures—hygroscopic, osmotic, and hydrostatic—are vital to the adequate function of intervertebral discs. The pressure within the nucleus is considerable because, if the longitudinal ligaments and annulus fibrosus are all divided in a postmortem specimen immediately after death, the vertebral bodies separate by a distance of 1 mm and a compression force of 100 lb is required to bring the vertebral bodies back again to the same width as before the ligaments were divided.

The turgidity of the nucleus pulposus is kept in check and balanced by the stretch of the annulus fibrosus, and upon this balance rests the integrity of the intervertebral joints. Other mechanical factors are of secondary importance. Even the integrity of the vertebral bony arches is less important. This does not mean that the integrity of the supporting ligaments, the vertebral arches, the muscles, the apophyseal joints, and the shape of the vertebral bodies and their relative positions can be ignored. Faults in any of these components of the intervertebral joints can lead to stress on the intervertebral discs. If the stress is sustained or repeated for long enough the cartilage will give way and then permanent damage results.

While it is possible for direct or indirect trauma to damage intervertebral discs, the amount of force required is considerable because forces sufficient to fracture vertebral bodies do not always damage the adjacent healthy discs. It is estimated that the normal adult disc will withstand a compression force of 1200 lb per sq. in. before rupturing. Less than 1000 lb pressure is enough to damage the vertebral bodies. Normal weight-bearing compression is in the order of 100 lb, but it is estimated that during stooping the compression force is increased to about 500 lb.[32] If now a load of 70 lb is lifted, using the spine only for bending, the compression force is increased to about 1000 lb, which is dangerously near the breaking limit. In spite of this a weight-lifter trained for the work can, with the proper techniques, lift as much as 374 lb without apparent damage. Herein lies the importance of the correct method of lifting, whereby the load is supported only by the spine in the erect position while the lifting is performed by arm and leg leverage.

When discs have undergone degenerative changes, trivial weights may be enough to cause rupture of the cartilage so that the processes of degeneration through which cartilage goes are vitally important not only for our understanding of the problem but also in order to take prophylactic measures to check or minimise the degenerative changes.

Several factors influence the degeneration of cartilage:

1 The inherited quality of the cartilage.
2 Developmental faults during growth and especially osteo-chondrosis in the spine.
3 Trauma, either isolated severe injuries or repeated minor injuries.
4 Sustained mechanical stresses.
5 Local circulatory faults.
6 Biochemical factors not yet determined.

The changes which accompany degeneration in cartilage are both structural and chemical. Softening, fragmentation, fibrosis, gas formation, haemorrhage, and calcification have all been observed. The chemical changes involve an increase in kerato-sulphate and chondroitin sulphate. The gel properties of the nucleus depend upon mucopolysaccharides, and these tend to break down with age. Imbibition of fluid diminishes and the nucleus pulposus becomes less turgid. The distance between the vertebral bodies diminishes and the annulus fibrosus bulges. Under some circumstances, and especially with trauma, the fluid content increases and the internal hydrostatic pressure rises so that the weakened annulus gives way. The disc herniates or prolapses through the annulus fibrosus in the weakest direction. If the annulus fibrosus is intact the pressure may expand at the expense of the cartilaginous end-plate to form a Schmorl's node, post-central disc expansion, or biconcave disc. The symptomatology of these various manifestations of disc degeneration will be discussed later.

Although it is the chemical changes which lead to weakening of the cartilage, mechanical factors are of considerable significance in the aetiology, the location, and the symptomatology of the derangements. The parts of the spine which are most subject to mechanical strains—the lower cervical and the lower lumbar regions—are the areas where spondylosis is most common. Episodes of acute pain from disc swelling and disc protrusion are almost always preceded by some trauma even though small. The direction and the degree of the protrusion depend upon mechanical factors and the sensitivity of the tissues which are affected by the displacements involve the patient in many and varied ways.

3 Synovial membrane

There is considerable doubt about the sensory nerve-supply to synovial membrane. Recent work by Wyke and others[33] has failed to show any sensory nerves in the membrane yet abundant nerves in the ligaments and capsules of joints. If this is so and the articular cartilage is also insensitive, it is difficult to explain the relief of pain which occurs immediately after the injection of a local anaesthetic into the joint cavity.

When mechanically sprained a joint produces more synovial fluid than normal, and quite large effusions can occur; the injury must therefore either stimulate the synovial membrane to increase its secretion or cause the absorption to be decreased. In normal conditions the formation and absorption of synovial fluid is properly balanced so that neither excess fluid persists nor does the joint become dry.

There is considerable elastic tissue in synovial membrane, and in joints where the range of movement is small the synovial membrane retracts away from opposing articular surfaces. However, where movement is very extensive—e.g. the knee and shoulder joints—there are folds in the synovial membrane which can get in the way of opposing surfaces, and in some circumstances these folds are nipped so that bruising or bleeding ensues, resulting in a synovitis or haemarthrosis. Whether this can happen in the spinal apophyseal joints has never been proved but it has often been postulated.

4 Mechanical strains in joints have a sensory component

Proprioceptive impulses reach the spinal cord and central nervous system from the capsules and ligaments. Wyke[34] reports that studies at the Royal College of Surgeons in London have shown that articular nerves contain a mixture of myelinated and unmyelinated nerve-fibres whose diameters range from less than $1\,\mu$ up to $17\,\mu$. There are three principal size categories which subserve different functions:

First, a large proportion (at least 45 per cent) of the total number of fibres in each articular nerve has diameters of less than $5\,\mu$. Most of these small myelinated and unmyelinated fibres, which are embraced in Group III of Table I, are afferent in function and subserve articular pain sensation; but a small proportion of the unmyelinated fibres in this group consists of efferent fibres of sympathetic origin that innervate the articular blood-vessels—that is, these latter are articular vasomotor nerve-fibres. Thus far, we have no anatomical or physiological evidence of the presence of secretomotor fibres in the articular nerves—or, indeed, of any direct nervous influence on the production of synovial fluid.

TABLE I

General composition of articular nerves

Group number	Diameter range	Structure	Function
I	13–17 μ	Large myelinated	Mechanoreceptor afferent (from joint ligaments)
II	6–12 μ	Medium myelinated	Mechanoreceptor afferent (from fibrous capsule and fat pads)
III	2– 5 μ	Small myelinated	Pain afferent
	$\angle$ 2 μ	Unmyelinated	Pain afferent Vasomotor efferent

Secondly, another large proportion (some 45 to 55 per cent of the total) consists of medium-sized myelinated fibres between 6 μ and 12 μ in diameter, and forms Group II of our classification. All of these fibres are mechanoreceptor afferents, innervating small corpuscular endorgans located in the fibrous capsules and fat pads of the joints.

Thirdly, a small proportion (some 10 per cent, or less) consists of large myelinated fibres between 13 μ and 17 μ in diameter, and forms Group I of our classification. These also are mechanoreceptor afferents, innervating *large corpuscular endorgans that are confined to the joint ligaments.*

These studies[35] have also shown that there are four types of articular nerve-endings:

Group I receptors are globular or ovoid, and are numerous in peripheral joints and in the apophyseal joint capsules. They occur in clusters of up to six corpuscles in the outer layers of the fibrous capsule, and are supplied by myelinated fibres (6–9 μ in diameter). These clusters are more densely distributed in those aspects of the joint capsule that undergo changes in stress during natural joint movement. They behave as low-threshold slowly adapting mechano-receptors responding to the mechanical stress obtaining in the part of the fibrous capsule in which they lie. Some of these receptors are active in every position of the joint. The resting discharge rate is 10–20 impulses per second. This is altered whenever the joint is moved passively or actively, whenever the tone in the related muscles changes isotonically or isometrically, or whenever the pressure gradient between the interior of the joint and the atmosphere is altered sufficiently. These type I receptors convey to the cord and brain *sensory impulses of static joint position, intra-articular pressure changes, and the direction, amplitude, and velocity of joint movements.*

Group II receptors are elongated conical corpuscles served by a single unmyelinated nerve terminal of about 5 μ diameter. They are found in all joint capsules in the inner layers of the fibrous capsule. They often lie alongside or coiled around the articular blood-vessels. They are distributed in each joint capsule in clusters of two to four, each member being innervated by a branch of the parent myelinated articular nerve-fibre (9–12 μ). Similar clusters are also found on the surfaces of fat pads in and around the joints. These fibres are inactive in immobile joints, but send afferent discharges at the commencement or cessation of joint movement. Their function is to indicate to the spinal cord and brain that the *joint is accelerating or decelerating.*

Group III receptors are confined to the joint ligaments and are structurally similar in appearance to the tendon organ of Golgi. They are served by axons up to 17 μ in diameter. They are found in the *spinal apophyseal joint ligaments but are absent from the longitudinal ligaments of the vertebral column.* These nerve-endings are inactive when the joint is immobile but *become active when the joint is reaching its limit of stretch.*

Group IV receptors are free nerve-endings or lattice-like plexuses linked by small unmyelinated fibres (2–5 μ) and distributed throughout the fibrous capsule, the adjacent periosteum, the articular fat pads, and the sheaths of articular blood-vessels. These are *the pain receptors* of articular tissues. They become activated only when there is marked mechanical deformation, or direct mechanical or chemical irritation. These fibres were entirely absent from the synovial lining of all the joints studied.

The investigators concluded that there is no mechanism whereby articular pain can arise directly from synovial membrane or from the intra-articular cartilage of joints. They also concluded that the mechano-receptors in articular tissues make substantial contributions to the perception of joint posture and movement, and are the main contributions to postural and kinaesthetic sensation rather than the sensory muscle receptors.

These important observations by Wyke et al. stress the role of the ligaments and capsules rather than the muscles as the sensory receptors. They convey impulses both at rest and in motion, both normal and abnormal to provide the central nervous system with complex information so that reflex muscle contractions can be co-ordinated during movement and during postural adjustment to change of position.

Abnormal afferent discharges result in corresponding abnormal reflex motor responses.

Most of the sensory impressions are intermittent but if sustained, because of persisting mechanical stresses, two reflex effects may follow: the segment of the cord which is constantly bombarded by the abnormal afferent discharge may become irritable so that a facilitated segment develops or, in time, reflex fatigue can set in so that the reaction to the stimulus diminishes. This is in line with the body's response to other sustained sensory impulses—e.g. a continuous noise will at first cause heightening of the sensitivity to it, but later the brain inhibits the noise and this may eventually lead to permanent inhibition in the form of deafness to those particular frequencies of sound. The same applies to the sense of smell, though olfactory fatigue sets in much more quickly than does auditory fatigue.

The effects of continuous bombardment on the central nervous system by abnormal sensory impulses from mechanically strained joints is important to the osteopathic concept and this will be discussed further, on p. 287, but in addition the muscles which move the affected joint are reflexly stimulated to contract to protect the joint from further injury. Sustained reflex contraction of muscle causes secondary pain. If the contraction is prolonged structional changes occur in the muscle itself (p. 88).

6 MECHANICAL EFFECTS ON MUSCLE

Excessive use of muscle will lead to hypertrophy; lack of use to atrophy. Separational stresses may be powerful enough to tear muscle fibres or their tendons. Continuous stretching at first evokes the stretch reflex; but if it is prolonged the stretch leads to loss of muscle substance because, in order to remain normal, muscle must contract intermittently. Continuous contraction may lead eventually to contracture and shortening. Contraction of isolated groups of muscle fibres when sustained is called 'fibrositis'. These contracted fibres can be palpated: they are tight and tender, and feel like cords running through the surrounding relaxed muscles. If contraction is sustained long enough, the muscle fibres undergo fibrous tissue metaplasia. The cause of most fibrositis is irritability of the nerve-supply to the muscle bundle. Elliott[36] found 'tender spots indistinguishable from the more benign forms of myalgia both in their clinical features and in their response to procaine in the muscles supplied by an irritated nerve root'. He considered that the myalgic spots were not inflammatory in origin but were caused by local muscle spasm. He confirmed this by electromyographic studies.

Discussing muscular pain in the spine, Strange[37] stated: 'These points of bundle spasm are palpable as well as tender. That they are indeed muscle bundles in spasm is confirmed by a number of other physical signs: the thickening is spindle-shaped; it lies in the line of the fibres of the muscle under examination; it moves at right angles to the line of those fibres; if it is pressed, a reflex flick of contraction of the whole bundle of which it is part may often be observed; it is almost invariably situated in one of the antigravity muscles.'

Further discussion on fibrositis will be found under 'soft tissue' Spinal Syndromes (p. 236).

Sustained muscle activity, as in strenuous exertion, leads to temporary swelling of the muscle, but this passes off unnoticed except in cases where the surrounding fascia is too tight—e.g. in the anterior tibial syndrome—or where the oedema of the muscle further embarrasses nerves which are under pressure already from other mechanical factors.

There are mechanical effects upon other tissues from changes in muscle tone. Weakness of muscle renders joints and their ligaments more vulnerable to strain. Generalised muscular weakness leads to poor posture. Conversely excessively powerful muscle action can damage bone—e.g. a fracture of the patella can occur from muscle contraction, and stress fractures can result from prolonged and excessive muscular activity.

7 MECHANICAL EFFECTS ON SKIN AND CONNECTIVE TISSUE

Intermittent pressure on the skin leads to cornification, and sustained pressure leads to atrophy, as in bed-sores. Continuous pressure on fat leads to loss of the fat beneath, as when elastic corsets are worn continuously and too tightly. Even the muscle below the fat will diminish to some extent, but muscle is more resilient to pressure compared with fat.

Connective tissue disorders are now grouped under the heading of the collagen diseases, and they are not discussed here because the aetiology of these diseases is chemical rather than mechanical.

COMPENSATORY MECHANISMS

The human body is remarkably adaptive. Reasonable health can be maintained in extremes of cold and heat. The digestive system can adapt to wide ranges of food from carnivorous to vegetarian and even vegan diets. The musculature will adapt itself to the habits of the individual so as to cope adequately with the average exercises which that person performs.

Adaptations occur, as already pointed out, to postural habits. If conditions are adverse enough, the adaptation breaks down and symptoms of protest warn us to change or reduce the stresses. If we do not take heed of these warnings, permanent damage results; but even then compensating mechanisms are brought in to keep the body function at least at survival level.

To give a chemical as distinct from a mechanical example, if alcohol is consumed regularly the liver in its detoxicating capacity learns to deal more efficiently with the chemical, and the body thereby adapts itself to a moderate amount of alcohol. If inordinate quantities of alcohol are taken, however, liver cells are destroyed and this damage is permanent; but even so there is compensatory hypertrophy of the remaining cells in an attempt to cope with the circumstances, and it is a long time before the cirrhotic liver gives up the ghost!

Our purpose in treating patients osteopathically is to help the body to adapt itself to the everyday mechanical stresses imposed upon it.

If a farmer comes complaining of backache, our first thought should not be to advise him to change his job and so reduce the stress on his back, rather should we improve the muscles, ligaments, and bones so that they can adapt themselves to his particular stresses. By correct use of his muscles, by improving his posture, by dividing the loads more evenly, and by correcting mechanical faults in his spine, we may well enable the man to continue with his occupation. This is our primary task. Nature has made an attempt and failed; but by understanding and treating the mechanical problem, we may restore the adaptive processes so that they can cope with these stresses. Only if we fail, or the body's tissues are not strong enough, should we then think in terms of compensation.

This is reflected in the osteopathic attitude, compared with the current orthopaedic attitude, to corsets. To the osteopath the corset is a last resort; it is an acknowledgement of the failure of treatment to restore normality or the failure of the tissues to cope with the mechanical stresses in that particular patient's spine. But a corset is often the first line of treatment prescribed by orthopaedic and physical medicine specialists.

Visceral adaptation is well recognised—for example, the hypertrophy of the remaining kidney after nephrectomy, the proliferation of marrow in menorrhagia, and the increase of haemoglobin in the blood when people live at high altitudes; but structural adaptation and compensation is less well recognised.

In scoliosis the muscles adapt to the extra load placed upon them on the convexity of the curve, but the bones and ligaments compensate for the imbalance by curving in the opposite direction further up the spine.

Electromyographic studies[38] in scoliosis have shown an increase of action potentials in muscles on the convexity of the curve.

In a patient who has one leg shorter than the other, compensation is often adequate even in the sacro-iliac joints, so that despite the shortening the sacrum is level and the spine straight. Compensation may also occur further up the spine. But sometimes the compensation is excessive, and this needs our attention. When treating the scoliosis we direct attention to the primary fault and not to the compensation. If the primary is corrected too rapidly, this sometimes upsets the compensation, and symptoms may result. In management of the short-leg syndrome, all this has to be taken into consideration: it will be dealt with in Chapter 3 (p. 132).

The difference of outlook between osteopathic and orthopaedic methods is well illustrated by the short-leg syndrome and its treatment. The osteopath will consider that even $\frac{1}{4}$ in. of discrepancy in the leg length is important, whereas the orthopaedic surgeon will ignore any discrepancy less than $\frac{3}{4}$ in. Perhaps it is a matter of emphasis. The osteopath who is preoccupied with the less serious locomotor problems pays more attention to detail. The orthopaedic surgeon who is preoccupied with serious fractures, gross scoliosis, tuberculosis, and neoplasms is apt to regard minor structural faults as unimportant. There may not be any symptoms at the time, but the cumulative effect of $\frac{1}{4}$ in. of leg shortening over many years is considerable, and this is a proven aetiological factor in backache of ligamentous origin as well as in pathological conditions of the disc.[39]

Nature appears to make more effort to compensate for gross structural faults than for minor ones. I have seen many patients with over 1 in. of shortening who are thoroughly compensated and symptom free, yet with $\frac{1}{4}$ in. of shortening other patients suffer from backache which can only be relieved by using a $\frac{1}{4}$ in. heel cushion.

Where there is a structural fault which cannot be remedied then our task is to help the compensatory mechanisms to give the best attainable functional response. When a corset is inevitable then one should also encourage movement and persevere with exercises to maintain muscle tone, rather than relying on this extraneous agency alone and allowing the muscles to atrophy from disuse.

Another example to illustrate the application of adaption first and compensation later is to be found in intervertebral disc disease. Our first task is to try to restore normality as far as possible. Normality in this context means restoration of normal position of bone and cartilage, restoration of mobility as far as is practicable, maintenance of good muscle power, and encouragement of normal activities within the capacity of the patient and his tissues. Most cases will respond well, but if these measures fail and the pathological process has gone too far to hope for restoration of normality, then we must (and the patient must) accept the limitations of the permanent damage, and treatment must be reviewed. Instead of mobilising the area, we must immobilise—i.e. use corsets, sclerosing injections, or operations to remove offending displacements and/or to ankylose the damaged joint. After these measures have achieved stability we must next encourage compensation in adjacent joints to enable them to take over the loss of function in the affected joint.

These basic principles must be kept clearly in mind when planning treatment. To recapitulate, our objectives are, in their order of preference:

1 Prophylaxis
2 Correction and adaptation
3 Compensation

To illustrate these principles with further reference to disc disease we ought, as a means of prophylaxis, to treat all predisposing mechanical problems, including ordinary osteopathic lesions, so that the degenerative disc changes do not ensue. If degeneration does take place, then we must correct as far as possible and help adaptation to the fault. If then, despite all our corrective efforts, the condition deteriorates, we must compensate for the permanent structural disability as best we can.

THE OSTEOPATHIC SPINAL LESION

So far the discussion has been on the general effects of abnormal mechanical stresses on separate tissues. Now we must particularise and dwell on a keystone of osteopathic practice—namely, the mechanical fault of the spine known as the osteopathic spinal lesion. *This is a condition of impaired mobility in an intervertebral joint, in which there may or may not be altered positional relations of adjacent vertebrae. But when altered position is present it is always within the normal range of movement at that joint.*

The keynote of this definition is 'impared mobility', and because impaired mobility in the intervertebral joint is a keystone of osteopathic practice, we must describe in detail both the lesion and the changes in mobility.

Why should such a lesion be so important? What evidence is there for its existence, and how does it manifest itself clinically?

A condition of impaired mobility in a peripheral joint is a nuisance but it is not of major importance, and it has no wide repercussions on the individual. This is because the individual can compensate well for the reduced movement, and as there are no vital nerves or blood-vessels in the vicinity the remote effects from it are negligible. Not so with the intervertebral joint.

Osteopathic spinal lesions always produce local signs, and the symptoms are predominantly local to the spine; but sometimes they cause remote effects because of the close proximity of the spinal nerves, the rami communicantes, the spinal blood-vessels, and the spinal cord itself. Furthermore, because spinal lesions are inclined to become chronic, they are of the greatest importance.

Restricted mobility in the knee is obvious, and the individual makes strenuous efforts (with or without medical guidance) to restore movement. Restricted mobility in a shoulder is less obvious and less spontaneous effort is made to restore movement; consequently adhesions in the shoulder are commoner and take longer to recover. Restricted mobility in spinal joints is not obvious even if two or three are involved; and, as pain may be minimal, little spontaneous effort is made to restore the ranges of movement and some restriction becomes permanent. I recall a patient with ankylosing spondylitis whose overall spinal movements were only about 10 per cent of normal, and yet he had long been unaware of the disability which had only recently become painful. He was a sedentary worker who was not interested in sport, and because the stiffness had developed slowly he had not noticed it. His limb joints had remained flexible, and he had therefore been able to pursue all his daily activities without difficulty.

On the face of it then, one or two spinal joint restrictions appear to be of little importance, but it is a fact that continuing loss of function in any tissue leads to deterioration in that tissue, so that degenerative changes take place in stiff joints earlier than they otherwise need to. Almost all spinal X-rays in people over forty years of age, whether suffering symptoms or not, show signs of degenerative change, particularly in the lower cervical, the mid thoracic and the lower lumbar areas. These degenerative changes were found to be much commoner in heavy workers than in light workers—e.g. 43 per cent of miners showed severe disc degeneration compared with 7 per cent in office workers in the same group.[40] The lower cervical and lower lumbar sites are the most vulnerable from mechanical stresses and injuries, because they are relatively flexible areas joined to relatively rigid sections of the spine. Leverage exerted on the neck is transmitted to the 5–7C joints, and these give way under strain rather than the upper cervical or the upper thoracic joints. The same applies to the lower lumbar region, where a mobile series of joints meets an unyielding pelvis.

A degenerating joint may be quiescent symptomatically but it is vulnerable, so that minor stresses provoke undue responses clinically.

This applies to any joint, but more so to weight-bearing joints and spinal joints. Spinal joints are the most vulnerable of all because of the prevalence of internal derangements in the discs. Inflammatory and further degenerative changes tend to follow from minor trauma. The cartilage is nourished by diffusion, and although it is slow to react to trauma the repair processes are also slow; once damaged, cartilage does not regenerate unless given absolutely ideal conditions, for example, over the head of the femur which is protected by a vitellium cup.

Damage to cartilage is repaired by fibrous-tissue metaplasia, and this is never as strong as the original cartilage. The nucleus of intervertebral fibro-cartilage becomes soft and the annulus fibrosus weakens. Minor trauma can then produce the clinical syndromes of herniation and prolapse.

Because osteopathic spinal lesions lead to pathological disc conditions, it is important to treat the lesion in the early stages before degenerative changes develop. Restricted mobility can, in most cases, be restored by manipulation. Normalisation of mobility restores the circulation, decreases the rate of degeneration, and minimizes any later pathological changes. To do this is eminently worth while, and on this basis the whole spine of any and every patient should be examined for lesions whatever the presenting symptoms are, and all the sites of reduced mobility should be manipulated.

This statement that all rigid spinal joints should be manipulated must not be misconstrued. Many rigid spinal joints are best left alone, and discrimination is required to decide which should be and should not be manipulated. This belongs to the realm of mechanical diagnosis. A section on indications and contra-indications to manipulation of spinal joints will be found in the Appendix, p. 279. All spinal joints should be examined for mobility; *if* restricted and there are no contraindications they should be manipulated. There is no point in manipulating a normal joint even though clicks can be obtained from it in the process: nothing is gained because normal exercise will maintain normal movements.

Normal exercise can maintain good overall general mobility, but it will not restore one or two isolated spinal joint restrictions. If anything, the adjacent normal joints will stretch a little more, and the stiff joint will remain. Manipulation when carefully and accurately performed can move the restricted joint without moving the adjacent mobile ones. This is where the skill of manipulation lies, and the details of procedure for achieving this with the appropriate ligamentous or facet apposition locking techniques are described in my *Manual of Osteopathic Technique*.

Features of the osteopathic lesion

1 Hypomobility (or hypermobility in some circumstances)
2 Positional faults
3 Pain and tenderness
4 Muscular tension
5 Reflex changes in skin and muscle; vasomotor and visceromotor
   changes.

An osteopathic spinal lesion is in essence a joint strain. It is a
functional entity (but not 'functional' in the psychological or derog-
atory sense) in which the dynamics of joint play are impaired. It is not a
pathological state. It could be described as a hyperfunctional or
hypofunctional state of the joint, but once pathological changes have
established themselves it is no longer a simple osteopathic spinal lesion.
It has then advanced or rather deteriorated into a spondylosis. If other
pathological processes are present, of course, the condition is not an
osteopathic lesion.

The border-line between physiology and pathology is not well defined. One would not describe a sprained ankle as a pathological state;
neither is a sprained spinal joint pathological, because both of these
conditions can recover and in the natural course of events both will recover, but the sprained ankle has a better chance of recovering fully
than has a sprained spinal joint, as explained earlier.

Because of this dynamic rather than pathological state, description
and proof are difficult. A sprained joint would—if examined histologically—show rupture of ligamentous fibres, some ecchymosis, and
some histamine-like changes in the blood-vessels, but that is all. These
are the responses to trauma anywhere in the body. The muscles surrounding the joint are reflexly on guard but they are not at fault
pathologically and no histological changes would be observable. This
must apply equally well to a spinal joint.

If a joint is under mechanical strain (rather than having just had a
recent sprain) it is doubtful if any histological changes could be demonstrated, but if the strain continues long enough, a joint lesion with
hypermobility or hypomobility will ensue, and eventually degenerative
changes will be demonstrable both microscopically and macroscopically.

But even though the osteopathic spinal lesion is not demonstrable on
a postmortem table or under the microscope, this does not disprove its
existence. The proof invokes other evidence which is clinical in nature.
This means that we have to rely on its physical signs for proof, and much
depends on the interpretation of those physical signs by the examining
physician. Physicians are fallible: physical signs are not always easy to

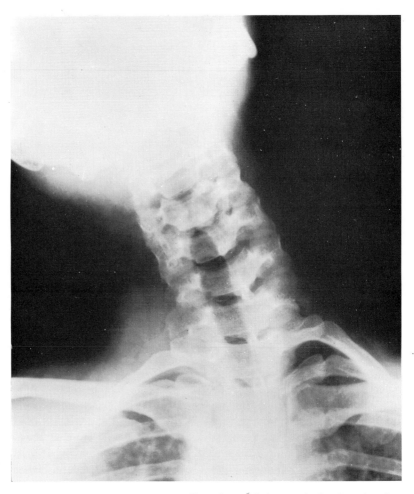

FIGS 1 AND 2 Side-bending mobility views of the cervical spine showing restriction of side-bending to the left at 4–5C. FIG 1 Side-bending to left.

demonstrate. Reduced mobility of 50 per cent in a knee is obvious because we can see it, whereas reduced mobility in a single spinal joint cannot be seen. The overall spinal movements may be full and compensation may be complete. A patient with a synovial effusion, say of 2–3C, has a complete range of overall neck movements; but if the single joints are tested individually then the restriction can be palpated. The gap between the spinous processes at 2–3C during flexion and extension is small. At maximum range there will be less than 5 mm of movement. If the range is 50 per cent it may be 2 or 3 mm in range. The physician has to take great care in palpation to distinguish between a normally mobile and a hypomobile or hypermobile spinal joint. Not only does it

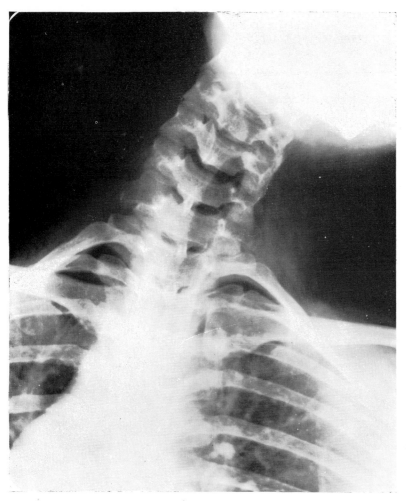

FIG 2 Side-bending to right showing normal mobility.

need care, but it needs practice. Confirmation of mobility can be obtained by taking *mobility X-rays* in flexion-extension. Side-bending mobility films (*figs. 1 and 2*) are useful, but rotational X-rays are usually so confusing to read that measurement is impracticable. Clinically, however, rotation can be palpable if the physician will take the trouble to improve his tactile skill.

From the clinical point of view it matters a good deal whether the 2–3C joint is mobile or not. It matters, too, for mechanical diagnosis whether we can distinguish between a lesion at 2–3C and at 3–4C. It matters because both the distribution of pain and the technique of manipulation will be different. To manipulate the ankle instead of the

41

knee would be considered ludicrous if the stiffness were in the knee joint. Why should not the same apply between 2–3C and 3–4C? Granted it requires more skill in palpation and more skill in the art of localising the forces of manipulation, but these skills are eminently attainable. Such finesse in techniques is possible in other medical spheres—witness, for example, the delicacy of a fenestration operation. Why should we not acquire an equivalent tactile finesse in palpation and manipulation? We all know of the incredible skill of the pianist and the remarkable delicacy of touch and tone which emerges from the grand piano. Our instrument—the human spine—is generally more robust than a piano, and it will stand rough handling when youth and elasticity are there, but it becomes a delicate instrument when old and frail. It is then that manipulations must be either delicate or not performed at all. Anyone without much musical sense can learn to play a simple tune, and anyone without much tactile sense can perform a few crude manipulations. But it requires a Rubinstein to bring out all the glory of a Beethoven sonata, and it requires a dedicated practitioner to obtain the best results from manipulation.

To manipulate a flail knee joint would be mere folly, yet often hypermobile joints in the spine have been manipulated because sufficient care has not been taken to examine them.

A spinal joint may be hypermobile:
1 Immediately after injury and before muscle guarding has set in.
2 Under continuous ligamentous strain.
3 In certain individuals in whom hypermobility is the norm.
4 In late degenerative changes of the intervertebral disc when the turgescence of the nucleus pulposus is lost and the stabilising effects of the annulus fibrosus cannot be maintained.

Details of mobility tests in individual spinal joints will be found in my *Manual of Osteopathic Technique*.

The ranges of individual spinal movements vary from patient to patient according to their make-up and the degree of habitual exercise taken. In adjacent spinal joints either there are approximately equal ranges of movement or there is a slow gradation of range from one area to the next. For example, in the thoracic joints the ranges of flexion-extension from above downwards are $3°, 3°, 3°, 2\frac{1}{2}°, 2\frac{1}{2}°, 2°, 1°, 1°, 4°, 7°$, and $9°$. The gap between adjacent spinous processes during flexion and extension can therefore be fairly well judged by comparing the range above and below the suspected lesion.

Mobility

The *mobility fault* may be in any range, including forward and backward-bending, side-bending, or rotation to either side, or in a combination of any of these movements. The fault may be a reduced range (hypo-mobility) or an excessive range (hypermobility), and either of these can cause symptoms.

Generalised stiffening arises from tightening of the capsules—which can happen with increasing age or disuse—but this is not regarded as an osteopathic spinal lesion. Individual restriction (especially in one range only) is almost certainly due to adhesions. Decreased movement in every range usually indicates an inflammatory or pathological state, and additional care must be taken over the differential diagnosis.

Generalised hypermobility is not in itself a fault, though patients in this category are more vulnerable to joint sprains. To be more accurate, such individuals when subject to a joint sprain react more severely than those who are stockily built, and their response to treatment is less satis-factory. Individual joint hypermobility occurs anywhere in the spine, but especially in the following sites: 4–7C, 9–12T, 4L–1S, and the sacro-iliac joints.

Testing spinal movements by recording the overall range is useful but often misleading, and it is not much guide to the level of the lesion. A common clinical pattern is the combination of two or three hypo-mobile joints and one or two hypermobile joints which are compensat-ing for the restricted ones. As both a hypomobile and a hypermobile joint can cause symptoms—often of a similar character—the mobility tests assume still more importance. More discussion on this point is presented in Chapter 3.

When defining an osteopathic lesion on the basis of its mobility we must first say whether it is hypermobile or hypomobile. Next, the range of movement which is affected must be stated; and, to avoid confusion over the exact meaning of flexion and extension, we use the terms for-ward-bending (F-Bg), backward-bending (B-Bg), side-bending (S-Bg), and rotation (Rn). Thus there are the following types of hypomobile lesion:

1 B-Bg restriction
2 F-Bg restriction
3 Rn restriction to right or left
4 S-Bg restriction to right or left
5 Combined restrictions

There are also hypermobile lesions in:

1 B-Bg
2 F-Bg
3 Rn to right or left
4 S-Bg to right or left
5 Combined ranges
6 Abnormal ranges, e.g. sheering movements

One must remember that the osteopathic spinal lesion is not a disc lesion. Disc derangements are discussed more fully in Chapter 3. Disc lesions pass through hypermobile and hypomobile phases during the course of their clinical manifestations. In defining such disc lesions we require a different terminology. The disc is 'herniated', 'prolapsed', 'degenerated', 'quiescent', 'recovering', 'stabilised', 'expanded', or 'lentiform', and one attempts to describe the pathological state of the disc when making a diagnosis. The term 'disc lesion' leaves the exact diagnosis open, just as does 'internal derangement of the knee'. Sometimes we have to be content with this simple uncritical diagnosis, but it is really not good enough.

The description of the osteopathic spinal lesion should indicate what physical signs are present. The position of the vertebra could be used, but as we shall see this is less satisfactory than describing its mobility.

Position

At one stage in osteopathic history the lesion was considered to be a bone displacement, and this arose from the fact that the relative position of one vertebra to the next was quite frequently altered. Also many patients described spontaneously the sensation of something moving abnormally in their spines. In addition, manipulation of such spines frequently brought about dramatic improvement in symptoms; and, as the manipulation was accompanied by a click, naturally the assumption was made that the bone had gone 'back into place'. Systems of manipulation were devised on this basis. The bone having been 'displaced' it must be put back and made to go in the direction from which it came out.

This 'bone out of place' conception is still upheld by many chiropractors and bone-setters, but the idea is losing ground amongst osteopaths, and in medicine the theory is superseded by discs going 'in and out of place'. That discs can swell and even burst, that they can herniate, and that fragments of disc can displace are undoubtedly true; but it is doubtful whether, once a disc has protruded, it can be completely replaced. Certainly, manipulation can often dramatically relieve pain, but the explanation is not always so easy of satisfactory proof. Disc herniations and prolapses are relatively terminal stages in disc disease, and when we talk about osteopathic spinal lesions, the joint has not reached that late stage.

The conception of a joint lesion (as distinct from a bone displacèment) is much more valid. The joint has been sprained and adhesions have formed—these are perhaps unilateral, binding it more on one side than the other, or affecting one apophyseal joint more than the other at the same level. The resulting restrictions of movement may be unilateral or unidirectional, and the adhesions may hold the vertebra more to one side, giving rise to minor positional variations. Another possible explanation is that joints get 'hitched' or 'jambed askew'. 'Joint bind' is another term useful in this context. Most of the sudden and dramatic results of manipulation must be in these conditions rather than in disc prolapses, because the pathological changes of disc degeneration take a long time to develop and a simple manipulation could not restore normality so quickly.

Peripheral joints can become 'hitched' and painful, and a sudden movement or manipulation can restore normal movement and stop the pain. The probable explanation here is that the articular cartilage has become roughened and irregular adjacent surfaces are awkwardly opposed. This can also happen in the apophyseal joints of the spine.

The click of a specific manipulation is certainly not the result of a disc being replaced. It is the sound of separation of two articular surfaces. Such a click in a normal joint means nothing at all. But, if the apophyseal joint has previously become 'hitched' and the click is followed by full movement at the joint, then something has been achieved by the manipulation, *but the disc has not gone back*. The only sound which has ever convinced me as being of disc origin is a very soft one—virtually inaudible, though palpable. This occurred once when I was applying traction in the flexed position in a patient with a history of recurrent attacks of low-back pain, who was in the recovering phase of one of his attacks, and my treatment was articulatory. He was lying prone (*Manual of Osteopathic Technique*, p. 254, fig. 153), with his feet strapped down at the end of the McManis table and holding on at the head end of the table, while I was articulating the lumbar spine in flexion, using a rhythmic movement of the lower leaf of the table. My left hand was palpating his lumbar spine when I felt a soft click; the patient was aware of it, and he compared it with other occasions when his disc had 'gone out'. On standing, the patient's pelvic shift had returned, whereas it had previously been recovering.

Another patient with persistent low-back pain received great relief from the application of traction in the prone position in a similar way to the above, but not until a click occurred did he feel relief. No doubt the click meant a separation of the articular facets. On one subsequent occasion, after performing this manipulation with evident satisfaction to the patient and to me, we heard a soft click; but this caused discomfort instead of relief, and quite soon afterwards sciatica developed which was obviously due to a disc prolapse.

Both these patients were made worse by prone traction in flexion, and this taught me to avoid the technique where disc disease is present or latent. It also taught me that the characteristic sound of a disc fragment moving is soft and virtually inaudible.

On many occasions I have been equally satisfied that after a similar soft click there has been a great relief of symptoms, and I have assumed that these sounds were of disc origin. The fact that the patient recovered, although satisfactory clinically, is not convincing proof that the disc displacement had caused the symptoms in the first place. They might have been caused by an apophyseal joint lesion, and the sound might have emanated from the facets.

The *positional* relationship between two vertebrae is by convention and convenience described with reference to the upper of two vertebrae. If the fourth lumbar vertebra is *rotated to the right*, it implies that the body of 4L is rotated to the right on the body of 5L in such a way that the spinous process of 4L is to the left of the 5L spinous process and the transverse process of 4L on the right is more posterior. It has a 'high side' on the right.

The term *tilted to the left*—say of the sixth thoracic vertebra—implies that it is tilted to the left on the seventh vertebra. The transverse process on the left is inferior and that on the right superior. The disc space is wedge-shaped and is narrower on the left.

The term *a flexion lesion of 4C* implies that the body of 4C is tilted forward on the body of 5C and the spinous processes at 4–5C are separated. The disc space is narrowed anteriorly compared with posteriorly.

Similarly an *extension lesion of 6C* implies a backward tilt of 6C on 7C and an approximation of the spines of 6 and 7C.

Although these positional appearances are visible on X-ray plates, and although it might be convenient to describe spinal lesions in this way there are several disadvantages:

1 Palpation alone of bony prominences is not a reliable guide to the position of the vertebral body or of the apophyseal joints. Spinous processes are notoriously irregular in shape; and even transverse processes can differ in their inclination on the two sides. (The transverse processes are, however, more reliable, and they should always be palpated for position in assessing a lesion.)

2 Even if there is a 'flexion lesion' and the spinous process of 4C is

approximated to the spinous process of 3C and separated from 5C, this does not indicate which joint is at fault, because either 3–4C or 4–5C, or both, may be in lesion.

3 The position of a vertebra is a static concept but we are not just dealing with bones, we are dealing with ligaments, muscles, nerves and discs. The whole concept of the spinal lesion should be of a living moving dynamic entity.

4 The position of a vertebra is not a reliable guide to the choice of techniques of manipulation, whereas the mobility is of utmost importance. Only if the joint mobility gives inadequate guidance in the choice of techniques do we need to consider the position of the vertebrae relative to each other.

5 The position of the vertebra is not a reliable guide to the site of a disc prolapse, and this again gives no help in the choice of manipulation or other treatment for disc lesions.

The position of a vertebra is significant where there is a pathological shift—that is, if the position is abnormal because it was produced by a movement which cannot normally occur. These are 'shifts', and they are of a sheering nature. Forward shift is a 'spondylolisthesis', and backward shift is a 'retrolisthesis'. Lateral shifts rarely occur, but when they do, serious internal derangement of the disc structure is implied. These shifts reflect serious derangements of spinal joints, and they are outside the limited meaning of the term osteopathic spinal lesion.

Though it is a mistake to describe lesions with reference to their position, this does not imply that the vertebral position is never important. The position of a vertebra depends on a number of factors which may be extremely important in any single case. The following factors govern the position of vertebrae:

(*a*) Posture—in this instance the position of a group of vertebrae may be altered.
(*b*) Anomalous shapes.
(*c*) Pelvic tilts—either lateral or antero-posterior.
(*d*) The internal architecture of the intervertebral disc.
(*e*) The shape of the articular processes and their facets.
(*f*) The length of the ligaments.
(*g*) The tension in the small muscles which move adjacent vetebrae.
(*h*) Pain.
(*i*) Adhesions.

For X-rays showing faulty position and corrected position after manipulation see *figs. 3, 4, 5, 6.*

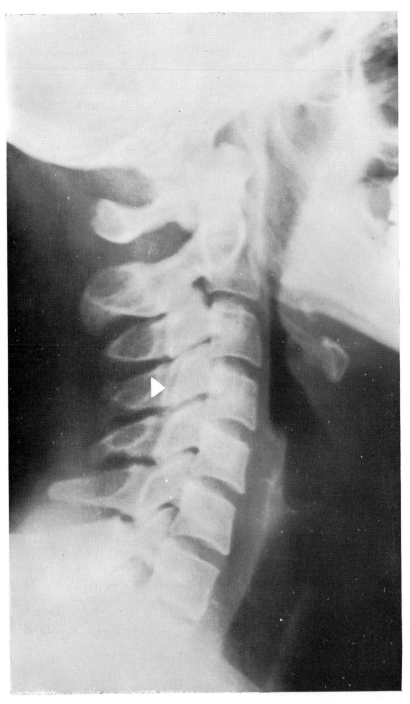

FIG 3 Lateral views of cervical spine showing overlap of the articular processes of 4C—indicative of rotation. There is no overlap of other articular processes.

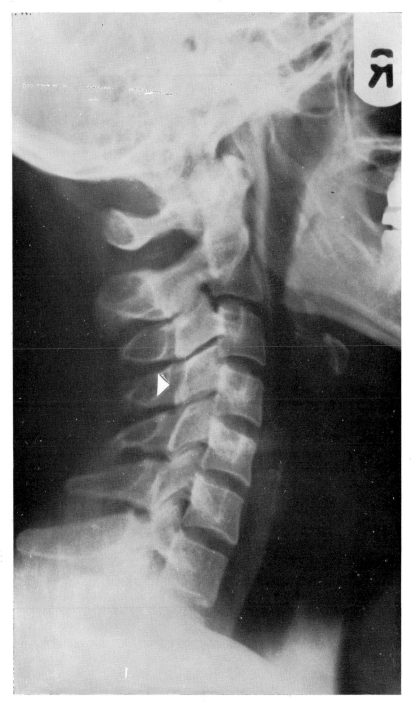

FIG 4 Cervical spine of the same patient immediately after manipulation. The articular processes of 4C are now in line.

49

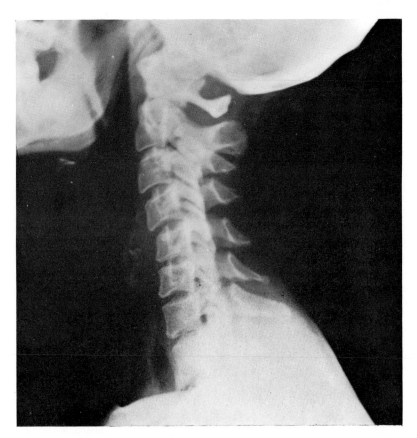

FIG 5 Lateral view of cervical spine showing posterior gapping at 4–5C.

When assessing a mechanical problem of the spine, the position of the vertebrae should be determined, and when faulty one should attempt to determine the cause of the displacement because this forms part of the mechanical diagnosis of the case.

Pain and tenderness

Although pain is not always present at the site of an osteopathic spinal lesion, *tenderness is a constant feature* even in chronic lesions. Tenderness is best elicited by comparing the site with other joints remote from the lesion. When palpating a normal spinal joint there is no tenderness over any of its components. It is, of course, possible to provoke tenderness if pressure is applied hard enough, but excessive pressure should be avoided. The site of tenderness is in the supraspinous ligament of the lesioned joint. The spinous process may also be tender, but normally

50

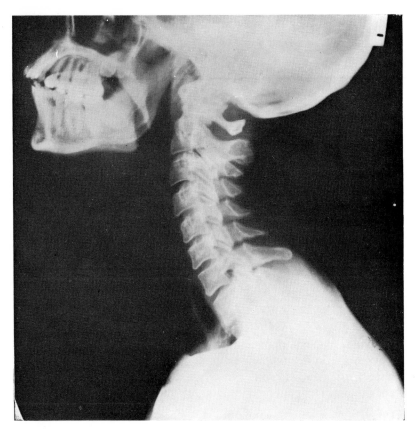

FIG 6 Same view showing correction of alignment at 4–5C.

it is less so. The transverse process may be tender, but, when this is the case, it is difficult to exclude tenderness in the overlying muscles. These muscles as well as the transverse process may be tender. Superficial to the transverse processes are the semispinalis, multifidi, rhomboids, trapezii, latissimus dorsi, and sacrospinalis muscles. Fibrositis in these muscles is a common accompaniment of the lesion. The small deeper muscles—longissimus dorsi and cervices—and the semispinalis and multifidi are attached to the transverse processes, and they may be tender at their attachments.

Differentiating between muscular tenderness, ligamentous tenderness, and bony tenderness is sometimes impossible because there is so much overlapping. But when muscle is 'stringy' in character and can be rolled over subjacent tissue producing tenderness at the same time, the tenderness must arise in these fibres because it can be abolished with with local anaesthesia. When possible these fibres should be pushed

51

aside and the deeper structures palpated for tenderness. Tenderness can be transient—for example, it may be present when the patient is prone and not when she is on her side. (In this book the patient is always feminine and the operator masculine—not for any Freudian reason, but for convenience of description!)

Pain arising from a spinal segment has a certain distribution; it is felt locally in the spine and/or referred to the dermatome, sclerotome, or myotome which is reflexly connected with that segment. Anatomy books must be consulted to give the reader the distribution, but it must be stressed that skin distribution of pain from deep structures is difficult to localise and that there is considerable overlapping of adjacent dermatomes.

When we consider the differential diagnosis of deep sources of pain in terms merely of its distribution, we find little help. It has been shown (by Lewis, Kellgren and others[24]) that if hypertonic saline is injected deeply anywhere in the spinal segment it produces pain of a segmental pattern. This somatically produced pain is also indistinguishable from viscerally produced pain if the sources of pain have the same neurological segmental level.

Although the distribution of pain is a guide to the level of its origin, it is no use in determining its exact source. Other evidence—e.g. the history, the relationship to movement and position, the relief by local anaesthesia, etc.—must be used to determine the source of pain more precisely.

Because the pain in a spinal lesion is deep and often diffuse, the localisation is poor. Its severity depends upon the acuteness of the lesion.

Nerve-root pressure from an apophyseal joint lesion, while theoretically possible because the intervertebral foramina are bounded posteriorly by the capsules of the apophyseal joints, is in my view extremely unlikely; and, if a patient presents with abnormal neurological signs and a root distribution of pain, I make a diagnosis of a disc prolapse or other more serious pathological process.

The pain of a recent sprain is continuous at first, but within a few days this subsides and then it occurs only if the sensitive ligaments are stretched. 'Stretching' pain and 'compression' pain are useful terms when describing a spinal lesion. A stretching pain is felt on the same side as the stretch, whereas a 'compression' pain is felt on the opposite side; but 'compression' pain does not occur in a simple spinal sprain.

There are two sources of pain in the simple osteopathic spinal lesion. One is ligamentous and it conforms to the above pattern: the other is a duller pain *arising in the muscles.* Any muscle which stays contracted long enough will ache—this has a 'burning' character and is relieved by muscle action, only to return again when the muscle is static once more.

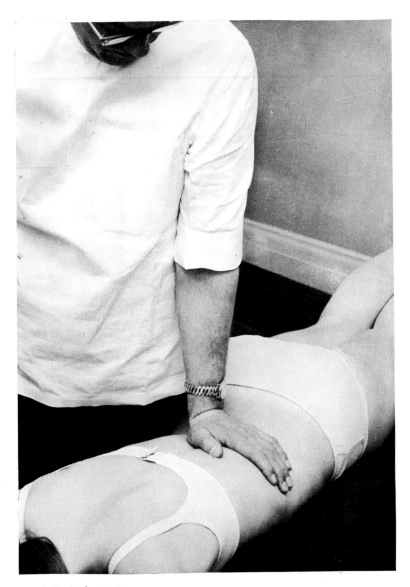

FIG 7 Springing test.

Reflex muscular contraction

The reflex contraction of muscles round a spinal lesion depends on the intensity of the pain. It can be intensified and provoked by the *springing test* (fig. 7): the patient is placed in the prone position, and a springing pressure is applied to the suspected lesion. If the lesion is acute the muscles surrounding the joint contract reflexly: they were already

53

contracted and at the ready, and the jolt of springing puts them on 'guard' to protect the sensitive joint against further pain. The time relationship is important with this test. Guarding occurs a fraction of a second after the pressure is applied; if it appears before the springing, then the patient is just apprehensive and is expecting to be hurt. If the contraction is delayed, the patient is trying to create an 'impression' and it is not genuine. If the contraction is sustained without variation during this test, there must be a severe continuous deep pain or the patient is not relaxing enough for the test to be effective.

The fact that the springing test evokes reflex guarding of muscle does not prove that there is a simple lesion present. It does not tell us any more than that a jarring movement in extension is painful and there must be some deep source of pain there. This deep source may be a simple joint sprain, or it may be a disc lesion, or it may imply disease.

In principle this test is the same as the one which we apply to the hip joint when we suspect early inflammatory changes. We suddenly jerk the joint in rotation with the patient relaxed. The jolt produces reflex guarding and pain. In the hip joint it may signify early osteo-arthritis or early tuberculous arthritis.

The springing test is the most sensitive of all the tests to apply to a vertebral joint, and it helps in the localisation of the level of the lesion. Any disproportionate response—i.e. if the guarding is excessive compared with the springing—should immediately arouse suspicion of pathological changes, and still greater care should then be taken to establish a diagnosis. An active tuberculous lesion of the spine would never be missed if this test was performed regularly in spinal examinations. Because it is such a sensitive test the practitioner should begin gently. If gentle springing does not evoke reflex guarding, then stronger springing can be used without risk, and without making the patient apprehensive.

Sustained contraction of paravertebral muscles implies a continuing source of deep pain. Muscular pain arises whenever sustained contraction is maintained long enough even in 'posturing' muscles. If the contraction is prolonged, internal changes take place in the muscle which we call contracture: the muscle becomes hard and 'fibrositic'. When palpating such muscle it is not only hard and stringy but there is tenderness. The fibres can be palpated separately from adjacent normal muscle which is soft when relaxed. Anyone who deals with musculo-skeletal problems and who does not believe in fibrositis has either not taken the trouble to examine muscles carefully or has a poor palpatory sense.

These irritable muscle fibres can be relaxed at least temporarily by infiltration with procaine. Sometimes there is lasting relief because the vicious cycle of spasm and accumulation of metabolites in the muscle, which leads on to more spasm, has been broken into, and the muscle ceases to contract permanently.

Because the source of the muscle irritability is usually in the faulty joint related to the muscle, we must correct this fault before lasting benefit accrues; but even if this is corrected the muscle changes may remain and will need treating as well. Local anaesthesia and deep frictional massage help to remove metabolites from the muscle and render the fibres less irritable.

Some patients are prone to 'fibrositis' without much provocation, and they usually have some generalised rheumatic, toxic, or gouty factor to account for it. Such patients have widely spread muscular pains which are not merely present at one site, as we should expect in mechanically produced 'fibrositis'. These 'trigger' points of muscle irritability are not confined to the immediate paravertebral muscles of the spinal lesion, but can occur at a distance. In fact any muscle in a myotome can be reflexly irritated by the spinal lesion.

The test of resisted isometric muscle contraction to elicit muscle pain is valuable where there has been muscle injury, but it is not valid for these local areas of muscle irritability. The fibres are already involuntarily contracted, and to make them contract voluntarily does not produce pain. If anything, there is a reduction in this type of muscle pain, because normal use of 'fibrositic' muscle relieves its pain. The probable explanation here is that contraction and relaxation facilitates the removal of metabolites and the 'P' substance postulated by Lewis.[41]

Reflex changes

At the level of the osteopathic spinal lesion motor changes in seg-mentally linked muscle have been described, but in addition there are frequently sudomotor, vasomotor and visceromotor changes. Most of these are shortlived and pass unobserved except when the patient is examined carefully within hours of the onset of the symptoms. These changes have already been discussed (p. 12).

The majority of reflex changes subside within hours or days of the onset of an acute lesion. If the lesion persists there is some chance that the vasomotor and visceromotor changes will persist also, but as I have stated already there must be some compensating and regulating autonomic mechanism to nullify these effects. In a small proportion of cases, however, the vasomotor and visceromotor disturbances last long enough to create persisting symptoms of a hyperfunctional or hypo-functional character (see p. 13).

MECHANICAL DIAGNOSIS

Mechanical diagnosis is the diagnosis of structural faults in the body, and the term is used to include procedures whereby we find and establish the source of mechanically produced pain or disability.

Mechanical diagnosis succeeds pathological diagnosis, and it is vital that this should be so because pathological states must be excluded before mechanical problems are assessed. This applies even if the mechanical problem has led on to the pathological state.

But diagnosis should not be an end in itself, however satisfying it might be to the physician; it should lead to correct treatment otherwise the treatment becomes empirical and misdirected, and perhaps useless or even dangerous.

The appropriate treatment follows from the pathological diagnosis and such has been the advance of medicine that the majority of diseases can be effectively treated. An immense armamentarium of treatment is available—drugs, surgery, diet, rest, hydrotherapy, etc., etc. Pathological diagnosis is the preoccupation of medical men, and so it should be. The earlier the disease is recognised the more effective is the treatment; but mechanical diagnosis has been given insufficient attention by the medical profession.

The attitude that, if disease is not present then the patient is suffering from some functional disorder which does not warrant serious consideration, is largely responsible for the neglect in this field of human suffering. It has led to such patients being relegated to the physical medicine and psychiatric departments of hospitals. A 'functional' diagnosis is almost a smear, as if the patient was at fault for bothering the doctor.

Infinite trouble is taken with patients suffering from obscure liver complaints. Vast sums of money are spent on artificial kidneys and hearts to try to restore patients who are all but moribund; and yet patients who suffer year in and year out from functional disorders are dismissed to the scrap-heap of medical care and considered merely as nuisances.

When disease has been excluded, the medical excuse—rather than the diagnosis—is often 'muscular', 'rheumatism', 'neurosis', or 'fibrositis'. But it is at this stage that the patients should be divided into those with mechanical problems and those with psychological problems. Most patients can be so allocated fairly easily, but where there is doubt a mechanical assessment should be made before assuming that the problem is a psychological one. Mechanical diagnosis should lead to the correct mechanical treatment. It is useless or only palliative to treat mechanical problems chemically with drugs.

The mechanical problem may be a displaced semilunar cartilage, a fractured scaphoid, an apophyseal joint fixation, or visceroptosis. Each has its appropriate mechanical treatment—namely, surgery to remove the fragment of cartilage, splinting for the fracture, manipulation to release the adhesions, and corrective exercises to restore proper muscle tone and posture for the visceroptosis. It would be useless to treat these mechanical lesions with drugs, with heat, light, and sound, or with psychotherapy—and surely no one will dispute this. It is when the mechanical problem is obscure that uncertainty arises. Furthermore, lack of attention to detail in mechanical diagnosis leads to errors of physical treatment even when the patient's problem is recognised as belonging to the musculo-skeletal system.

Let us now proceed to describe some of these diagnostic procedures for mechanical diagnosis. The patient must be 'assessed' before detailed diagnosis, and there are several considerations, both general and detailed—body type, occupation, sporting and other physical activities or lack of them, injuries, and congenital defects or developmental errors. All these have a bearing on the problem even before detailed considerations are made in the assessment of local symptoms.

GENERAL CONSIDERATIONS

Body types

The stocky type of patient usually has a short broad body and strong muscles. The range of joint movements is less than average but normal for his type. The ligaments are strong, and when strained they recover well. The limbs are large, heavy, and shorter than average. The neck is thick set, the chest is broad, and the antero-posterior spinal curves are less than average. The vertebrae are large and heavy, and there may be only four lumbar vertebrae. The processes are thicker and larger than average.

These patients are less liable to have musculo-skeletal problems than are the slender type, but degenerative changes in the spine are common

and the spondylosis is marked by larger osteophytes and the proliferation of bone. The disc spaces are wide rather than deep.

According to Goldthwait,[42] these people are more susceptible to
chronic bronchitis and emphysema, hypertension, arteriosclerosis and
myocardial degeneration, chronic nephritis, and gall-bladder disease.

Manipulative treatment of the stocky type sometimes presents
difficulty because of their inability to relax and the natural shortness of
their ligaments. It is useless to aspire to obtaining a full range of all
movements, and such patients are in any case accustomed to some
degree of general stiffness.

The slender type is usually taller as well as thinner than average.
The muscles and ligaments are weaker than average and these patients
are more inclined to develop a sway posture with accentuation of the
lumbar lordosis, thoracic kyphosis, and cervical lordosis. The vertebral
bodies are small and the processes are thin, yet the intervertebral discs
are deeper and lentiform in shape. The thoracic cage tends to be flat
and the ribs less horizontal, reducing the subcostal angle to less than
70°. There may be a cervical rib, and the tenth rib may be floating as
well as the eleventh and twelfth ribs. There may be six lumbar vertebrae.
The abdominal contents tend to droop into the pelvis, and the epigastrium is very flat.

This is the asthenic type, and they are more prone to peptic ulceration,
colitis, spastic constipation, hormonal disturbances, hypotension, and
peripheral vascular dysfunction. The autonomic nervous system is more
labile and is readily upset.

Treatment of this type is sometimes difficult because of the longer
leverages involved, and because the poor muscle tone often leads to
relapses after corrective manipulation. Improved muscle tone and
correction of posture is vital for them.

The intermediate type is really the average person with no particular
idiosyncrasies. But even though the dimensions are average such patients
may well fall into one or other of the categories below.

The obese type may be too heavy from over-eating or from some
hormonal or water imbalance; but the obesity itself creates mechanical
problems such as lumbar lordosis, spondylolisthesis, and osteo-
arthritis in the weight-bearing joints. Heavy breasts may drag the shoulders down and cause brachial plexus traction symptoms. Such patients
may be active and alert but more often they are inactive so that their
muscles tend to weaken, and this accentuates the mechanical problems
still further.

Manipulative treatment of the obese is rendered more difficult because palpation is less accurate, and the sheer weight of the patient can prevent the operator from reaching far enough round to be effective. Localisation of forces is more difficult because the fat can get in the way before sufficient tension is exerted. The operator too is at greater risk from straining his own back! One of my patients who had an enormous belly yet was not excessively fat elsewhere actually suffered from lower rib and costo-chondral junction pain because of the mechanical pressure of the fat everting the lower part of the rib cage. These symptoms subsided completely when his weight reduced.

In the obese the lumbar lordosis has to be compensated for by a thoracic kyphosis which in turn leads to cervical lordosis. This causes the cervical intervertebral foramina to diminish in diameter and thereby increases the risk of nerve-root irritation. The anterior margins of the thoracic vertebrae grow osteophytes from the greater mechanical load taken anteriorly.

Breathing is embarrassed by the fat in the abdomen and thorax. The diaphragm is depressed and its excursions are reduced causing orthostatic dyspnoea as distinct from the orthopnoea of cardiac failure.

Premiums for life insurance are higher for the obese because their life-span is usually shorter.

The hypermobile type shows excessive laxity in ligaments all over the body. This is characteristic of the acrobatic dancer and the successful devotee of Yoga; and, although lax ligaments may be an advantage in the acquisition of some of those skills, they are a distinct disadvantage to the ordinary mortal. Such people are inclined to sustain persistent ligamentous strain which is difficult to overcome.

An assessment of the ligaments should be made in all patients with backache. It is very easy to do this because the hypermobile subject shows excessive movements in the metacarpophalangeal joints and at the elbows and knees. Hypermobility of a spinal joint can occur in any type of person, but it is ten times more likely if the subject belongs to the hypermobile group.

This problem should be suspected in any patient who complains of backache and yet has a complete range of movements. The ache is characteristic in that it develops after a sustained position of strain, especially in flexion, although free and full movements are possible through that range. Once such ligaments are overstretched their capacity for recovery is poor, and any sustained subsequent stretch will provoke pain.

The function of a ligament is to withstand intermittent stretching of a limited character. Ligaments will give way if continuous stretching is sustained for long enough; they will also give way when subjected to a severe stretch which is beyond their elastic limit.

After an interval, continuous stretching causes pain, depending on the load and the initial strength of the ligament. If the ligament is abused often enough, the pain threshold diminishes and the latent period before pain asserts itself decreases until the time arrives when any stretch of the ligament hurts and pain is felt instantaneously. At this stage there is difficulty in differentiating ligamentous pain from pain of other origin, but a careful enquiry during history taking will establish the above sequence of symptoms.

When ligaments have become so sensitive to stretch that pain comes on within seconds of moderate stretching, they are so irritable that even compressing them hurts. Both stretch pain and compression pain develop at the same time and at the same site. This is exemplified in the lower lumbar spine when the joints have reached this stage of ligamentous irritability: forward-bending (stretch) provokes pain and backward-bending (compression) causes pain as soon as the spinous processes impinge on each other enough to compress the supraspinous and interspinous ligaments. Both types of pain can be temporarily eradicated by infiltrating procaine into the appropriate site.

A tearing stretch of a ligament causes instantaneous pain because of its rich sensory nerve-supply. In the normal course of events such a sprain will repair provided the tear is not complete and the opposing fragments are close enough together, and provided the part is rested while the fibres knit together. The repaired ligament can recover fully and become just as strong as before, but in hypermobile subjects the repair is usually less strong and they are prone to further sprains at the same site.

If ligaments are used to excess during repair, the repair remains incomplete and the resultant ligaments are permanently elongated, so that a hypermobile joint results. Such a joint will be vulnerable to lesser strains in the future.

Physiological hypermobility develops during pregnancy and the normal state returns soon after parturition, but during the hyper-mobile phase the patient is at risk in the ligamentous sense, and permanent overstretching is common in the lower lumbar and sacro-iliac joints.

The hypomobile type is stiff before he is thirty years old. He may be stiff in childhood, and if so irreparable damage may be done to his ligaments by excess of zeal on the part of the gymnasts at school and elsewhere, who try to make such subjects conform to the normal pattern of mobility. This type has short ligaments and tight capsules, and often the muscles are also short and tight; they tend to become progressively tighter with age. Hypomobile subjects are often of a stocky build, but not necessarily so. They are perfectly comfortable and usually perfectly happy with their short ranges of movement: what they lack in mobility they make up for in strength. Their ligaments do not sprain easily, and if they do, repair is prompt and efficient.

Of the two types—hypermobile and hypomobile—the hypomobile have the advantage over the hypermobile symptom-wise.

The muscular type frequently conforms with the stocky and hypomobile types, but this is not necessarily so. There are no disadvantages in having more than average strength, but if such people become inactive fatty degeneration tends to affect their muscles.

The flabby type may be slender or obese; poor muscle tone is inevitable when insufficient exercise is taken. The person whose muscular tone is poor is much more vulnerable to mechanical strains than are normal or muscular types. The office worker who allows his spinal muscles to get slack during the week and then suddenly exerts himself at golf or gardening at the week-end is much more vulnerable to strains and sprains. Yet by contrast a ballet dancer patient of mine who had a complete defect of both partes interarticulares of 3L was able, by dint of continuous and strenuous daily exercise, to hold her own on the stage for thirty years before she developed any symptoms. Both the spinal ligaments and intervertebral discs are better supported and will stand far more stress when accompanied by a good set of spinal muscles.

Slack musculature leads to poor posture because the ligaments are made to take undue strains—this is the basis of the 'sway' posture. These individuals rely on the iliofemoral ligaments at the hip joints and the longitudinal spinal ligaments to prevent themselves from falling over. Eventually the ligaments elongate, and further abnormal mechanical stresses produce still more symptoms.

Thermosensitive, hormonal imbalance, and neurotic types are seen in practice, and they are included under this discussion not because of a mechanical aetiology but because their symptoms have a strong bearing upon the musculo-skeletal system:

Thermosensitive types are not necessarily diseased nor are their symptoms severe enough to be classified under Raynaud's syndrome, but usually their peripheral circulation is poor and in cold weather the hands and feet go blue because the total surface circulation is diminished. This affects the muscles, and such patients are liable to develop 'fibrositis' and muscular rheumatism in the winter. They cannot stand the heat either, and are often distressed by temperatures of over 80°F.

The hormone-imbalance types are common, but the water retention which occurs in some forms of obesity, in myxoedema, and in pituitary dyscrasias may lead to mechanical and postural difficulties not only in the spine but in the limbs too. As these disorders are not easy to treat, some degree of mechanical trouble might have to be accepted as that patient's norm.

The neurotic types are legion, for anxiety has a profound effect on the physical body in chemical terms (as seen in the various stress syndromes) and also on the musculature. Nervous tension begets muscular tension. The commonest site for this is in the cervical muscles at their attachment to the skull. Tension in the splenius capitis, semispinalis capitis, and trapezius gives rise to headache, neck ache, and shoulder ache. If the tension is sufficiently sustained it will lead to joint restrictions and to more neck ache, and so a vicious cycle is established. Even cure of the neurosis may not clear up these secondary changes, and local treatment of the neck muscles and joints may well be an essential part of relieving the neurosis. On the other hand, to treat the neck alone and not to cope with the anxiety state will bring only temporary benefit.

There is a particular type of neurosis which is almost confined to osteopathic practice. I call it the 'positional' or 'bone out of place' neurosis. The patient comes in, having made a careful examination of the bones in the mirror, demonstrating that this part of the iliac crest is high, that part of the clavicle is prominent, or the knee turns in. Such patients are temporarily pleased with a few clicks of their joints, but they are back again in no time having found something else 'out of place'.

We have to admit that some of these neurotic subjects have been made so by the over-zealous osteopath who is himself almost obsessed with the 'bone out of place' theory! These patients are best reassured and not treated.

Occupational and outdoor activities

Postural influences have considerable bearing on body mechanics. It matters a great deal what work people do for eight or ten hours a day—the posture adopted, the muscular effort required to perform these duties, and the mechanical stresses with which the body copes. It matters also what sleeping posture is adopted for another eight hours of the day—the type of bed, the height of the pillows and the attitude of the body. Even the exercise in bed can matter mechanically as well as in other ways!

Extra-occupational activities can also be very significant—gardening, tennis, rock-climbing, polo, etc. These occasional uses and abuses of the body can lead to symptoms which seem to be out of proportion to their apparent cause.

Trauma

The history of injury is important in considering any mechanical problem in the body, but it should be assessed carefully because the mere fact of injury does not in itself mean that it was causal. There may have been some predisposing factor which the injury brought to light, or the injury may have affected another part of the body and have no bearing on the presenting symptoms.

Another misleading point is that an old forgotten injury can in fact be aetiological. It is surprising, on first being questioned about injuries, how often a patient will deny any, but on reflection will remember an incident long since dismissed as unimportant. Spinal injuries are particularly liable to be forgotten because they do not cause pain at the time. The shock-absorbing properties of healthy discs is considerable, and even if some damage occurs, immediate pain is slight because of the absence of sensory nerves in the discs. In addition the effects of trauma on cartilage develop slowly: a delay of 24 or 48 hours after injury is usual because cartilage takes that long to swell and only when such swelling stretches adjacent sensitive structures do symptoms develop. The patient—and sometimes the doctor—fails to realise this, and the symptoms and injuries may remain unconnected in the patient's mind. Careful questioning may help to restore the link.

To prove that injury was aetiological in any one case is extremely difficult, because most people can remember or conjecture a history of injury. However, if early in life one joint in the spine or an extremity shows signs of degenerative changes compared with the rest of the joints, there is strong presumptive evidence that an injury was the cause, for otherwise degenerative changes would also have occurred in several joints.

The injury may not be an isolated one. There may be many minor traumata, and when repeated several times the effect may be equivalent to a major traumatic episode. Occupational mechanical stresses come under this heading as in the miner, the farrier, the ballet dancer. Where there is a clear-cut history of injury and the symptoms follow without any doubt, then the nature, the degree, and the direction of the trauma must be ascertained because this may well give a lead to which tissue has been damaged. When examining a spinal lesion, it is often very important to know whether the patient twisted to the right or to the left.

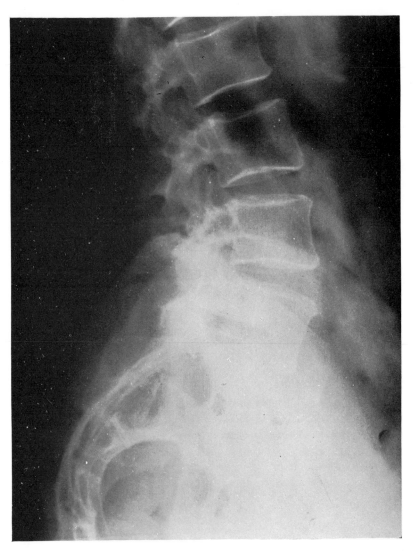

FIG 8 Lateral view of a lordosis showing increased bony density in the posterior vertebral arches of 4 and 5L.

Gross mechanical disorders

A further general consideration in assessing any patient is the presence of gross structural faults like scoliosis, kyphosis, lordosis, congenital and developmental defect, short legs, gross restrictions of limb mobility, or paralysis and paresis.

These are major overriding considerations when assessing the mechanics of the body. They lead to excessive mechanical strains and

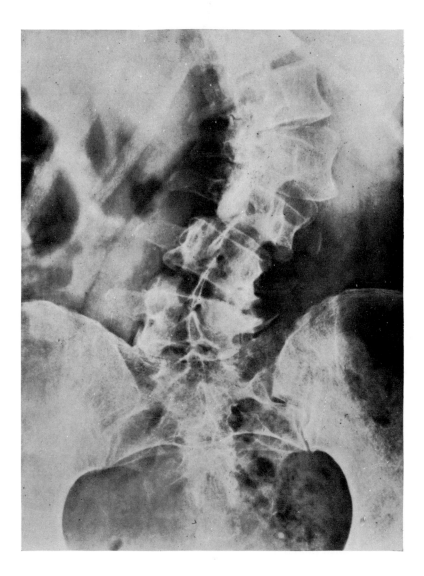

FIG 9 A scoliosis of the lumbar spine showing osteophyte formation on the concavity of the curves where most weight bearing takes place.

render some sites more vulnerable than others. The effects cause increased compression, usually at the sites of increased weight bearing, as in the spinal apophyseal joints in lumbar lordosis (*fig. 8*) and on the concavity of the curve of a scoliosis (*fig. 9*). This leads to sclerosis of bone and narrowing of joint spaces, while on the convexity of the curves there is stretching of ligaments and sometimes osteophyte formation.

DETAILED CONSIDERATIONS IN THE DIFFERENTIAL
DIAGNOSIS OF MECHANICAL LESIONS

The signs and symptoms of pain, tenderness, paraesthesiae, hyper-aesthesia and anaesthesia, hypomobility and hypermobility, locking, displacement, muscle tone, and soft-tissue and skin changes all have to be considered and interpreted in the differential diagnosis of mechanical lesions of the spinal column.

Pain

Some basic principles of pain production are helpful here. The localisation of pain depends upon whether the source is deep or superficial. Superficially produced pain is well localised and sharp in character. Deeply produced pain is less well localised and usually of a duller quality, though its intensity depends upon the severity and cause at its source. Superficial pain can best be compared with pinching the skin, and deep pain with strong squeezing of a normal muscle (Lewis[43]). Superficial pain is felt at its site of origin. Deep pain is felt in the dermatome, myotome, or scelerotome which is segmentally connected with the source, and therefore it is poorly localised and is often felt at a distance from its source. This is called 'referred' pain, and the distribution of this reference is segmental whatever the source of the deep pain. Deep pain from somatic structures is indistinguishable from pain derived from viscera if the sources are linked with the same segment. Deep pain may cause variations in sudomotor, visceromotor, and myotome activity, but it does not cause loss of power, loss of reflexes, nor loss of sensation. These latter signs indicate loss of nerve conduction either from mechanical pressure on a peripheral nerve or on the spinal cord, or from disease of nerve tissue.

Pain receptors are found in ligaments, capsules, muscles, tendons, periosteum and bone, dura mater, blood-vessel walls, fascia and fatty tissue. (Pain receptors are also found in other tissues but only the above are relevant to musculo-skeletal problems.) Mechanical causes of pain are stretching, displacement, and pressure involving these tissues. Muscular spasm causes pain when contractions are sustained.

Direct pressure on nerves causes pain in their distribution. Pressure can arise from hard tissues like bone, but oedema, inflammatory exudates, and muscle tension can cause mechanical pressure on nerves in some circumstances. Distension of the venous system can also cause pain if the back-pressure is sufficient and is maintained.

Pain thresholds vary from patient to patient. This has been tested by applying pressure of varying intensity to evoke a painful response. Only 61 per cent were considered normal, 22 per cent were hypersensitive, and 16 per cent were hyposensitive to this test.[44]

Spinal pain—i.e. pain felt in the vicinity of the vertebral column—can arise in the following ways:

1 By mechanical irritation of any of the pain-sensitive structures enumerated above.
2 By mechanical irritation of the nerve-roots.
3 By reflex spasm of the paravertebral muscles.
4 By chemical irritation of pain-sensitive tissues by the constituents of inflammatory exudates.
5 By oedema and vascular distension.
6 By referred pain from viscera.

These generalisations are at first sight confusing, but tissues behave in characteristic ways and certain points are worth mentioning because they often enable the clinician to identify the source of the pain. For example, the pain arising in *fatty tissue* (as in panniculitis) can be localised precisely because the fat is near the surface and it can be picked up separately from the deeper muscles. Squeezing the tissue involved will evoke a painful response, whereas squeezing normal fatty tissue elsewhere will not evoke pain.

The pain arising from a *muscle injury* can be elicited by making the muscle contract against resistance without allowing movement of the adjacent joints. This test, while helpful in differentiating pain in muscle from that of other sources, is not absolute because it is not always possible—even with the greatest care—to avoid some indirect pressure or stretching of adjacent structures. In addition pain from a chronic contracture of the muscle is not increased by contracting the muscle further.

Pain due to sustained contraction of muscle is ischaemic in nature. Lewis[45] has shown that pain develops if exercise is carried out with the circulation occluded, but as soon as the circulation is restored the pain disappears: some 'P' substance probably forms in the muscle and this is removed by the blood when the circulation is restored. During sustained contraction relative ischaemia develops because normally blood flows only during relaxation. Sustained contraction impedes blood-flow so that 'P' substances form and pain ensues. This is the probable explanation for the pain of 'fibrositis' in which some fibres contract chronically.

Pain in damaged tendons usually arises when the muscle attached to the tendon is contracted, but the pain of a tendinitis is often superficial. It is a tenosynovitis, and this pain is only evoked by moving the tendon to and fro in its sheath.

Pain is evoked from irritable ligaments by stretching them and by finger pressure over them. The ligaments—even deep ones—can be stretched by passive stretching of the joints to the limit of their range. When accessible to palpation, an irritable ligament is tender on pressure, and it is possible to squeeze such a ligament and evoke pain—for example, the interspinous ligaments can be squeezed by approximating the spinous processes to produce pain.

Pain arises from adhesions because, during movement, they stretch the sensitive tissues which adhere together. In adhesive capsulitis of the shoulder, for example, the joint cavity can be infiltrated with a local anaesthetic which will reduce the pain of stretching but only partially so, because there may be extra-capsular adhesions which are not reached by the anaesthetic.

The concept of 'stretch' pain and 'squeeze' pain is useful in differential diagnosis. If, in designing our tests, we move the joints passively and thereby avoid the complication of muscle pain, we can stretch or squeeze the soft tissues according to which way we passively move the patient. Depending on which tissues are being stretched or squeezed, this gives added information. For example, if testing side-bending of the neck to the right causes pain on the right, then we are squeezing some sensitive structure or structures on the right, such as opposing apophyseal joint surfaces or intervertebral foramina. On the other hand, side-bending the neck to the right which causes pain on the left means that stretching evokes pain in some sensitive structure on the left, such as the capsule of an apophyseal joint or an irritable muscle.

Pain only arises from cartilage when it is displaced or swollen, thereby stretching adjacent sensitive ligaments. A cartilaginous loose body will cause severe pain if it is squeezed between opposing surfaces to force them apart or when it blocks a joint. Cartilaginous thickenings or chondrophytes are sensitive, and pain arises from them when adjacent surfaces are squeezed together: they are also sensitive to firm palpation. If any tissue is irritable enough, both stretching and squeezing it will cause pain.

In bone the pain depends on whether the structure is of compact or cancellous type, and whether any increased pressure is involved. Compact bone is relatively insensitive, whereas cancellous bone is pain-sensitive. Covering bone is an exquisitely sensitive periosteum.

Viscerally produced pain is indistinguishable from deep somatic pain except for colic. A distended viscus can produce intermittent regular pain, sometimes of severe degree, which is characteristic and quite unlike intermittent pain produced in other somatic structures.

Blood-vessels are sensitive when inflamed and over-stretched, as when veins are becoming varicosed or distended.

Many tissues which are not normally sensitive become so when inflamed because the inflammatory exudates, which contain histamine, acetyl choline, potassium ions, plasma kinins, and hydroxytryptamine, lower the threshold of pain production.

Pain is felt centrally in the brain, but it is conveyed via the free nerve-endings in the affected tissues. The nerves themselves are not inflamed. Pain actually arising in nerves (as distinct from their endings) implies inflammation in the nerve, because peripheral nerves are insensitive to normal movements and pressure. For example, the ulnar nerve at the medial epicondyle of the humerus is insensitive if palpated in the normal way. One can only evoke a painful response if it is tapped very briskly. On the other hand, in the presence of ulnar neuritis, the nerve will ache spontaneously and even light pressure will evoke more pain. The pain of neuritis is not severe at the site of the swelling, rather it is felt proximally and distally: we know this happens in the median nerve when it becomes inflamed from intermittent compression in the carpal tunnel.

When a nerve-root is compressed by a prolapsed disc at the inter-vertebral foramen it becomes swollen and congested (Herlin,[46] as well as others, has demonstrated this many times).

Normal nerves will stand a tremendous amount of mechanical irritation before they become irritable and inflamed, but if other factors are associated—like vitamin-B deficiency and hormonal or water imbalance, then much less mechanical irritation will produce neuritis. A combination of factors is common in peripheral neuritis, and all factors must be treated to produce a cure. This is why the responses may be confusing in syndromes like nerve-root compression and median-nerve compression.

Partial and intermittent compression of a nerve causes pain, but if the pressure becomes complete and continuous the conduction of the nerve ceases and the initial pain stops.

Compression probably causes pain in nerves because it interferes with the blood-supply, and as compression is likely to be greater in a confined space than in an open space, the site of compression matters. In other words, nerves are more vulnerable to compression in the intervertebral foramen and carpal tunnel, for example, than they are along their main tracks.

Judging by clinical patterns, the initial pain of a very large disc prolapse is so severe that it may be relieved only by morphine: but within twenty-four to forty-eight hours the nerve conduction ceases and lasting damage then occurs in the nerve, leading to paralysis with loss of sensation and deep reflexes. If the compression is insufficient to cut off all the blood-supply, the pain may be severe and persistent. The nerve becomes irritable, so that sub-threshold stimuli are enough to provoke pain, paraesthesiae, and hyperaesthesia. Ischaemia probably produces metabolic changes in the affected nerves, but the nature of these changes is not known.[47]

The pain which arises in a nerve is felt in the area of its distribution, and it is much more clearly defined than is a segmental referred pain involving a similar area of the body. This point alone can be helpful in reaching a conclusion about the source of pain.

Pain has quality (sharp, dull, or burning), but it also has intensity, distribution, and periodicity. All these help one to assess the individual problem.

Intensity of pain is one of the most difficult qualities to assess because it is purely subjective and because individual responses vary. The personality of the neurotic patient accentuates the pain, while the stolid patient's mind diminishes it. Fatigue causes accentuation of pain and rest relieves it. Some measure of intensity can be made by the response to drugs: if morphine relieves it and aspirin does not, then it is severe. If none of the analgesics relieves the pain then it is not of a physical nature. The behaviour of patients during pain gives a fair measure of its intensity: if they can concentrate on something else it is not a severe pain, and if they are able to continue normal activities the pain may be a nuisance but it is not severe, even though words like 'agony' and 'torture' are used.

In these various ways the physician builds up a picture of how much each patient is suffering; but it is axiomatic that for a doctor to appreciate pain he has had to suffer it himself. The physician should never assume that a patient does not suffer even though the description is light-hearted or the pain is demonstrably psychogenic in origin. Sympathy for the patient is never misplaced except in sheer malingering. Suffering is not the same as pain. The degree of pain from a fracture may be greater than that of angina of effort; but the suffering is greater with angina because the patient is also anxious about his future, whereas the patient with a fracture knows that the pain will soon cease and he will recover fully.

Severe pain produces other signs—namely, an increase in heart-rate, breathing, sweating, and vasomotor tone, a rise in blood-pressure, and sometimes nausea and vomiting.

Although almost universal in patients with musculo-skeletal problems, pain must not be assumed to be present. Patients must be allowed to describe the symptoms in their own way, though the words used may be misleading. For example, 'numbness' is frequently used incorrectly, and if one asks the patient if absence of sensation is implied, the usual reply is 'No, I don't mean that, I mean a dull ache.'

It is inevitable that patients have difficulty in describing pain because there is no yardstick to measure it by. The commonest comparison is the toothache, on the assumption that everyone has suffered from this! Picturesque and dramatic phraseology when describing pain usually implies an underlying neurosis.

The site of pain is one guide to its source, and a knowledge of standard anatomy is necessary for its correct interpretation; but the distribution of deep pain is variable because:

1 Dermatome and myotome areas do not correspond—myotomes are usually at a lower level than the corresponding dermatome. Gough and Koepke[48] have shown by electromyographic examination of erector spinae muscles in twenty-one cases of complete transverse spinal cord injury 'that the innervation of an anterior myotome by a spinal nerve is within two segments of the corresponding dermatome but in the posterior myotomes the innervation was usually lower. The cervical and lumbar posterior myotomes were in almost all cases several segments lower, as many as six in some cases'. Their method could not demonstrate the upper extent of the posterior myotomes.

2 The recurrent spinal nerve supplies areas of the posterior longitudinal ligaments for two segments above the level of re-entry of the nerve.

3 There is overlapping of the dermatomes, some areas of skin having a nerve-supply from adjacent spinal nerves.

4 There are pre-fixed and post-fixed plexuses in the cervical, brachial, lumbar, and sciatic plexuses.

5 There is often irradiation of pain on the ipsilateral and even on the contralateral side when the pain is severe.

6 In herpes zoster the skin eruption is often across several dermatomes and tends to be horizontal rather than oblique as one would expect if the rash followed the distribution of a single nerve.

7 Pain in the dura mater is poorly localised and spreads over several dermatomes. Within the spinal canal the anterior dura mater has a richer nerve-supply than has the posterior dura mater.

These factors lead to poor localisation of pain which arises in deep structures. Atlases of dermatomes, sclerotomes, and myotomes, which are compiled by anatomists, are valuable for study so long as we realise that the areas portrayed are very approximate. Only when the cause of the pain is in the skin or immediate subjacent tissues can there be any real accuracy in the localisation. The more severe the pain the more widely does it spread via reflex action and internuncial neurones to adjacent segments of the cord. This spread may be ipsilateral when the pain is moderately severe but contralateral when it is very severe. In a severe capsulitis of the shoulder the pain will radiate right down to the hand, but as the inflammation subsides the pain becomes localised to the deltoid insertion areas.

There is considerable evidence that pain is conveyed not only by neurones of the central nervous system but also by neurones of the autonomic nervous system, and because the sympathetic and parasympathetic nerve distribution is diffuse and difficult to map out, such pain is diffuse and poorly localised: 'Continuous discharge of nerve impulses along efferent sympathetic nerve fibres can set up afferent impulses in adjacent pain nerve fibres.'[49]

Then there is the question of the curious distribution of rashes in herpes zoster. The pain is probably due to hyperalgesia induced by products of inflammation in the posterior nerve-roots, because a profuse lymphocytic infiltration of the affected ganglia and nerve-roots, together with petechial haemorrhages and necrosis of one or two spinal nerves has been demonstrated; and yet the distribution of the rash does not conform with the anatomical distribution of those nerves. I have often seen the herpes rash spread half way round the body in the lumbar region in a horizontal manner, whereas the anterior primary rami run obliquely. The horizontal pattern of herpes vesicles is the rule rather than the exception, and the area may spread over four or five oblique dermatomes.

Tenderness

Tenderness in the sense of being sensitive to pressure implies hyper-algesia of the tissue which is being palpated. It is not synonymous with hyperaesthesia, which involves the skin only.

The tenderness is of necessity superficial, otherwise it would not be accessible to finger pressure. It may be subjective or objective—i.e. the patient may be aware of tenderness from the pressure of clothing, etc., although this is not in itself very well localised—but palpation can help to localise it more accurately, and it then becomes an objective sign.

Tenderness can be obliterated by infiltrating the appropriate tissue with a local anaesthetic, and in this way the tender tissue can be identified, though of course this does not imply that the cause of the tenderness is in that superficial tissue. The real cause may be deeper. For example, manipulation of a spinal joint can disperse tenderness in the interspinous ligament without that ligament being treated in any way. Similarly the tenderness of 'fibrositis' in muscle can be dispersed if the underlying cause in the joint is corrected.

The technique of testing for tenderness should be carefully performed, because if excessive pressure is applied at any site it will hurt. Examples of extra sensitive sites are the transverse processes of the atlas, the tendo-achilles, and the testis. It is desirable always to compare the tenderness of one site with that of another—preferably the identical site on the other side of the body—or, if in the mid-line, the spinous processes or the supraspinous ligaments can be compared with adjacent processes or spaces so long as the same amount of pressure is used. If this simple precaution is not observed false impressions are created in both patient and observer. When this precaution is observed the sign is reliable. The mere fact of tenderness does not imply that that tissue is at fault, but it does give a segmentally reliable guide as to the source of the trouble. Tenderness at, say, the 4–5T interspinous ligament is a reliable indication that the source of the trouble is segmentally connected with the 4–5T level. Tenderness at the acromio-clavicular joint capsule meant that there is some inflammation in that joint.

Another point to be taken into consideration is the subjacent tissue. If bone is subjacent, less pressure will be required to elicit tenderness than would be required if muscle were subjacent, because the tissue compression is greater against bone. Tenderness diminishes gradually away from the maximum site, but our object is to find the maximum site because this more accurately marks the level of the lesion.

When tenderness in soft tissue is caused by changes in that tissue, it implies that some inflammatory or irritative change has occurred in it. For example, a boil is tender to touch, and the cause is obvious; in urethritis the wall of the urethra is tender to palpation; in a semilunar cartilage injury the joint line is tender at the site of the coronary ligament attachments; and in myositis the muscle belly is tender. But when the source of the tenderness is not obvious, then other tests are necessary to ascertain the source: for example, sacro-iliac tenderness in fact often arises from the lower lumbar joints; tenderness in the costal margin is more likely to be coming from a cholecystitis than from the costal cartilage, and so on.

The warning implied by these facts is that tenderness as an isolated sign is unreliable, but that in conjunction with other positive signs it is of considerable aid to diagnosis.

Paraesthesiae

The term paraesthesiae means disturbed skin sensation, and it embraces the terms hyperaesthesia and anaesthesia. Increased sensitivity of the skin is a manifestation of irritability of the nerve-supply to that area of skin. Loss of sensation—numbness or anaesthesia—means that the sensory supply has been blocked or cut off from that area of skin, and it implies loss of conduction somewhere along the sensory track of that nerve. However, the sensation may be neither increased nor absent, yet it is altered, producing paraesthesiae. Patients frequently have difficulty in describing accurately the sensations they experience in the skin. Other sensations—like burning and loss of temperature sense, diminished vibration sense, and deep pressure senses—can all be altered by disturbances of nerve-supply to the periphery. Interpretation of these symptoms and signs belongs to the realm of neurology, and they need not be discussed in detail here.

The sensation of pins and needles is sometimes misleading because it might be of nervous or vascular origin. Temporary ischaemia followed by a return of the blood-supply leads to tingling during the recovery of circulation. Tingling in the presence of a good peripheral circulation must be of neurological origin.

Mobility

In testing a peripheral joint, one of the most important signs to elicit is its ranges of movement. If the joint is large and the bones are long, the assessment is relatively easy; but in testing spinal joint mobility the problem is more complex, and the assessment of an individual joint is more difficult though none the less important.

The first step is to test the over-all ranges of movements in each area of the spine. This should be recorded, not only because it helps with the clinical picture but because the patient's subsequent progress can thus be gauged better.

The ranges of movements in several peripheral joints should be tested, even though these are symptomless, in order to ascertain the individual's type of ligaments—i.e. whether it is normal for that patient to have long or short ligaments. If all the peripheral joints are extremely loose one expects that spinal mobility will be above average.

A state of relative hypermobility and relative hypomobility can be normal for one individual, but comparative hypermobility and hypo-mobility in the same individual is significant in mechanical diagnosis.

A combination of hypermobility and hypomobility in the spine is common because hypomobility is compensated for by hypermobility in joints above and below the restricted area. Because of the frequency of hypermobile and hypomobile joints in the same patient, the overall spinal movements are not sufficient evidence of individual joint function for mechanical diagnostic purposes.

Detailed mobility tests are described in my *Manual of Osteopathic Technique*. In principle the tests depend upon the palpation of adjacent spinous or transverse processes during the separate movements of flexion, extension, side-bending, and rotation. At most levels the spinous processes of two adjacent vertebrae can be spanned by the palpating thumb or finger, while the operator uses his other arm to move the area passively. It is essential to avoid the influence of gravity in these tests; while it is feasible, say, to test individual cervical joints with the patient seated, it is more satisfactory and a more reliable index of movement if the patient is supine during the tests.

Where bony points are inconspicuous—for example, the transverse process of the axis, which is hidden under the thick sternomastoid muscle and is very short compared with the transverse process of the atlas— accurate palpation is impossible and one has to rely upon a *sense of mobility*.

In palpating adjacent spinous processes three features should be observed: the gap between; the resistance of the supraspinous ligaments to palpating pressure; and the degree of approximation and separation during extension and flexion. A fourth observation—its tenderness—is subjective.

When the supraspinous ligament is weak and the space dips in during palpation, it gives the immediate impression of hypermobility; but this is not always so, and a separate observation must be made as to the degree of approximation and separation during flexion-extension tests. Equally the mere observation of firmness in a supraspinous ligament is no criterion of the range of movements at that joint.

Flexion-extension is the easiest of the mobility tests because palpatory skill only is required, but rotation and side-bending call less for a sense of palpation than for a sense of tissue tension. By this I mean the feeling of 'give' or the elasticity of the joint as compared with the sense of resistance and the unyielding nature of a restricted joint. Acquisition of this 'sixth sense' is not difficult but it requires practice. This tissue-tension sense is also essential for accurate manipulation after the mobility tests have been performed.

Palpatory skill is vital in examination of the abdominal and pelvic organs, and such skill is not acquired rapidly. Some doctors are better at it than others by virtue of the sensitivity of their fingers, but it is a skill which anyone can acquire with practice. The approximation and separation of the 4–5L spinous processes is obvious to the beginner once the test is demonstrated; but the sense of rotation in the 6–7C joint requires practice before it can be assessed relatively, yet this is as essential to the mechanical diagnosis of conditions of the 6–7C joint as is the assessment of mobility in an internal derangement of the knee joint.

Practice in testing for mobility can be obtained by feeling peripheral joints, graduating from the larger to the smaller ones. It is not only the movements under voluntary control which are tested but also the movements of 'joint play' that give essential information: J. B. and J. McM. Mennell[50, 51] have both stressed the significance of these movements in diagnosing joint dysfunction. In testing the metacarpophalangeal joints, for instance, we are not only concerned with flexion, extension, adduction, and abduction (which are under the control of voluntary muscles) but also with the degree of rotation and antero-posterior shearing move-

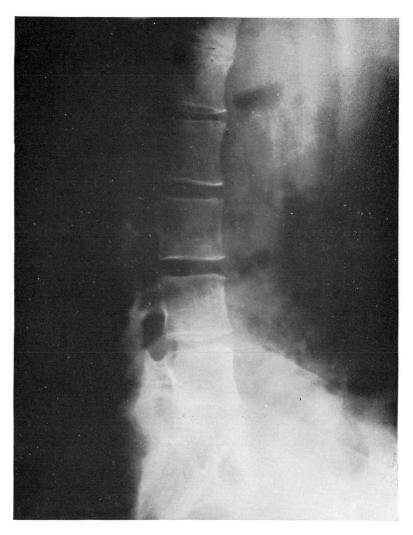

FIGS 10 AND 11 are mobility views showing flexion (FIG 10) and extension (FIG 11). The 4–5L shows instability—in forward bending the 4th lumbar vertebra shifts anteriorly on 5L—as well as gapping posteriorly to an excessive extent.

ments which can be palpated passively. Any restriction of these ranges by adhesions or tightness of the capsules adversely affects the voluntary movements, and it may only be possible to restore normal movements by manipulating in rotation and shearing directions.

Similarly for spinal conditions we can apply passive movements to test the joints and similar passive movements to manipulate them in a

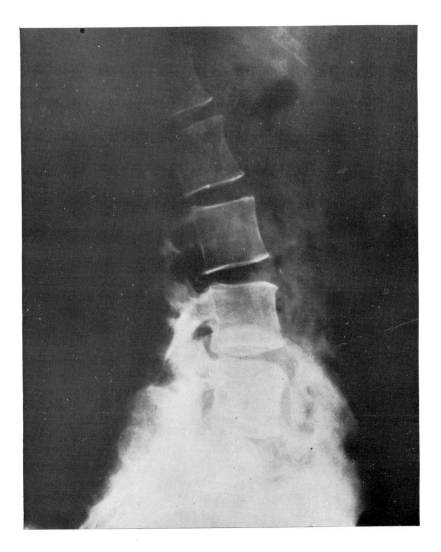

FIG 11

way which is quite outside the patient's voluntary performance.

Following on this point is the question of exercises for improving spinal mobility: these may be essential in restoring full ranges of movement, but if a patient has a hypomobile joint the other joints in the area may become overstretched and hypermobile, without the restricted one being normalised. The outcome may well be worse than the original condition in this case, and the correct sequence of treatment is to restore mobility by manipulation specifically to the affected joint until sufficient

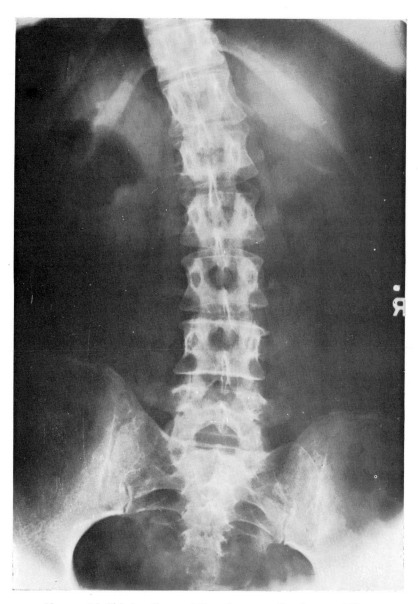

FIGS 12 AND 13 Side-bending mobility views revealing hypomobility at
12T—2L especially to the right.

improvement has taken place, and *then* to use exercises to continue the
improvement.

An isolated flail peripheral joint is obvious, whereas an isolated hypermobile intervertebral joint is not, but it would be equally foolish to

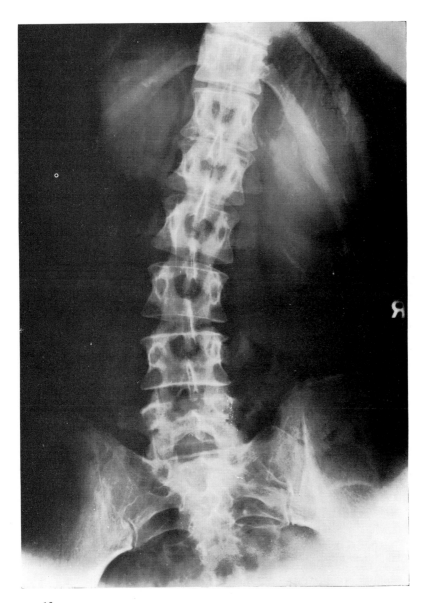

FIG 13

manipulate the hypermobile vertebral joint as it would to manipulate the
flail peripheral one. This adds further weight to the importance of
detailed examination of individual spinal joints. It also shows the
importance of specific manipulations because, if a hypermobile joint is
present within a hypomobile area and if that part of the spine is forcibly

79

manipulated as an area, then surely the weak joint must give way first, and the outcome will be worse than the pre-existing condition.

In completing the examination of the spine for mobility, special *functional X-rays* (figs. *10, 11, 12, 13*) should be taken to assist the examiner in confirming his palpatory mobility tests. Films should be taken in full forward-bending and full backward-bending, and also in side-bending to each side; and they should all be taken in the horizontal resting position otherwise the passive range will not be recorded. In theory it would be helpful also to use rotation X-rays for assessing degrees of rotation, but in practice these films are so confused that they are unhelpful.

The study of mobility is, in its uncomplicated form, the study of ligaments. Where no disease or structural derangement is present, the range of movements is a function of the confining ligaments, but the range of movements is not governed by the ligaments alone. It can be influenced by weight-bearing and by the muscles, and this is why functional X-rays should not be taken vertically except to observe the influence of gravity on the spinal column. The tone of the muscle influences the movements, and if there is pain then reflex muscle tension will prevent the full range of movements even though the ligaments are normal. These points must be taken into account when testing for joint mobility. Moreover, inflammatory changes and any internal derangement, such as chondrophytes, displaced cartilaginous fragments, or loose bodies, will all reduce mobility.

During the 'softening phase' of disc degeneration the disc ceases to be a turgid resilient structure and abnormal movements take place, resulting in excessive ranges and abnormal shearing ranges (see later in the chapter on disc lesions). If fragments are displaced, the intense reflex muscle guarding comes into play, with reduced mobility and sometimes locking of the joint.

Even in the absence of disease and degeneration there can be hyper-functional or hypofunctional states of a joint. We do not need to envisage pathological changes whether of the discs or apophyseal joints when we find excessive or restricted movements. These may be consequent upon mechanical considerations alone, and in these cases the appropriate mechanical treatment is indicated.

Extraneous factors which influence joint mobility are usually obvious, such as the large belly preventing full flexion of the hip and spine! Collagen diseases, diseases of the central nervous system, and neoplasms may interfere with joint mobility, but these again are usually obvious and in any case here the joint condition is of secondary importance.

Locking

As a physical sign *locking* in a joint is a special form of hypomobility. There is a sense of blockage—something solid in the way—stopping further movement in that direction. When testing the joint either actively or passively the movement may be free and painless up to a certain angle, and then suddenly no more is possible. Such locking occurs in the knee joint with a displaced semilunar cartilage, and it occurs to a more variable extent when a loose body gets in the way of opposing joint surfaces. Locking is not the same sensation as that produced by adhesions or tightness in the capsule, because the blockage has a solid unyielding feel to it; it is not ankylosis either, because ankylosis implies no movement in any direction. Ankylosis may involve bony or soft tissue, but all movements are blocked. With locking some of the ranges of movement may be quite free, but in another range the movement is arrested, and this is not by pain or muscle protection, although in the early stages both of these may accompany the blocking. The sensation of blocking is quite different from the sensation of adhesion restrictions, and it is not easily described; but once felt there is no real difficulty in distinguishing between the two types of restriction. With adhesions there is elastic resistance—the joint will go a bit further even though pain is accentuated—but with locking any attempt at further movement is blocked and has a solid feel to it. Adhesions can be so dense and strong that the distinction may be difficult. The sense of movement restriction from adhesions depends upon their density and duration. Recently formed adhesions are stretchable but very painful because inflammation is present. Long-established adhesions which have become brittle are not so stretchable and not so acutely painful unless the force used is enough to break them; the joint movement is then suddenly released so that a very sharp pain is felt at the moment of separation, though this pain soon subsides. If early adhesions are stretched enough to tear them, the pain is intense and persists for hours or days after the manipulation has been performed; furthermore they tend to re-form unless diligent efforts are made to maintain movement.

These observations are based upon the shoulder joint which is easier to assess than the intervertebral joint, though the same sort of rules apply. The majority of vertebral manipulations which are accompanied by a click are not painful, and the breakdown of adhesions cannot account for the sound. Rather it is the sudden release of 'joint binding' which makes the noise. Normal joints have some degree of cohesion, and if the articular surfaces are separated a clicking sound is produced and the sound means nothing more than that. However, a joint can become bound by extra-cohesion rather than by adhesions. So far no

satisfactory explanation has been brought forward for this form of
'joint bind', and although it is most common in intervertebral joints it is
by no means confined to these joints. Patients themselves often demonstrate this by just stretching the joint or joints in question, when popping
sounds are produced. An increased range of movement and a greater
sense of freedom ensues. Such popping could not be explained on the
basis of adhesions.

The cracking of metacarpo-phalangeal joints has been studied by
Roston and Wheeler Haines,[52] who found that on applying a pull of
8 kg to the finger a sharp cracking sound occurred. An X-ray taken
immediately after the crack showed a space between the two bones.
They found that a similar sound could not be repeated straight away but
that it could be repeated after an interval of twenty minutes. Their
interpretation of the sound was that a partial vacuum is created by the
separation.

Blocking of an intervertebral joint almost always implies a disc
protrusion. Some of the movements are free and yet one range—perhaps
side-bending to the right—is blocked. Such blocking of an intervertebral
joint is characteristic and can be easily recognised not only in active
movements but in passive testing; although it has an unyielding quality
this often has to be sought for by mobility tests. The overall range of
side-bending is only partially limited because the other intervertebral
joints bend sideways quite satisfactorily in a chronic disc herniation.
In the acute phase the movements may all be reduced by muscle spasm,
making it difficult to localise the level of the disc lesion. In that event
other criteria must be used to diagnose the level of the lesion.

The osteopathic spinal lesion has not this quality of locking. It may
feel tight in one or more directions, but there is no solid resistance to
movement. It is conceivable that other causes exist for 'locking' of
an intervertebral joint, such as the nipping of synovial fringe in the
apophyseal joints, but there is little evidence for this. Opposing irregular
surfaces from osteo-arthritis of an apophyseal joint could lock against
each other, just as happens in osteo-arthritic peripheral joints. 'Joint
mice' or loose bodies may be found in peripheral joints, but I cannot
find evidence that they occur in spinal facet joints.

The physical sign of locking in a spinal joint therefore becomes an
important differential point in diagnosing disc protrusions from
adhesions and joint binding. This is discussed further in the chapter on
pathological conditions of the disc.

Displacement

In this connection I do not wish to discuss gross deformity, which is well covered by orthopaedic textbooks, but rather the minor positional faults and alterations of contour which are sometimes missed and where the significance is either lost or exaggerated according to the school of thought and training of the practitioner.

One of the key points in examining any patient for any condition is to observe the contour and shape first of the patient as a whole and secondly of the part of the body in question. Before a joint has been palpated its outline will give useful information as to the anatomical landmarks and swellings, the state of the muscles, and the shape of the bones.

Spinal joints cannot be observed individually, of course, but the outline of the body, the contours of the buttocks, shoulders, and chest wall, and the carriage of the head, give useful information about posture and the shape of the spine. The central spinal groove is not such a reliable guide to the shape of the spine as one would wish, and many a scoliosis is missed by too casual observation about the mid-line appearance. Some scolioses are represented more by rotation than by lateral deviation, and the spinous processes are then no guide to the severity of the deformity. In these cases the scoliosis is more obvious when a tangential view is taken of the spine, either looking downwards from above with the patient erect, or more conveniently after asking the patient to flex forwards so that one may look horizontally to observe the symmetry of the two sides of the spine and to note whether one side is 'higher' than the other. In a structural scoliosis the 'high' side is always on the convexity. The tangential appearance of a spine is worth observing in every patient because even single lesions can sometimes be detected in this way.

Fat patients are a problem because the underlying shapes are obscure. The folds of skin in the loins should always be noted: asymmetrical folds imply some variation in the level of the pelvis or of the contour of the lumbar spine.

In the past, great importance has been attached to the position of one vertebra relative to the next; but we now realise that the position of a vertebra is no criterion of function, and that an 'apparent displacement' is quite compatible with normal joints above and below the 'displacement'.

Merely examining the spine by noting the levels of the pelvis, the contours of the body, and the shape of the spinous and transverse processes is obviously incomplete. Yet I have seen this done to the apparent satisfaction of the practitioner.

The shape of the spinous processes is extremely variable. They can be deviated to either side and they can be 'tilted' without a corresponding alteration in the position of the vertebral bodies. About half the spinous processes in the thoracic area are asymmetrical in most patients. Usually one or two of the lumbar spines have an alteration in shape; and the bifid spines of the cervical area are always asymmetrical, so that these are obviously no guide to the position of the vertebrae.

Symmetry of transverse processes, on the other hand, is the rule rather than the exception, and some reliance can be placed on the findings on palpation. They are more deeply placed, of course, so that fat and muscle can interfere with accurate palpation. The length of transverse processes in the lumbar spine is rather variable; but, apart from the fifth lumbar where anomalies are common, prominence of one transverse process, say at 3L, means in most cases that the vertebral body has rotated to the prominent side. The transverse processes in the cervical spine are difficult to palpate because they are small, divided into tubercles, and covered by scalene muscles between which run the emerging spinal nerves. Pressure over them, even when normal, causes dull pain, and they should not be relied on as a test of position. However, the articular processes of the cervical spine are relatively superficial, they are almost always symmetrical, and they are part of the formation of the apopyseal joints above and below, so that these bony landmarks can be used to define positional relationships.

One source of error in assessing position in the cervical spine is that the margins of the articular processes become thickened either from inflammatory change or from the formation of chrondrophytes and osteophytes. The bulge is taken to be a displacement, and manipulation is then performed inadvisedly. Sometimes an enlarged lymphatic gland lying directly over the articular processes can mislead.

When a positional fault is observed and the practitioner is confident that this is true, this of itself still does not signify any serious lesion. The other tests of mobility and of soft tissues must be performed. If the mobility tests are normal and there is no local tenderness or other functional disturbance, then the positional fault should be ignored.

But we cannot ignore a positional fault in the pelvis, even in the absence of other physical signs, because this base line of the spine is vital to the whole body, not only laterally but anterior-posteriorly. A young patient who had had pain in his mid-thoracic spine for three months was cured within a week of using a heel cushion to correct his pelvic tilt: nothing else was done and there were no local signs in the pelvis other than the tilt. The position of the pelvis depends upon the lower extremities, the shape of the sacrum and ilia, the state of the sacro-iliac joints, the tone of the spinal, pelvic, and abdominal muscles, and the general posture.

When a positional fault is diagnosed clinically it is desirable to confirm it radiologically, and for this weight-bearing X-rays are more significant than standard views.

The two films (*figs. 14, 15*) illustrate this point. The one taken supine shows little significant change, but the same patient on the same day taken standing shows a pronounced tilt of 4L to the left on 5L. When reading X-rays for positional faults due regard must be paid to all components of the vertebrae—the bodies, transverse and spinous processes, and the facets. Oblique views are important because they often reveal features which are not obvious in the anterior-posterior and lateral views. The intervertebral foramina of the cervical area are best seen in oblique views. In the lumbar area the apophyseal joints and partes interarticulares are only properly seen in oblique views. In the thoracic area there is less need for oblique views but even there the costo-vertebral joints are seen better.

Muscle tone

As a diagnostic aid, the testing of muscle tone is important not because muscles per se are often at fault but because they are reflexly linked with all the deep structures. They act as a kind of barometer, reflecting the state of the internal weather of the related segment.

In this context muscle power and tone are distinct entities. Power is an easily measurable quantity, and in all cases the testing of power, comparing one side with the other, should be part of the routine of muscular, skeletal, and neurological examination.

The concept of tone is more difficult to understand, but an attempt must be made to describe it. A person with flabby muscles has poor tone, and a person with excessive strength has excessive tone; but tone is not merely a quality of strength or bulk. It is a quality of elasticity and resilience, and this state is created by regular exercise. Feeling the muscle and sensing its size and resistance to palpation gives one some idea, and the constant practice of palpation enables the practitioner to sense poor tone, normal tone, or an excess of tone.

The physiological state of muscle tone has been defined as 'a state of partial tetanus maintained by an asynchronous discharge of impulses in the motorneurones which supply the muscle'.[53] 'It is considered to be a function of the small γ efferent nerve-supply to the muscle which is permanently active but does not necessarily set up movement through the α motorneurones. It is the motorneurones which contract muscles either when reflexly stimulated or by voluntary activation.'[54]

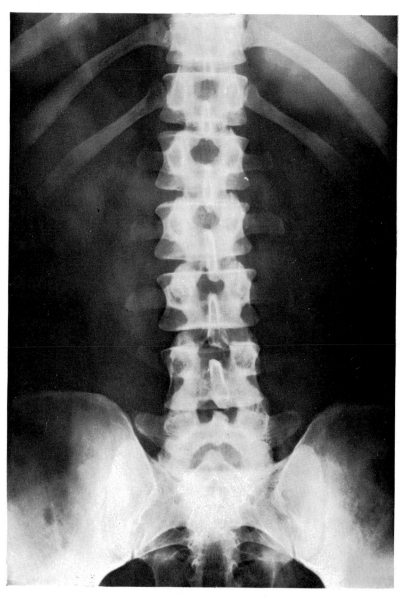

FIGS 14 AND 15 Both of these lumbar X-rays were taken of the same patient on the same day. FIG 14—the supine X-ray gives information of bone structure but it is misleading because the erect view (FIG 15) shows considerable weight bearing deformity.

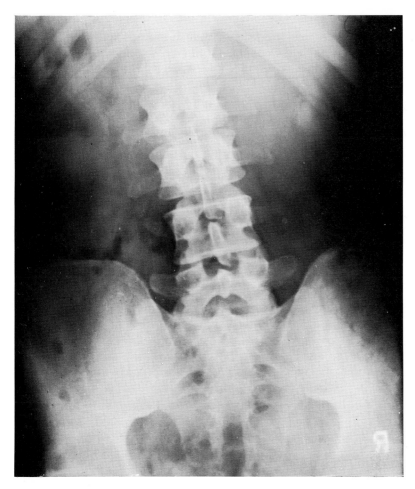

The clinical variants of muscle tone are as follows:

1 Flaccid muscle without any tone, as in paralysis.

2 Relaxed muscle yet with a small amount of tone. The muscles feel soft but not flabby as in a denervated muscle.

3 Contracted muscle, with continuous increased tone such as is found around a faulty and painful joint. When contracted muscles persist they develop a 'stringy' feeling because some fibres which are continuously contracted lie between more relaxed fibres. They can best be felt by palpating the muscles transversely. The contracted and relaxed fibres lie parallel with each other, and this produces long lines of tight fibres. Such muscle contraction has been called fibrositis, and although there are differences of opinion as to its cause this type of contraction is very common.

4 Muscle guarding is a reflex contraction of muscle which is evoked when the source of the guarding is stimulated. It can best be elicited by the springing test (see pp. 53, 95, *fig. 7*) over the spine with the patient prone.

5 Muscle contracture is persistent muscle contraction which has led to permanent shortening of the muscle.

6 Cramp is a sudden painful contraction of the whole muscle.

Continuous contraction of any muscle causes fatigue and eventually pain, and in cramp, when the whole muscle contracts violently, pain is severe. Normal activity involves alternating contraction and relaxation which is painless, but sustained contraction—except in the posturing muscles—gives rise in due course to an ache which is caused by the accumulation of metabolic waste products which should be dispersed during relaxation.

'Fatigue occurs owing to the change in the muscle induced by anoxia and accumulation of metabolites. Both these changes are offset by blood-flow, but there are mechanical problems in maintaining blood-flow during sustained contraction for the rise in intra-muscular tension tends to prevent the passage of blood.'[55]

Voluntary muscle becomes fatigued when contraction has been stimulated for too long. Eventually the muscular response ceases altogether, but this does not necessarily apply to the posturing muscles. The clinical impression is that prolonged contraction leads to fibrous change in the muscle.

In the spine it is possible that continuous contraction involves the γ type of fibres—the 'slow red' posturing muscle fibres—whereas reflex contraction and voluntary contraction involve the α fibres —the 'fast pale' fibres—in the erector spinae group. It is well known that posturing muscles require less oxygen and can continue to contract without fatigue, but even these have a limit, and they will ache if contracted for long enough. This is why fibrositis is a painful condition itself irrespective of its source.

Muscle guarding is always significant, because it implies some acute internal derangement—either of mechanical or pathological origin— and it is a warning of something seriously wrong. It is always present in tuberculosis of the spine and in osteomyelitis, and it is diffusely present in osteoporosis of the vertebral column where the severity of the guarding is a measure of the severity of the osteoporosis. Muscle guarding occurs with disc herniations and tends to disappear when the disc prolapses. It is not present with osteopathic spinal lesions except in severe recent spinal joint sprains.

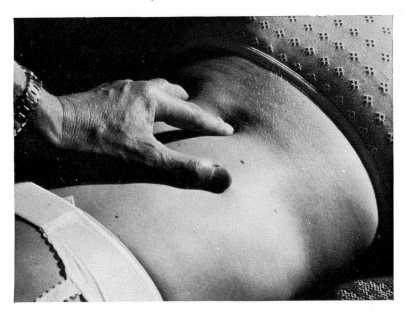

FIG 16 Skin puckering test for the subcutaneous tissues.

Soft-tissue changes

These include panniculitis, fatty nodules, oedema, and swellings.

Recent advances in knowledge of the collagen diseases have shed light on conditions of the soft tissues of the skin, the fat, the areolar tissue, and fascia. It is of course extremely rare to find dermatomyositis or scleroderma in association with osteopathic spinal lesions, but undoubtedly some soft-tissue changes accompany the lesion. The skin changes have been referred to already (p. 55).

In testing the areolar tissue it ought to be possible to pick up the skin from the subjacent fat and muscle and move it about freely, and if this is not possible then the elasticity of the skin or areolar tissue is in doubt. The skin is tethered more tightly in some sites than in others, but the texture of the areolar tissue can be readily compared with that of other sites in the body or with that of other people. In dermatomyositis the skin is sufficiently adherent to the subjacent muscle to reduce movement in the limb or the spine, but this is a diffuse process and not localised. In some osteopathic spinal lesions, especially the chronic ones, the area of the lesion has thickened areolar tissue and it is tender. There are two tests for this. The *first* (*fig. 16*) is to press the subcutaneous tissues along with the tips of the fingers at about 20° to the surface, applying sufficient pressure to stop merely sliding along the skin yet insufficient to arrest the movement of the. fingers along the skin, when a slight

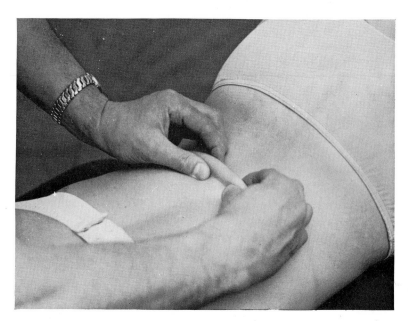

FIG 17 Skin rolling test for the subcutaneous tissues.

puckering effect will be noticed and a sense of resistance to the moving fingers as compared with nearby sites. Where there is thickening and tenderness it frequently coincides with the level of the lesion. The *second test* (*fig. 17*) is by 'skin rolling'. Starting a few inches away from the level of the lesion, pick up the skin into a roll between the fingers and thumbs of both hands and gradually roll the skin towards the lesion site. If the areolar tissue is normal it will roll easily and painlessly, but if a lesion is approached the resistance to rolling will increase and tenderness will be apparent. These two physical signs are by no means consistent, and they are not in themselves a guide to the existence of a lesion, but when positive the increased resistance and tenderness is felt over the level of the lesion.

Panniculitis is a condition of the *panniculus adiposus* in which there is diffuse thickening and tenderness in certain areas of the body. The skin tends to pucker when the surface layers are lifted and squeezed together to give the *'peau d'orange'* effect. The commonest sites for this are over the deltoid and over the medial condyle of the tibia below the knee joint; and, if panniculitis is suspected in the spinal areas, these two sites should be palpated also. In the spine, panniculitis mostly affects the trapezius area but any and all spinal areas can be involved. Dercum's disease is an accentuated form of panniculitis and does not concern us in mechanical lesions.

Other fatty lesions are the *nodules* which commonly appear in the sacro-iliac and gluteal areas of the lower back. Readily palpable and sometimes tender, they are quite distinct from trigger points or fibrositis of muscle, because they are round and firm in texture. They move easily under the skin and over the subjacent muscle and fatty layer. They comprise a very definite clinical entity and can be excised surgically. Their significance is disputed, and tenderness is no criterion that they are causing symptoms because that tenderness may be an expression of a deeper source of pain. However, these nodules have some sort of fibrous capsule, especially if they have been present for a long time, and this capsule can be stretched by changes in the quantity of fat enclosed and by the water balance of the body. When the capsules are stretched they are painful, and the pain is well localised. That they are causing pain can be easily proved by infiltrating the nodule with a local anaesthetic and then pounding it with something hard, which will relieve the pain permanently. If the pain had been arising from a deeper structure and merely causing tenderness of the nodule, such treatment would merely have a temporary anaesthetic effect and the pain and tenderness would return in a few hours. The fat content can often be dispersed in this way, but sometimes it is necessary to puncture the capsule in several places with a thick needle before the fat can be squeezed out. But even this may not be sufficient, and then it may be worth while to excise them surgically. If after dispersing the nodule the same nodule re-forms, the likelihood is that its capsule will be tougher than before and it will be impossible to disperse it by pounding.

Oedema of the soft tissues of the spine is rare in my experience. The only likely explanation for swelling which pits on pressure in the spinal area would be inflammatory changes, as in cellulitis or gout.

Effusion of apophyseal joints is impossible to detect clinically except in the cervical apophyseal joints where the capsules are almost subcutaneous. Acutely inflamed joints in the neck exhibit swelling of these capsules which can be exquisitely sensitive (see p. 208). Such swelling usually subsides in two or three days. It should not be mistaken for a displacement, and manipulation of such a joint will merely accentuate the pain and effusion.

By analogy, apophyseal joints in the thoracic and lumbar areas must become acutely inflamed and this probably accounts for many misdiagnosed disc lesions. The differential diagnosis of these conditions will be dealt with later (p. 137).

Skin changes

The following skin changes may be relevant in mechanical problems of the spine:

A pilonidal dimple, a naevus, or a patch of hair in the lumbo-sacral area usually implies that a congenital anomaly is present in the area.

Hyperaesthesia, hypoaesthesia, hyperhidrosis, and dryness in a local area of the spine implies altered vasomotor activity in the subjacent spinal segment. The significance of this is discussed on p. 11.

Hyperaesthesia and hyperhidrosis usually go with an increased 'red response' to scratching and a decrease in electrical skin resistance (see p. 288).

Clinical examination and procedure

History-taking The anamnesis of every medical condition is vital to diagnosis, and by itself may sometimes be sufficient to lead to an accurate diagnosis, but in any case the history will direct the practitioner towards a diagnosis. The least we can expect from a history is guidance as to which system of the body to examine in detail.

Clinical examination should ideally involve all the systems—loco-motor, central nervous, alimentary, genito-urinary, cardio-vascular, respiratory, and psychological—but such detailed examination is impracticable at a first consultation. In practice, essential basic observations should be made in all the systems but only the system directly involved need be examined in great detail. In osteopathic practice the locomotor and central nervous systems obviously command our closest attention, but a general examination is always desirable lest signs of disease are unaccompanied by symptoms in the other systems. By so doing errors of diagnosis by omission are unlikely.

History-taking is an art in itself which needs constant practice. The standard methods in medicine have stood the test of time and need not be elaborated here. There are two stages: the first stage when, after initial questions like 'What are your complaints?' or 'Would you like to tell me your story?', the patient can explain in his or her own words what is wrong; and the second stage, when specific points need further questioning by the doctor.

Sufficient time must be allocated for careful history-taking. In the first instance it is wise always to give full rein to the patient's own description of the symptoms, their duration, and their intensity. It is only legitimate to interrupt spontaneous history-giving if the patient is too garrulous and is side-tracking from the symptomatology, though even then it is better to allow the patient to explain everything without interruption. If the history is confused, the practitioner is gaining insight into the patient's mentality and background however irrelevant the remarks may be. A poor witness and particularly one with inadequate vocabulary, will need bringing back to the salient points. The patient who never replies directly to a question is mentally confused and advice should be sought from a psychiatrist.

During the second stage of the anamnesis special enquiries need to be made about injuries because so often they are forgotten, sometimes until the patient's second or third visit. The patient's occupation, hobbies, and sporting activities always need looking into because of their relevance to body mechanics. The patient's posture in the consulting room is not always the habitual one, and questions about the manner of sitting, standing, or lying are usually important. The relationship of position and activity to the symptoms can be vital to the diagnosis.

Errors in history-taking can creep in:

1 When the patient has a preconceived idea of the diagnosis. The patient who interprets symptoms all the time needs discouraging from such interpretations otherwise undue emphasis can side-track the history towards the diagnosis already in the patient's mind.

2 When the patient has had a previous examination and a previous diagnosis has been made. It is the duty of the practitioner to form his own conclusion irrespective of any antecedent diagnosis.

3 When the patient unwittingly suppresses symptoms—not necessarily because of a desire to mislead, but because such and such a symptom seems to have nothing to do with the pain which is the presenting complaint. The other symptoms may, unknown to the patient, be very relevant. It is therefore vital in all cases to enquire about general health and any other symptoms whatsoever.

4 When the practitioner is biased towards a particular diagnosis—as, for example, the osteopath who favours structural faults and structural diagnosis. I well remember a patient who complained of backache but who failed to respond to my treatment of a minor lesion, and it was not until her anaemia was corrected that the backache subsided. A similar bias occurs in all specialities—e.g. gynaecological procedures have been performed in the hope of relieving backache which is subsequently found to be of structural origin. This practitioner-bias occurs in every speciality and derives from over-specialisation and a desire to make the patient conform with the practitioner's own preconceptions. One must guard against this.

Inspection Clinical examination commences with inspection—which we should be doing from the moment the patient enters the room—but detailed inspection of the unclothed patient, comparing one side with the other, gives more information. The feet, the rotation of the femora, the level of the iliac crests, the contour of the spine, and the general posture should all be noted; these can be observed in a few moments. The carriage of the head and shoulders should be watched when standing and walking. The gait gives useful information, but a self-conscious gait is not always a reliable guide. Inspection of the patient's shoes gives clues about habitual weight-bearing and walking which the self-conscious gait might hide. It may not be until late in the consultation that the patient feels relaxed enough to adopt his or her usual posture. The advantages of examining the naked body are clinically obvious, but a patient who is shy will adopt all sorts of misleading distorted muscular tensions under such circumstances, so that brief garments are best for such patients. I learned a salutary lesson when I missed a carcinoma of the breast merely because I did not examine the breasts. The patient complained of backache, and my examination and X-rays eventually led to a diagnosis of secondary growths, but if I had had the patient unclothed it would have been obvious at a glance. The patient knew about her breast, but avoided the subject and left me to find out.

Contours should be observed in all positions, standing, sitting, supine, and prone.

Following inspection, the overall *active ranges* of movements should be tested and recorded, preferably using the standard methods of recording and best described in *Joint Motion*: *Method of Measuring and Recording* published by the American Academy of Orthopedic Surgeons[56].

While testing the active mobility ranges the *passive ranges* can also be assessed by an extra stretch of the movement, to observe whether the patient can go further with passive stretching and whether there is any resistance to additional movement. However, the ranges of individual spinal joints must be tested separately. The detailed examination of each joint is described in my *Manual of Osteopathic Technique*.

Testing the overall active and passive ranges gives some indication as to the area of the lesion or lesions. For example, side-bending the lumbar spine to the right may show uniform movement down to 12T, then a straight section say to 3L, and then good movement again below 3L. This indicates some mechanical fault at 12T–3L, and only detailed mobility tests will enable the practitioner to decide which of the three joints are causing the symptoms.

Rotation restriction in the cervical area suggests upper cervical lesions, whereas side-bending restriction suggests lower cervical lesions. This is not invariable, but it is a useful guide before the individual mobility tests are performed.

Flexion-extension restrictions can be noted, and when not extensive the level of the restrictions can be seen within one or two segments.

Palpation is the next logical step in clinical examination, but we need to know what to palpate for and how to distinguish the normal from the abnormal.

Palpation of the components of the locomotor system is by no means easy, and much practice is needed before one can obtain the maximum information possible. We can use the whole hand or the tips of fingers and thumbs. In the '*springing*' test (*fig. 7*, p. 53), which helps so much in localising the level of the lesion in the thoracic and lumbar areas of the spine, we use the whole hand, applying pressure to the spinous processes with the back of the hand. For this test (p. 57, *fig. 12*, in *Manual of Osteopathic Technique*) the table should be low enough for the practitioner to be able to lean over the prone patient. His arms should be kept firm with the elbow fully extended so that the springing sensation is derived from his whole arm and body rather than just from his hand. The practitioner leans on the patient and exerts a springing movement to the spine once or perhaps twice in quick succession. It should be done gently at first and if there is no protest from the patient the force of springing can be increased.

The test gives information about the 'give' of the joints, and with practice the exact level of the restriction of movement can be detected, though the other tests of flexion, side-bending, and rotation are necessary to confirm the details of the mechanical fault.

The amount of pressure needed to evoke a response is also a measure of the sensitivity of the joint. Sometimes restrictions of springiness occur without symptoms and without subjective tenderness, but this is unusual. There may be undue 'give' in the spine, and if symptoms are present then a hypermobile type of lesion is probable.

If the springing test evokes *reflex muscle guarding*, there must be some acute internal derangement of the joint. Protective guarding by paravertebral muscles may be continuous. In this case we call it *sustained muscular tension*, and this can be present without the guarding response. If slight, guarding may only be evoked when the joint is jarred. Even slight guarding is significant, and it means that the practitioner should himself be on his guard—i.e. on guard about the diagnosis—because serious pathological lesions of the spine always show guarding during the springing test. Tuberculous, infective, and neoplastic lesions and osteoporosis can be picked up by this clinical test more quickly than by any other. A positive springing test can indicate an acute mechanical lesion—e.g. a disc herniation. This in itself is not serious but these cases still require cautious handling, even though the general health of the patient is not in jeopardy. Thus muscular guarding is a vital observation in every case.

The test itself does not make a diagnosis but it does warn one that an acute internal derangement or pathological process is present, and in my view this is *one of the most valuable diagnostic aids in the osteopath's armamentarium*. A similar test for the neck, which gives a sense of

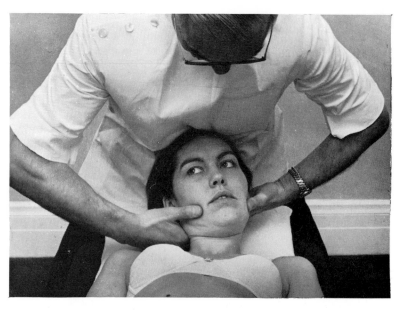

FIG 18 Lateral mobility test of the cervical spine

springiness of the cervical joints, helps to localise the level of the lesion (*fig. 18*). The patient lies supine and the practitioner stands at the head of the table. The patient's vertex is supported by the practitioner's abdomen at about 20° flexion: the pressure should be sufficient to hold the head off the pillow without additional support of the hands, and yet not so much as to compress the cervical spine uncomfortably. The patient should in fact be able to relax the neck and shoulders in this position. The practitioner is then free to apply the radial border of each index finger to the area of the articular processes in the mid cervical region. At this stage there is a tendency to support the patient's head in the operator's hands, but this should be avoided. The hands should be free and the elbows out sideways, as shown. The next step is to press the side of the neck laterally while still retaining the vertex of the head in the mid-line in order to 'buckle' the neck into side-bending. This must be performed gently and must not cause pain, otherwise the patient will resist and the operator will be unable to feel the movement properly. The 'buckling' to each side is done alternately, and the level of the lateral pressure altered by moving caudally or cranially. In this way the sense of give or resistance is felt anywhere between 2C and 7C. When the resistance is located it should be repeated several times for confirmation, and it is useful if, say, there is resistance at 3–4C on the right to apply several springing movements on the right rather than alternating between right and left.

The springing test in the cervical area is of course a measure of side-bending, just as springing the thoracic and lumbar areas is a measure of extension; but individual side-bending tests in the cervical area can also be carried out by moving the whole cervical spine laterally and palpating at each level. The essence of the springing tests, whether cervical, thoracic or lumbar, is the sensation of 'give' which it imparts. If the area does not 'give' there is something wrong, and more detailed study and palpation is required to complete the mechanical diagnosis. Following the 'springing test' detailed mobility tests should be performed to test the degree of flexion, extension, side-bending, and rotation. Such mobility is best felt with the tips of the fingers or thumbs, because adjacent spinous processes can be spanned by one digit.

The palpation can next be directed to any 'displacement' of the bony landmarks; to test whether the spinous processes are approximated or separated in the neutral position; and to observe whether the transverse process on one side is more or less prominent or more caudal or cranial compared with adjacent ones.

In palpating spinous processes with the patient prone both index fingers and both thumbs should be used to run down each side of several processes in order to note deviations. Not much importance can be attached to individual deviation, but the general contours can be ascertained in this way.

The transverse processes are more reliable as guides to positional faults because they are not so subject to anatomical variations in shape as are the spinous processes. The transverse processes are best palpated by applying the thumbs and rolling gently up and down over them (*fig. 19*). (This contrasts with moving the thumbs medially and laterally for palpating paravertebral muscle tension (*fig. 20*)).

After testing mobility and bony landmarks, the palpating hand should be directed to feeling the skin and soft tissues.

The skin may be rough or smooth, warm or cold, sweaty or dry, and anaesthetic or hyperaesthetic. A frequent accompaniment of the osteopathic spinal lesion is an area of hyperhidrosis at the same level, which can best be detected by the very gentlest touch—i.e. just stroking the skin over a series of spinous processes. If there is increased sudo-motor activity, resistance to the stroking is increased and it feels slightly rough instead of beautifully smooth. Of course other palpating tests may have set up an erythema over the lesion, especially in a histamine sensitive patient, and then this skin test is useless; to be of much value this skin-stroking must be the first palpatory observation.

The areolar tissue of subcutaneous fat is palpated by the skin-puckering test and the skin-rolling test (*figs. 16, 17*).

Muscle tension (as distinct from muscle guarding and muscle tone)

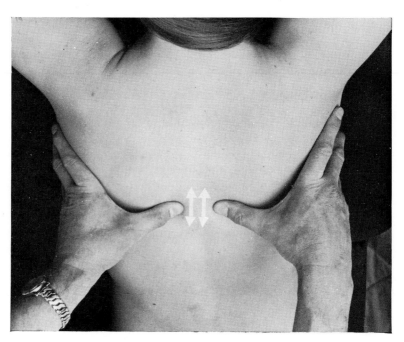

FIG 19 Palpation of the transverse processes. Arrows indicate the up and down movements of the thumbs.

is palpated by rolling the fibres at right angles to their course. Localised muscle tension (fibrositis) has a stringy feel. The fibres run longitudinally, and so the palpating fingers or thumbs must move laterally over the fibres. By palpating longitudinally one would miss these tensions. Excessive pressure should be avoided because any tissue is sensitive if sufficient pressure is applied and a contraction may be provoked merely by hurting the muscle. In fact a much lighter pressure is applied transversely to muscle as compared with the up and down movement already described in palpating transverse processes.

Apart from the above objective tests of palpation, the fingers can be used to elicit tenderness but this is essentially subjective, and it is accurate only if we can rely on that particular patient's testimony (see p. 72).

The refinements of palpation are, as already indicated, a matter of practice and concentration. Some 'ham-handed' individuals can never palpate, however good they are as doctors. The practitioner must visualise what tissues are under his fingers, and he must have much practice with normal tissues before attempting to recognise abnormal tissues. The veriest tyro can feel a firm superficial lipoma, but it requires experience and a delicate touch to feel an enlarged spleen. The same

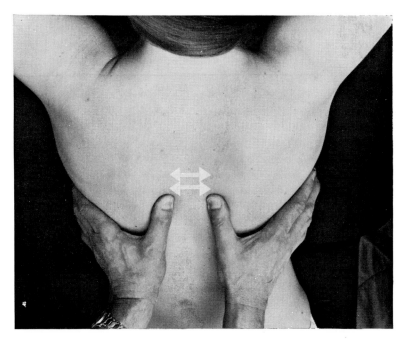

FIG 20 Palpation of the erector spinae muscles. The arrows indicate the direction of to and fro movements of the thumbs.

tyro can appreciate muscle spasm, but minor soft-tissue changes have to be carefully palpated to be detected.

To obtain the maximum information from palpation requires concentrated attention while observing one structure at a time. A good system of palpation is to proceed from the most superficial to the more deep—first the skin, then subcutaneous tissue, then muscle, then ligaments, and finally bony landmarks. If each structure is observed separately the emerging pattern will be greatly clarified.

Further examination is usually necessary to establish a complete mechanical diagnosis. The standard methods of examination of the central nervous system and other systems in the body will help to eliminate pathological changes there.

Radiological examination

X-ray investigations using standard techniques are of little help in mechanical diagnosis. They may be important in the negative sense of excluding bone and joint disease, but X-rays can be invaluable in confirming clinical observation if they are used correctly. 'Functional' X-rays give more information. There are two types of functional films:

1 *Erect X-rays* give information about weight distribution and levels. Leg-length discrepancies can be determined accurately this way (*fig. 25*, p. 133), and scoliosis can be studied with full-length views (*fig. 55*, p. 254.) Lordosis (*fig. 53*, p. 158) is best assessed in erect lateral views.

2 *Mobility* X-rays (*figs. 12, 13*, p. 78, *figs. 22, 23*, p. 124, *figs. 36, 37*, p. 164) give information about ranges of forward- and backward-bending and side-bending. When two films are compared and measured they give information about hypermobility and hypomobility. They may show abnormal shearing movements which are indicative of the unstable hypermobile phase of the disc lesion. Mobility films should be taken horizontally. It is misleading to combine mobility and weight-bearing at one and the same time. Weight-bearing/mobility films do not show the full ranges of passive movements.

Myelograms and *tomograms* may be necessary as final analyses in difficult cases, and further laboratory tests of the blood, urine, cerebrospinal fluid, etc., may be required as ordained by medical practice.

Interpretation of symptoms and signs relative to the spine

The previous section gives a picture of what to expect when isolated faults occur, but in clinical practice it is rare for a patient to have a single simple problem. Patterns of symptoms and signs emerge during the anamnesis and clinical examination. Each of the signs and symptoms helps to build up a pattern from which a reliable diagnosis can be made. When the condition is simple a spot diagnosis can be made, e.g. a fall causing a dinner-fork deformity at the wrist means a Colles' fracture without more ado. When more involved—e.g. a fall causing a pain in the shoulder—it may well require careful testing of the shoulder and neck before a diagnosis can be made. When still more involved, the history and examination may point the way but an X-ray or blood-count is needed to establish the diagnosis. There are, of course, patients with syndromes which are mild and transient or so involved that a precise diagnosis is not possible; but each and every symptom means that something is wrong, and all signs when properly elicited should give positive information that the tissue is normal or abnormal.

Groups of symptoms and signs which occur frequently can be recognised as *syndromes even though an exact interpretation may not be possible*, and for this reason I have tried in the next chapter to describe syndromes, to ascribe a logical meaning to them, and to point the way to treating them.

Some symptoms have obvious origins, but many have not. A cough is a sign that the larynx is being irritated and if the cough produces some sputum we do not need to enquire further for the irritant; but an un-productive cough may be due to wax in the ear or some other obscure lesion of the recurrent laryngeal nerve. Similarly with the locomotor system, a pain in the shoulder may be obviously due to a supraspinatus tendon strain or it may be due to some obscure lung or diaphragm lesion.

A complete discussion on the interpretation of signs and symptoms would require a whole book and will not be attempted here, but certain observations are well worth making because they are apposite to our subject.

Positional pain Pain which alters with variations in position (standing, sitting, lying, or bending) is probably mechanical in origin—i.e. it involves the musculo-skeletal systems rather than the visceral systems—and pain which is unaffected in any way by alteration of position is unlikely to be of mechanical origin.

Positional pain which has been present consistently for months or years without exacerbation or remission is always mechanical in origin and not due to disease. Mechanically produced pain arises from stretching or compressing a sensitive structure.

Pain which develops during *compression* suggests that the tissue being compressed is sensitive. Compression may be merely weight-bearing or it may be from squeezing of the tissues as in side-bending or backward-bending.

Pain which develops when the tissues are *stretched* implies that those tissues which are being elongated are sensitive.

Pain which develops during side-bending is either compression or stretch pain. If the pain is on the opposite side to the side-bending (contralateral side), it implies stretch pain. If the pain is on the same side (ipsilateral side), it implies compression pain.

All spinal movements involve stretching or compression of several structures; but the distribution of the pain, its character, and its intensity are further guides to its source.

Pain produced by standing and relieved by movement and rest suggests compression of a disc with bulging which stretches the longitudinal ligaments.

Pain produced by forward-bending with free side-bending and backward-bending suggests the protrusion of a disc; but, if the forward-bending causes pain only after the delay of some minutes, this implies weakness of ligaments. This is *delayed stretch pain* and, although this type of pain can arise in the degenerating disc, that pain is still likely to be ligamentous because of course the discs are not themselves sensitive.

Pain produced by continuous forward-bending could be muscular in origin—i.e. fatigue pain—but this can readily be distinguished from ligamentous stretch pain by the adoption of a stretched position of the ligament while the muscles are relaxed, as when slumping in a low chair.

Painless forward-bending followed by pain during the return to the erect position suggests that during flexion there is an alteration of position of either the vertebrae or the disc between and that during extension there is a painful realignment. This in turn implies an unstable joint and weak ligaments. Crisp[57] claims that in these circumstances a fringe of synovial membrane can get in the way and block the extension of an apophyseal joint.

Stretch pain occurs with adhesions, but the pain is immediate and not delayed as with relaxed ligaments. Furthermore adhesions produce hypomobility whereas relaxed ligaments produce hypermobility.

Pain produced by backward-bending only, with free forward-bending and side-bending, suggests compression of the facets or partes inter-articulares or spinous processes, and is part of the lordosis syndrome (see p. 156).

Sometimes with a disc protrusion forward-bending as well as side-bending to each side may be relatively free and yet backward-bending is painful; but in these cases there is a lower lumbar kyphosis and not a lordosis, and X-rays show a wedge-shaped disc (wider posteriorly than arteriorly).

A patient who is unable to extend after free forward-bending may have weak erector spinae muscles, or if at the same time there is acute pain, as in 'lumbago', then there is a strong probability that a disc has herniated.

A painful arc of movement, whether in forward-bending or side-bending, strongly suggests a protrusion of a disc with a nerve-root riding over the bulge.

When pain is accentuated by coughing and sneezing this is a sign of its acuteness, and it implies that compression is increasing the pain though it is *no* guide to the source of the pain.

When pain is relieved by traction this suggests that the apposition of adjacent structures is causing pain, as in arthritis where opposing facets are sensitive or in nerve-root irritation when there is insufficient room in the intervertebral foramen for the inflamed nerve. Relief by traction suggests that this is an appropriate form of treatment.

In inflamed nerves pain can be evoked either by compression or stretching, but nerve pain can usually be distinguished from pain arising in ligaments, muscles, and bone if paraesthesiae are also present. None of the other structures produces paraesthesiae, and the paraesthesiae arising after ischaemia are readily distinguished from those of nerve irritation by observations on the circulation.

An example of nerve pain evoked by compression and by stretching is seen in the cervical spine with a prolapsed disc. Many of those suffering pain in the normal position of the neck are relieved of the compression by traction of between 30 and 40 lb. The pain then subsides, but if the traction exceeds 40 lb the pain comes on again.

The above observations apply to symptoms related to position. There are in addition *signs* which depend on position—for example, the straight leg raising (S.L.R.) test.

The *S.L.R. test* should be performed with the patient supine. The lower extremity should be elevated with the knee kept extended, and the patient is asked at what stage pain comes on. The angle which the leg makes with the plinth should be recorded and compared with that on the other side.

Straight-leg raising can be restricted by pain, or painless restriction can be due to tightness of the hamstrings. If both occur they can be distinguished by modifying the S.L.R. test. After the leg has been raised to the angle of pain it should be lowered a few degrees again to the point at which pain ceases, and then the foot should be dorsi-flexed. This has the effect of stretching the sciatic nerve without putting an additional stretch on the hamstrings. If pain recurs on dorsi-flexion of the foot it is likely to be due to tethering of a nerve-root (4 or 5L or IS) rather than just painful tightness of the hamstrings. Charnley[58] has shown on the cadaver that during the first 30° of the straight-leg raising the nerve-roots remain stationary and only move between 30° and 70°. Very little movement occurs beyond 70° of flexion.

Sometimes the S.L.R. test evokes pain in the other leg. This contra-lateral pain implies that torsion of the lumbar spine is part of the pressure mechanism.

If both legs are raised together, the pull on one sciatic nerve ceases and a bilateral effect is produced on the lumbar spine, but it is very difficult to perform this test passively. The patient always wants to help, and by contracting the psoas muscles on both sides a lordosis is automatically created which is painful if a lordosis syndrome is present. If both legs are elevated still further the lordosis is lost and lumbar flexion takes place. These latter observations are useful in themselves, but they must not be confused with the single S.L.R. test.

The S.L.R. test is a guide to the degree of pressure on the nerve-root (4 and 5L, and IS); an angle limited, say, to 10° implies that there is virtually no room left for free movement of the nerve within the inter-vertebral foramen. This test assumes importance in prognosis and treatment, and further discussion of these points will be found on p. 178.

The *neck-flexion test*, when it evokes pain or paraesthesiae in the lower extremities, indicates that the appropriate nerve-root is being tethered because during neck flexion the spinal cord rises within the spinal canal. This effect increases caudally—i.e. cervical flexion only pulls slightly on the cervical nerve-roots, pulls moderately on the thoracic roots, and pulls strongly on the lumbar roots. The cauda equina rises 2 in. during full neck flexion in the normal subject.

The neck-flexion test can be applied in the standing or lying position provided the additional factor of weight-bearing or non-weight-bearing is taken into account. Occasionally neck rotation may evoke a response when flexion does not. If neck flexion evokes paraesthesiae only (without pain), then the more probable explanation is that the cord is being compressed in the cervical spine rather than that nerve-roots are being tethered.

Sometimes a combination of the S.L.R. and the neck-flexion tests can be useful. The maximum possible stretch may be necessary to evoke any response: this is best done with the patient standing and flexing the torso fully forwards, then subjectively flexing the neck too. If this test is negative, then all the nerve-roots in the whole spinal column must be free to move in their intervertebral foramina.

In the cervical spine backward-bending causes pressure on the nerve-roots in the intervertebral foramina, but the compression on one side is maximum when combining backward-bending and side-bending to the affected side. This is the *foraminal compression test* of the cervical spine.

Sometimes when there has been a large disc prolapse in the lumbar spine the patient is kept in a kyphosed position and it becomes impossible to lie supine except with the knee flexed. This interferes with the S.L.R. test because the pain creates an angle of 'fixed' flexion of the hip so that the test can only start, say, at 30°. Further raising of the leg may be free to 50°, giving only about 20° of painless movement. This 20° gives an indication of the greatly reduced space in the intervertebral foramen.

When the second or third lumbar nerves are compressed at the intervertebral foramina the S.L.R. test is negative because, of course, the femoral nerve is not stretched in this test. In this event the patient is tested (Ely's test) when lying prone by extending the hip with the knee flexed to a right angle. It is important not to flex the knee beyond 90° because this always puts an undue stretch on the quadriceps and is uncomfortable except in the very flexible young patient. The angle which the thigh makes with the table when pain is provoked is the one that should be recorded.

Activity pain The influence of activity on pain of skeletal origin can be of some guidance in diagnosis—e.g.:

Pain which develops only with exertion and disappears immediately with rest is called intermittent claudication; it is due to relative ischaemia and the need of the muscles for more oxygen during exercise. As the arterial disease progresses, further impairment of circulation may cause pain on trivial activity or even at rest, but this confusion in symptomatology is unlikely if one enquires into the history of the syndrome carefully and at an earlier stage.

Pain which develops with rest and is relieved by activity is not so easily explained. It may be of vascular origin in so far as the rest might lead to slowing up of circulation and accumulation of metabolites: this is the probable explanation in gout where pain is at its worst in the early hours of the morning.

In osteo-arthritis, pain sometimes increases with rest and then after a few movements (e.g. on starting to walk) the pain diminishes, but this pattern is distinguishable because stiffness accompanies the pain. Pain plus stiffness after rest is probably due to sustained reflex muscular guarding of the affected joint. Stiffness alone (without pain) after rest can probably be best explained on the same muscular basis though its intensity is less.

Fatigue sometimes produces muscular pain, or at least muscular fatigue can be severe enough to be painful. General fatigue after a busy day can accentuate any pain just as can anxiety, because the pain threshold is presumably lowered with fatigue and anxiety.

Backache of muscular origin, as for example the backache of gardening, which is merely from unaccustomed muscular exertion, passes off quickly. This is the experience of most people who only engage in gardening occasionally.

Muscular pain—or rather the aching stiffness in muscles—which follows unaccustomed exercise sometimes comes on with trivial amounts of exercise. This leads to the suspicion that focal sepsis is present, or that the serum uric-acid level is raised, or that the electrolytic balance in the muscles is on the acid side of normal.

Pain which is accentuated by heat suggests neuritis, whereas pain relieved by heat suggests that the origin was muscular tension. Throbbing pain implies vascular congestion—perhaps inflammation or Paget's disease—or the arterial pulse may be stretched over a tight structure.

Pain which is unaffected by activity or rest or position is likely to be visceral or due to neoplasia. It can of course be psychogenic in origin but psychogenic pain is unrelieved by analgesics. If pain persists despite analgesics, it may be because the pain is too severe for the analgesic to be effective; but in these cases there are other indications of the severity of the pain.

Pain at night which is relieved during the day may have a positional explanation, but on the other hand it may be gouty or due to bone disease. Anxiety states which are worse at night often increase pain of other origins during the night.

Interpretation of deformity and posture It is sometimes necessary to elicit signs of deformity in cases where the fault is not obvious.

For example, a *short leg* of moderate amount (say $\frac{1}{4}$ in.) is not obvious at first glance and yet may be an important factor in the aetiology of backache. The patient should be observed from behind, preferably without garments; the iliac crests are palpated and compared; the posterior superior iliac spines are palpated, and for this the thumbs should be placed below these spines and pressed upwards against their lowest pole, rather than wobbling about on top of the spines; the gluteal folds are noted; and the posterior knee creases are compared. (The greater trochanters of the femora are of little use in this regard.) Then if one is still in doubt, the patient should be asked to flex the spine. If a short leg is present, the lower back on the short side will look lower: a tangential view will further assist this observation.

Sometimes kyphoses, lordoses, and scolioses are not very obvious, particularly in the obese patient or in powerful muscular types. Flexion of the patient in the standing position will show deformity. The high side of rotated lumbar and thoracic vertebrae can be observed by looking tangentially along the flexed spine. Deformity of the thorax may be less obvious from in front as compared with the posterior aspect.

The position of the pelvis, the relationship of anatomical landmarks— and particularly the anterior and posterior superior iliac spines— are carefully checked in standing, sitting, and lying; the relative alterations of position are noted, but undue importance must not be attached to minor variations in symmetry because the shape of the innominates on the two sides is rarely perfectly symmetrical. Tests which depend on circumducting the hips one way or the other to show apparent alterations in leg lengths are of limited value, and in my view they are not reliable enough for diagnostic purposes.

It is always useful to enquire whether the patient is in the habit of standing more on one leg than the other, because years of this habit can alter the contour of the pelvis and lumbar spine.

Positional observations relative to deformity and posture should be confirmed radiologically in the standing position. This is the only accurate way of measuring discrepancies of femoral leg lengths and sacral tilts (see p. 131).

Local anaesthesia as an aid to diagnosis

In spite of taking the utmost care in mechanical diagnosis, the exact source of symptoms may still remain in doubt. In these circumstances the use of a local anaesthetic may clarify the diagnosis on the grounds that if pain is present before the injection and it ceases after the injection, then the local anaesthetic must have reached the local source of pain.

Clinical examination will have revealed the probable source of pain. Then if the suspected structure is infiltrated carefully, the pain will either cease or persist. If pain is relieved then the diagnosis is confirmed, but if the pain is not relieved or only slightly relieved then the diagnosis is still in doubt.

The practitioner using local anaesthesia must have not only a detailed knowledge of anatomy but also know the depths to which he must penetrate to reach the suspected tissue; and he must know the structures through which the needle passes before reaching the site of the intended injection.

A sudden increase of pain as the needle enters the sensitive structure is likely, and further pain occurs when the fluid is being injected. Although these pains are regrettable in themselves, they are satisfying to the patient and doctor alike because the exact site of the pain source has been reached and identified. If referred pain is produced during the injection, similar to the pain which the patient has been describing, then the referred pain is segmentally linked with the injection site and at least one cause of the reference of pain has been located.

3

CLINICAL SPINAL SYNDROMES
AND THEIR MANAGEMENT

In the following pages the reader will find my attempt to classify, identify, describe, and treat the common and some of the less common syndromes which affect the spinal column. I have tried to make the approach as balanced as possible, so that the various syndromes are seen in perspective. Most authorities on spinal problems tend to over-emphasise certain aspects of this complex subject. For example, Cyriax[59] stresses the importance of the discs in their role of spinal symptom production. The treatment he advocates is largely directed to the disc component. Hackett[60] emphasises the importance of the ligaments, and tends to blame weak ligaments for most of the symptoms arising in the spine. Williams[61] dwells on the importance of lumbar lordosis as a cause of low-back pain, and his book revolves around the correction of lordosis. Mennell[62] points to the importance of the small uncontrolled movements of joints and blames joint dysfunction for many spinal problems. Goldthwait[5] concentrates on body mechanics and the correction of faulty posture. Schmorl and Junghans[63] describe in great detail the late stages of spinal pathological changes and draw conclusions from the morbid anatomy of the spine.

All these authorities have made valuable contributions to the subject, yet none is completely comprehensive. Although in these pages I have attempted to be comprehensive, it is in fact an impossible task. The emphasis here is the osteopathic emphasis upon the earliest clinical manifestations of spinal symptomatology, and the role of mechanical factors in health and disease. It is unwise and even misleading to attribute all symptomatology to one aspect of this involved subject. The majority of patients who have spinal problems do not die from them, and post-mortem findings in recent spinal syndromes are not available. Furthermore, because surgery is indicated in very few cases, we have little direct living macroscopic evidence of what goes on in spinal lesions. X-rays—even with the help of mobility views, weight-bearing views, tomographs, and oblique views—reveal only bones. Myelograms only show outlines and shapes, and all the other components—muscle, cartilage, nerves, meninges, lymphatics, blood-vessels, and ligaments—are not available to our inspection.

Because of these considerations and the imperfections of our knowledge, it is often impossible to state with conviction what has happened to the spine in the past, what is its present state, or what effects our treatment will have on its future. We have to rely largely on the symptomatology and signs to make a diagnosis, and we have to apply the appropriate treatment on the most rational basis. It is essential for the practitioner to take the utmost care, and constantly to increase his knowledge, experience, and practical techniques. Only in this way can he give his best in the light of modern knowledge of the subject.

Because an exact diagnosis cannot always be made, I have attempted here to diagnose the *syndrome* rather than the exact pathological process. The cause of the syndrome may be obvious but this is not always so, and only the probable explanation for these latter syndromes has been indicated. The management of the various syndromes follows from the diagnosis, and I have tried to be as helpful as possible in a practical way by setting down the details of treatment as carefully as possible.

One redeeming feature about spinal problems is that many patients recover whether treated or not, and some recover in spite of treatment rather than because of it! When a patient recovers it does not follow that the treatment brought about the recovery, and this false assumption has led many astray. It is vital to remain detached when observing the results of any form of treatment. We all know that treatment—whether it be a bottle of medicine or a click of the spine—has powerful suggestive effects.

In the course of my own medical career with its osteopathic bias, my outlook has changed. My interpretation of physical findings and my conclusions therefrom have altered as my knowledge and experience have increased.

The observations which follow are based upon thirty years of critical analysis—being critical of myself as much as anything. I have taken the view that if the patient recovered it *might* have been due to my treatment; but if the patient was worse then the treatment was almost certainly responsible, and I must therefore seek the cause of my errors to avoid repeating them in the future.

If the patient gives the credit for his recovery to the practitioner it is very pleasant for his ego; but this credit is not always valid, and in any case the practitioner is merely being instrumental in helping Nature to do what she has been trying to do all the time—namely, to restore the function and the structure to normal.

The only cases in which the practitioner can be sure of the efficacy of his treatment are those in which symptoms rapidly subside when they have been present for a long time and have shown no signs of spontaneous recovery. If the patient's symptoms are static or increasing and then suddenly remit after treatment, the credit can justly be attributed to the treatment.

Because there are an infinite number of variables in nearly all the syndromes here described, the usual research methods are either not applicable or the problems are too complex for precise assessment. Admirable as they are, clinical trials which treat in a standard manner a large number of patients with the same condition and an equal number of controls for comparison have only limited value (see p. 283). Because even a simple manipulation cannot be exactly repeated by different operators, and no two patients are alike, it will always be impossible to be as sure about manipulative trials as one can be with, say, drug trials. The variables are so numerous that even with a computor the task would be formidable.

We must learn therefore from our mistakes rather than our successes, and from quick responses in chronic conditions rather than from good responses in acute or recent conditions.

Before describing the syndromes of spinal origin a list of possible causes is appended, not because such a list is of much use for diagnostic purposes but because it is helpful to realise the multiplicity of causes, and to see them in some sort of order on an aetiological basis. Some conditions, though rare, are linked together because of a clinical or pathological resemblance.

LIST OF CAUSES OF SPINAL PAIN

1 Ligamentous strain from injury, congenital anomalies, and occupational or postural faults which lead to hypermobility (relaxed ligaments) or hypomobility (adhesions and tightened capsules) or displacements and subluxations at all levels of the spine and pelvis:
   Pelvic tilts (laterally and antero-posteriorly)
   Kyphosis (postural, juvenile, senile)
   Lordosis (habit pregnancy, obesity)
   Scoliosis (idiopathic, congenital, paralytic)
2 Injuries in addition to ligamentous damage—e.g. fractures, dislocations, periosteal bruising, and muscles tears.
3 Disc degeneration:
   Herniation: prolapse: Schmorl's nodes: narrowing
   Ballooning and post-central disc expansion
   Calcification and vacuum phenomenon

These in turn may lead to further ligamentous strain, secondary apophyseal joint lesions, and spondylosis.

4 Spondylosis, with the attendant changes of osteophytosis, narrowing of disc spaces and intervertebral foramina, overlapping facets, and enlargement or splaying of the vertebral bodies.

5 Osteo-arthritis of the apophyseal joints and costo-vertebral joints, and of the sacro-iliac and sacro-coccygeal joints.

6 Spondylolysis, spondylolisthesis, retrolisthesis, and 'kissing' spines.

7 Anomalies and congenital faults—synostoses, cervical ribs, pseudo-arthroses, hemi-vertebrae—which lead to pathological joint conditions and nerve irritation.

8 Muscular and soft-tissue lesions: tension states, 'fibrositis', focal sepsis, muscular rheumatism, gouty rheumatism, collagen diseases, panniculitis, and fatty nodules.

9 Osteochondrosis—early and late.

10 Ankylosing spondylitis: osteitis condensans ilii: stiff back syndrome.

11 Osteoporosis—nutritional, menopausal, senile, steroid, thyroid, hyperthyroid, immobilisation.

12 Infection and general diseases:

Osteomyelitis, spondylitis secondary to focal sepsis, tuberculosis of vertebral bodies, discs, and sacro-iliac joints.

Typhoid fever, brucellosis, actinomycosis, influenza, smallpox.

Gout—muscular and sacro-iliac.

Blood dyscrasias and alkaptonuria.

13 Paget's disease and other rare bone diseases.

14 Neoplasms: secondary carcinoma, angioma, myelomatosis, osteitis fibrosa cystica.

15 Visceral diseases causing referred pain to the spine or pressure erosion.

16 Central nervous system diseases: meningitis, poliomyelitis, syringomyelia, tetanus, spinal subarachoid haemorrhage.

17 Psychogenic causes.

18 Iatrogenic causes: unskilled manipulation, inappropriate and ill-timed manipulation, myelography, surgery with subsequent adhesions, ill-fitting or too prolonged use of corsets, plaster-of-Paris jackets, casual use of the term 'arthritis' in diagnosis.

This is a formidable list, and an exact diagnosis is not always possible. In clinical practice, those cases which cannot be accurately diagnosed are better described as syndromes, a list of which follows.

LIST OF CLINICAL SPINAL SYNDROMES

1 Adhesion syndromes (p. 114):
  The hypomobile types of spinal lesions including 'joint bind'
2 Ligamentous strain syndromes (p. 119):
  The hypermobile types of spinal lesion
  The 'short leg' syndrome is included here, though there may be no
  hypermobility.
3 Acute episodic syndromes (p. 136):
  Traumatic
  Disc protrusions
  Muscular
  Inflammatory
  Miscellaneous acute spinal pain—e.g. gout and herpes
4 Chronic degenerative syndromes (p. 150):
  Spondylosis of the vertebral bodies
  Osteo-arthritis of the apophyseal joints
5 Lordosis syndromes (p. 156):
  'Kissing' spines
  Apophyseal joint overlap and arthritis
  Partes interarticulares faults, sclerosis, spondylolysis, spondylo-
  listhesis
  Intervertebral foraminal compression
  Secondary remote effects in the sacro-iliac joints and the knees.
  Visceroptosis
6 Nerve-root syndromes, with and without abnormal central nervous
  system signs (p. 168):
7 Peripheral nerve lesions of the lower extremity. (Though not of
  spinal origin these are included for completeness) (p. 183):
  Meralgia paraesthetica
  Peroneal nerve lesion
  Tarsal tunnel syndrome
  Metatarsalgia
8 Sacro-iliac syndromes (p. 184).
  Hypermobile lesions
  Subluxations
  Sacro-iliitis
  Osteitis condensans ilii
9 Ankylosing spondylitis. Stiff back syndrome (p. 190)
10 Coccygeal syndromes (p. 193).
11 Thoracic and rib syndromes (p. 194):
  Hypomobile thoracic lesions

Disc protrusions
Costo-vertebral lesions
Spondylosis
Intercostal lesions
Costo-chondral, interchondral, and sternal lesions
Tietze's syndrome

12 Brachial syndromes (p. 203):
Acute apophyseal joint lesions
Hypermobile lesions
Disc protrusions
Foraminal compression syndrome
· Thoracic outlet syndrome
Peripheral nerve lesions of the upper extremity

13 Occipital and upper cervical syndromes (p. 219):
Hypomobile lesions
Nervous tension states
Semispinalis capitis 'fibrositis'
Osteo-arthritis of the apophyseal joints
Headache syndromes
Ear syndromes
Facial syndromes
Eye syndromes
Klippel-Feil syndrome

14 Cervical myelopathy and amyotrophic neuropathy (p. 234).

15 Soft-tissue syndromes (p. 236):
Muscle and tendon
Areolar and fatty tissue

16 Osteochondrosis syndrome (p. 240).

17 Kyphosis syndromes in the adult (p. 244).

18 Scoliosis syndromes (p. 252).

19 Spinal gout (p. 255).

20 Spinal osteitis: tuberculous and non-specific (p. 260).

21 Neoplastic syndromes of bone and nerve (p. 261).

22 Miscellaneous and rare spinal diseases (p. 264).

23 Visceral backache syndromes (p. 265).

24 Psychogenic syndromes (p. 267).

From the preceding list it will be seen that the causes of spinal pain are legion, though certain well-defined patterns emerge time and time again. These patterns will now be described, probable explanations offered for them, and the appropriate treatment indicated at the optimum phase. *The time factor is of considerable importance because most of these syndromes are NOT static.* They all tend to increase or decrease, and even when chronic there are variations in their intensity from time to time.

The characteristic symptoms and signs will be stated, and the most significant features outlined. It must be remembered that there is considerable overlapping in these syndromes so that any one patient may present features of two or three syndromes. In addition there may well be a progression or deterioration from one syndrome to another. In choosing the order of description I have tried to adopt a reasonable sequence so that any merging of one into the next is also described in adjacent sections.

Some of the syndromes have obvious clinical subdivisions, and these will also be described, depending on the site, age-group, intensity, duration, and so forth.

1 Adhesion syndromes—the hypomobile type of spinal lesion

The chief characteristics are:

Reduced mobility at the one joint (if more than one joint is involved we call it a 'group' lesion), together with good general spinal mobility.
Pain evoked by stretching, but only at the limit of movement.
Local tenderness in the supraspinous ligament.
Muscular tension.
Positional faults.
Reflex changes.
Good response to manipulation.

This is the osteopathic spinal lesion *per se*. It follows an acute spinal joint sprain which is described under the heading of acute episodic syndromes (p. 136).

The joint has recovered from the initial sprain but instead of getting better it goes on to adhesion formation and reduced mobility. The movements are not all reduced in all ranges (except when the lesion becomes chronic), and the pain is only evoked by stretching the adhesions. This sign may be difficult to elicit, but careful attention to detail with mobility tests will demonstrate several or all of the above features. A lesser form of this lesion is called 'joint bind', in which restricted movements and slight tenderness are the only features (see p. 81). There is a 'stretch' pain rather than 'compression' pain, when adhesions are present—i.e. when the patient is side-bent to the right the pain is felt in the left. There is no pain at rest and the lesion may be asymptomatic, largely because the joint is not stretched far enough to evoke pain or because stiffness is the only symptom and this is dismissed as unimportant or disregarded altogether by the patient or doctor. When stiffness occurs in a spinal joint without accompanying pain or tenderness it suggests that the capsules of the apophyseal joints and the other ligaments of the vertebral joint have tightened, just as can occur in the shoulder joint from lack of use. In single lesions the overall spinal movements of the group may not be restricted at all. There may even be an excessive overall range because of hypermobility in adjacent joints. These lesion restrictions can only be detected by careful passive mobility tests (see *Manual of Osteopathic Technique*, p. 40).

In addition tenderness can be elicited over the spinous process or transverse processes and adjacent ligaments. There may well be a positional fault, and this has been described already (p. 83). As a rule there is some muscular tension in the immediate vicinity, but there is no reflex muscle guarding even with the springing test (see pp. 53 and 88). There are reflex changes in the skin (see p. 11). The pain is local rather than referred, and when referred there are no abnormal signs in the central nervous system. The pain is not of the 'compression' type which is felt on the side to which the spine is side-bent.

The standard mobility tests for individual lesions already mentioned are sufficient in most cases, but the stretch pain of adhesions may only be detectable by traction. In the absence of foraminal compression signs and abnormal central nervous system signs the *traction test* is useful, and when positive this suggests that the adhesions are longitudinal ones. These may be missed by testing the joints only with flexion, extension, side-bending, and rotation.

The traction test (fig. 21) is carried out by placing the patient supine on the table with the feet tethered by cuffs round the ankles. The 'slack' is taken up by a preliminary stretch of the patient, which consists of pulling on the axillae so that any looseness of the ankle straps or of the body on the table is taken up. The patient's head is now grasped firmly and comfortably by the operator taking hold of her occiput in his right hand and her chin in his left hand. (To facilitate description the patient is always assumed to be female and the operator male.) It is important to ensure that the operator's grip is not causing any discomfort, otherwise the patient's attention is distracted from the test. As this test is essentially subjective, any pain felt when the final stretch is given must be reported. The next step is to stretch the whole spine by a firm pull on the patient's head, taking up the elasticity of the spine. It is surprising how much the neck will elongate, and this should be quite painless. A firm strong stretch may be sufficient to elicit pain, but usually it is necessary to give an extra tug. If pain occurs it may be felt at any level of the spine, and this implies some fault at that level. Normal joints are elastic and painless. If pathological change or a disc lesion is present the initial stretch may relieve an existing pain and an extra tug then may provoke it, but the test is not primarily designed to help in the

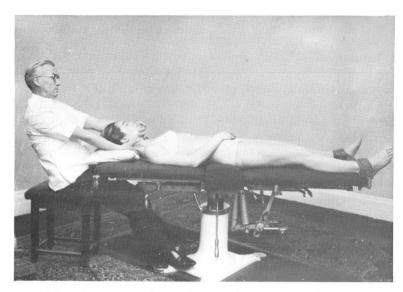

FIG 21 Traction test or technique for adjustive manual traction.

diagnosis of other conditions for which there are other tests, but rather to ascertain whether longitudinal adhesions are present in the simple hypomobile type of spinal lesion.

If the operator is satisfied about the diagnosis and there are no contra-indications to manipulation, an actual adjustment can be made to follow the test by giving a still stronger tug, as described under the heading of 'Rhythmic Adjustive Manual Traction' (p. 235, *Manual of Osteopathic Technique*).

As a single diagnostic and treatment procedure this method is one of the most useful if not the most useful of all techniques of manipulation. It is applicable as a test in every patient, and it is safe for the majority. It is not a specific manipulation in the sense that only one joint is being manipulated because the whole spinal column is involved, but it is specific for longitudinal adhesions. Many patients having had careful specific adjustments fail to respond until this technique is used because the longitudinal adhesions have not been released.

Apart from pathological contra-indications to the use of this technique, the chief contra-indication is hypermobility—i.e. if hyper-mobility is present at any level of the spine the technique ought to be avoided because any traction applied to the whole length of the spine will exert its stretch first on the hypermobile and weak ligaments before it stretches the hypomobile capsules or the adhesions.

The technique may be disconcerting to the type of patient who relaxes to perfection because there is a sense of separation at all levels, but no

116

risk is involved—only an unpleasant sensation, and this pitfall can be avoided by giving several preliminary gentle tugs before the final one. If there is an unexpected amount of stretch with a moderate pull then it is not advisable to pull harder.

Adhesions in planes other than the longitudinal one are best treated by articulatory and specific techniques. These tests reveal the direction of limitation, and the choice of technique is governed by this mechanical diagnosis. Detailed descriptions of these specific techniques for specific lesions are to be found in my *Manual of Osteopathic Technique*.

The *time factor* in *any* spinal problem is important, and this applies no less in the single hypomobile lesion. The fact that adhesions have formed implies that the lesion has been present for at least ten days. It takes seven to ten days for adhesions to form in any joint, and manipulation of these lesions is appropriate at any stage after these ten days. It is debatable whether specific manipulation is needed in the earlier stages of simple vertebral joint sprains because the majority will recover anyway, and it is reasonable to allow this time to elapse before performing any specific manipulation. It is quite in order to do some soft-tissue relaxation and some gentle articulation in the early stages, but strong adjustive manipulations are contra-indicated except where there is an actual subluxation. This latter condition is discussed more fully on p. 222.

Simple hypomobile osteopathic lesions which have been present for only a few weeks should respond to two or three specific manipulations and there should be an improvement in symptoms even after the first adjustment. The immediate reaction should be a sense of freedom and of greater range in movement, and often this response continues; but a painful reaction lasting one to two days is to be expected if strong adhesions have had to be released. Any painful reaction to manipulation which lasts longer than two days suggests one of several causes:

(*a*) That the manipulation was too forcible.
(*b*) That the manipulation was incorrectly applied or that the exact mechanical diagnosis was misconstrued and the wrong technique was chosen.
(*c*) That the joint was inflamed or the soft tissues too irritable.
(*d*) That the patient resisted and the adhesions were merely stretched painfully.
(*e*) That the manipulation provoked a late reaction in a degenerated disc (see p. 137).
(*f*) That the joint was hypermobile already.

It is better not to try to achieve full release of all movements at one manipulation if considerable force is involved. It is far better to graduate the manipulations and in the first place only to use the gentlest of specific movements. The principles of using the *minimum of force* consistent with achieving one's objective should be a guiding principle in every technique.

On the occasion of the patient's *first visit,* when the primary purpose is diagnosis, it may be desirable to go on straight away and give treatment. This is most appropriate in simple lesions where little in the way of soft-tissue relaxation and no articulatory techniques are needed. However, if the symptoms have been long-established and a course of treatment is required, then it is better not to begin treatment on the first visit, but to give a full treatment on the second visit.

The advantages of treating the patient on the first visit are that the patient feels something has been done and therefore recovery has commenced with no time being lost; but the disadvantages are that a first consultation is almost always accompanied by anxiety, nervous tension, and muscular tension. If the diagnosis which is made on the first visit is uncomplicated, and the practitioner can confidently and conscientiously predict a good response, then this reassures the patient, so that on the second occasion he or she will attend in a more relaxed and receptive frame of mind, and greater attention can be given to the details of treatment.

Although the first visit is the most significant in that a diagnosis has to be made and confidence shown, the second visit is the most vital in establishing the 'rapport' between physician and patient. More physical contact between physician and patient then takes place during the administration of treatment. The confident picture established on the first visit is translated into action, and the patient feels that progress is being made.

The second visit should be fairly soon after the consultation but not too soon—say within two or three days, if this is possible—so that the anxiety of the first visit has had time to subside but there is not too much delay before beginning treatment.

The second visit gives the opportunity for answering questions which have arisen in the patient's mind since the consultation. Often the patient is too worried to understand all of what has been said on the first visit, and some further explanation and reassurance may be needed.

Full co-operation from the patient can only be expected if a proper explanation is given and an adequate diagnosis established. Therefore sufficient time for full history-taking and thorough examination must be given on the first visit, otherwise the patient cannot be imbued with the necessary confidence to accept the treatment wholeheartedly. However correct the diagnosis and however good the treatment, it will not succeed and will not be accepted by the patient until this is done. The best results can only be achieved under these conditions.

Simple uncomplicated osteopathic lesions should yield quickly to appropriate manipulation, and it is my practice to make the appropriate adjustment there and then without preliminary soft-tissue and articulatory preparation; but I would not urge practitioners with little experience to do this. On the second and third visits attention must be given to soft-tissue treatment, and as a rule the relaxation of muscles by deep kneading, followed by the articulatory treatment, should take ten to fifteen minutes. Articulatory techniques, as distinct from specific ones, may be sufficient to release the restricted movements by themselves, but more often than not a specific adjustment must be given to obtain a quick response. At least some relief of symptoms is desirable by the third visit so that the original confidence expressed by the physician is translated into fact. Relief of pain always reinforces the confidence that the patient places in the practitioner, particularly if his predictions turn out to be true.

A rapid succession of treatments is undesirable in most cases because the tissues must react to the manipulation and sufficient time must be allowed for this. Two days at least should be the interval between treatments where specific adjustments are needed. If the patient insists on getting on with treatment, then soft-tissue and articulatory treatment only should be given during the following day or two.

If a painful reaction occurs on the second or third day after manipulation then more care is required because this is the reaction of cartilage to trauma and disc changes must be suspect.

The techniques of manipulation which follow the mechanical diagnosis of the osteopathic lesion are described in my *Manual of Osteopathic Technique* and will not be repeated here. The fact that a whole book is devoted to them indicates the importance of these lesions in clinical practice.

2 Ligamentous strain syndromes—the hypermobile type of spinal lesion

The *characteristics* of the single hypermobile spinal lesion are:

The individual faulty joint is hypermobile.
There are full painless general spinal movements.
Pain only begins after an interval during which the ligaments are under load or continuous stretch, i.e. the onset of pain is delayed. It is usually a dull ache and diffuse in character. It is accompanied by muscular stiffness which takes several minutes to subside. This is due to sustained muscular contraction to protect the joint.
There may be generalised hypermobility, and in any case these lesions

are commoner in hypermobile subjects. Exercise relieves the muscular stiffness and the dull ache.

The ligaments are tender if they are accessible to palpation. When not accessible, pain may be evoked by compression of the tender ligaments as well as by sustained stretching of them.

A history of injury is uncommon, but pregnancy is a predisposition. The soft flabby asthenic types are more likely to be affected than those of stocky build. There is an adverse response to manipulation. Forced movements merely accentuate the hypermobility.

Ligaments are supportive in function and will accept a great deal of mechanical strain before protesting, but if the load is heavy and sustained for long enough, then the fibres will elongate or tear. A sudden stretch beyond the elastic limit of the ligament will tear the fibres—this is the characterisitic of a sprain—but a sustained stretch short of this elastic limit will eventually lead to elongation of the ligament. In the process of elongation, pain is produced in the ligament—this is Nature's warning that damage is being done.

After a tear repair will take place, and provided sufficient time is given to the process, the repair will be complete, the ligament will grow as strong as before, and it will be restored to the same length as before injury. But if the tear is repeated before full recovery or if the tear is severe, then the fibres will not unite strongly, and a permanently weak elongated ligament will remain.

During the repair of a torn ligament pain occurs on stretching, but as normality returns the pain of ordinary stretching will subside. The ligament remains tender and swollen during repair, but the tenderness will disappear when normality is restored. The duration of repair depends upon several factors—namely, the degree of injury, whether the adjacent ligaments are intact and unruptured, the amount of use put to the joint during recovery, the support provided externally, and the site of injury. A severe sprain, say, of the lateral ligament of the ankle takes six weeks to recover. The time taken can be reduced by adequate support by infiltration with procaine and/or hydrocortisone, by passive movements within the painless range, and by normal use of the joint so long as this does not evoke too much pain. A minor sprain may take merely a few days to recover. A sprain of a joint which is not subject to much strain recovers quickly. Where a sprained joint is supported too much— i.e. if no movement is allowed as with plaster-of-Paris splinting—then repair takes place well but at the same time excessive fibrous tissue is laid down in the form of *adhesions*. These adhesions may be intra-capsular or extracapsular depending upon where the fibrinogen is released at the time of injury. Sprained ankles, sprained wrists, and sprained knees are not normally complicated by adhesion formation because movements are obligatory during normal activities, but shoulder joints and spinal joints are frequently complicated by adhesion formation because full movements of these joints are not necessary during ordinary activities.

Adhesions—in the sense of adherent fibres—are a part of the process of repair, and excess fibres are later absorbed on normal use of the joint, just as excess callus is absorbed after a fractured bone has consolidated and the limb can be used normally again. If adhesions persist after the normal recovery-time has elapsed, then the joint will remain stiffer than before and there will be pain upon stretching these adhesions.

The point of time when repair adhesions persist unnecessarily for the normal functioning of that joint is the time when manipulation is appropriate, not by forcible manipulation, but by firm passive stretching techniques. Exercises and active movements by the patient will achieve a response similar to that of articulatory techniques, and this is naturally desirable. However, the appropriate exercises are not always possible, and if the patient is unable or unwilling because of pain to stretch the adhesions then passive movements should be instituted.

The point of time mentioned above may not be easy to determine, but with a sprained ankle, if pain persists after six weeks then the pain is due to adhesions. If the pain at the ankle and restriction of movements persist for several months, then the adhesions must be tough and they will need to be forcibly manipulated to free the joint.

With spinal joints the time factor is shorter because the injury is often less severe and the ligaments are smaller. Most simple spinal joint sprains recover symptomatically in seven to ten days. Pain ceases and only tenderness persists for a further week. This is the pattern of the normal response to a sprained spinal joint. Such joints recover spontaneously. They do not require treatment apart from analgesics to relieve pain and care to avoid further mechanical strain at the site of injury during the fortnight of recovery. If pain persists after three weeks, then adhesions or displacements have occurred and the appropriate manipulations are indicated. For the diagnosis of the local mechanical fault, spinal mobility and spinal positional tests should be performed as described in my *Manual of Osteopathic Technique*. The appropriate technique is chosen according to the diagnostic findings. If a displacement has occurred then the sooner the manipulation is performed the better. If hypomobility is present the manipulation in the correct direction will release the adhesions and free the movement of the joint. If, however, instead of hypomobility and/or subluxation there is hypermobility at the joint in question, manipulations are contraindicated.

The *differential diagnosis between adhesions and hypomobility on the one hand and overstretched ligaments and hypermobility on the other hand* is not always easy because the symptoms are similar—both types of patient suffer from 'stretch' pain, both have a history of injury, and both have tender ligaments on pressure. Some help can be obtained from the history of the length of time which has elapsed and the severity of the injury, but the chief reliance must be placed on mobility tests, and the practitioner should be familiar with normal ranges of movements and must be able to distinguish between hypermobility and hypomobility. The distinction is obvious enough in large joints like the knee or ankle, but not so easy in spinal joints until the techniques of mobility tests are mastered.

The time factor is again important in differential diagnosis because pain from adhesions occurs at the moment of stretch, whereas pain from relaxed ligaments is delayed—i.e. the stretch requires to be sustained before pain starts. Another time consideration is that ligaments become more irritable when subject to repeated strain. The length of time of the delayed pain becomes shorter and shorter until eventually the pain may be felt at the moment of stretch, just as if adhesions were the cause of the pain. This can be confusing but the history will be helpful. For example, the patient who sits badly in a slumped position overstretching his supraspinous and interspinous ligaments in the lumbar area may initially experience pain after sitting, say, for three hours. The back becomes stiff and uncomfortable. Then a few weeks later sitting for one hour is enough to provoke the same response. Later a few minutes will bring on the pain, and still later immediate pain occurs with slumping.

The *treatment* of overstretched ligaments consists of (1) support during recovery, (2) strengthening exercises for the surrounding muscles to minimise the mechanical load on the ligaments, and (3) sclerosing injections of ligaments which are permanently overstretched.

A *recent spinal joint sprain* should be supported where practicable. In a whiplash injury of the neck either or both of the anterior and posterior groups of ligaments may be torn, and the neck should be supported in a collar for six weeks or more. The only way to clinch the diagnosis of ligamentous tears in the cervical spine is to take functional X-rays—i.e. lateral views, with the neck in full flexion and full extension. Tears of the anterior longitudinal ligament are even more important than are tears of the posterior longitudinal and supraspinous ligaments, partly because the damage is not usually recognised, but also because the anterior longitudinal ligaments provide the only anterior support for the vertebral bodies. Tears of the longitudinal ligaments are always serious because they lead to instability and later to disc displacements.

The standard X-rays taken in the mid position are usually not sufficient because they may show no abnormality whatever, yet a backward-bending film will show undue gapping anteriorly (*figs. 22, 23*). Even quadriplegias have resulted from severe cord damage without any apparent bony injury.[64] In these cases functional mobility X-rays provide the only means of establishing the diagnosis.

Severe tears require immobilisation of the neck in a plastic neck splint for six to eight weeks, and after this interval further mobility tests should be arranged. Without this precaution the lower cervical joint will remain permanently unstable, and subsequent disc degeneration, together with its attendant miseries, will be inevitable.

Pure flexion-extension injuries do not normally involve the apophyseal joints. There needs to be some element of side-bending and/or rotation to involve the capsules of these joints. When injured the swelling of the capsule is readily palpable in the neck because these joints are quite superficial. The row of articular processes should be palpated in the posterior triangle of the neck—for position in case of a subluxation, and for swelling in case of a recent sprain.

The initial treatment of simple apophyseal joint sprains *without* subluxation consists in soft-tissue massage, gentle articulation, and the avoidance of further mechanical strain. It is not usually practicable to provide strapping support for the neck, and such sprains seldom require a collar.

If a subluxation or 'joint bind' has occurred, the joint should be manipulated and then treated as a simple sprain. It should not be repeatedly manipulated—'Find it, fix it, and leave it alone' is a good old osteopathic maxim.

Thoracic spinal joint sprains occur less frequently than do cervical and lumbar joint sprains, and because of the firm support of the ribs there is no risk of hypermobility in joints between 1T and 10T. *Lumbar joint lesions*, on the other hand, are frequent and these joints often become hypermobile.

The *aetiology of hypermobile lumbar lesions* involves:

(a) severe initial sprain caused by hyperflexion injury;
(b) habitual ligamentous strain from faulty sitting posture, habitual standing on one leg, or an anatomical short leg;
(c) degenerative processes involving the discs and the ligaments of the vertebral complex (see p. 130).

(a) Severe flexion sprains of the lumbar spine tear the supraspinous ligaments first and then the posterior longitudinal ligaments. Because the ligamentum flavum is rich in yellow elastic fibres it is unlikely to

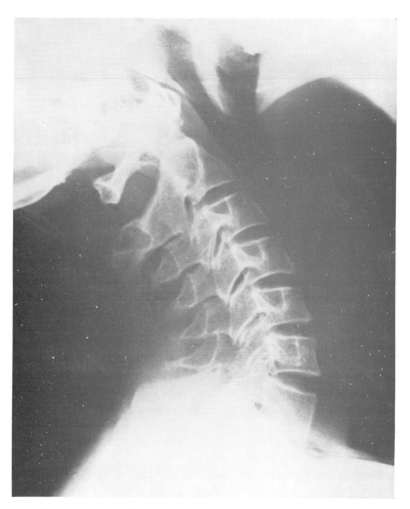

FIGS 22 AND 23 Mobility views of the cervical spine showing hyper-extension at 6-7C. This is strong presumptive evidence of a tear in the anterior longitudinal ligament.

tear, and the interspinous ligaments are not tough enough to consider in this context. Severe extensor sprains of the lumbar spine may well tear the anterior longitudinal ligament, but the clinical manifestations are more those of compression of the posterior components of the joint complex, with jambing together of the facets, damage of the partes interarticulares, and contusion of the interspinous ligaments.

(b) Chronic ligamentous strain of the posterior ligaments of the spine occurs with a habitual slumping attitude when sitting in a chair. The faulty posture starts in childhood unless parents and teachers insist on

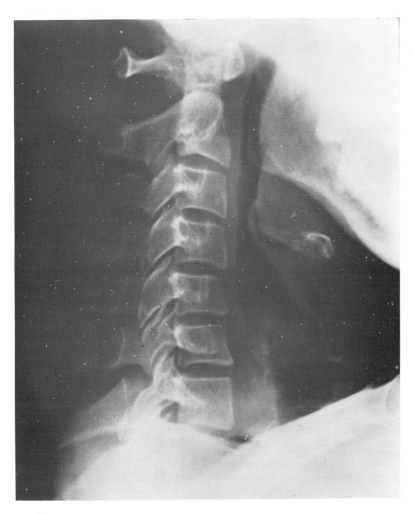

FIG 23

an upright sitting posture. Often blame can be laid against the design of chairs and desks, but the poor example of parents and teachers in their own slouching posture is also blameworthy.

During growth, ligaments elongate without causing pain. The child therefore does not receive any warning of the damage. It is only when some sudden additional flexion strain occurs that pain arises and the fault is recognised.

The lateral ligaments are strained and gradually elongate when there is a lateral pelvic tilt. The ligaments on the convexity of the curve elongate and those on the concavity shorten. This is the normal adaptive response during growth to a pelvic tilt, and there is no pain. Only later,

125

when the ligaments are stretched beyond their elastic limit, does pain develop.

The pain at first is subliminal as far as conscious awareness is concerned, but sufficient noxious afferent impulses will reach the cord to evoke reflex contraction of the surrounding muscles, and then a sense of stiffness rather than pain is produced.

Stiffness in the muscles after sitting badly, standing badly, or bending over for an hour or so is the first indication of ligamentous strain.

The *treatment* of hypermobile ligaments in the lumbar spine consists of correction of posture, restoration of the pelvic balance either by manipulation of the pelvis or the use of heel lifts, and of strengthening exercises of the erector spinae, abdominal, and psoas muscles. If these measures are not sufficient by themselves, then a lumbo-sacral corset must be worn until posture has improved and the tone of the muscles has recovered sufficiently to dispense with the corset. Sometimes additional help is required in the form of sclerosing injections.

Corsets The prescription of a corset in the treatment of hypermobile ligaments of the lumbar spine gives relief, but reliance on this measure alone is poor treatment. Such patients, who are not taught correct posture and whose muscles are allowed to weaken still further, will grow to rely entirely on the corset, and eventually they will have backache in spite of the corset. The task of rehabitating such patients and weaning them of their corsets is a slow and tedious one.

Generally speaking the use of a lumbo-sacral corset is permissible as a temporary expedient during the treatment of weak ligaments, but the continued need of a corset implies that the patient's tissues have failed to recover. This may genuinely be the fault of the patient's tissues; but if it is the fault of the physician because he has not taken the trouble to advise the patient about posture and exercise, then it is reprehensible and inexcusable.

It is true to say that a corset never cured any back problem, but its use may be desirable to prevent further damage. The prescription of corsets for all and sundry backaches, without proper indications and proper diagnosis, is retrograde and slipshod. It leads to unnecessary expense, unnecessary discomfort, and unnecessary invalidism in many cases. On the other hand, extremists in the reverse direction who condemn all corsets to the waste-paper basket are also making a mistake. The only proper advice is based on a proper assessment of the mechanics and a proper estimate of the patient's potential recovery.

Sclerosants The sclerosing treatment of hypermobile ligaments consists of injecting fluids into the affected ligaments to stimulate the formation of fibrous tissue within the ligament. Hackett[60] advocates the use of Sylnasol or of a phenol-glucose solution, but in my experience ethanolamine oleate is a more effective agent.

When the diagnosis of relaxed ligaments has been made, and this depends on the three criteria mentioned already—hypermobility, local tenderness, and 'delayed stretch' pain—1 ml of ethanolamine oleate, mixed with 1 ml of 2 per cent procaine, is injected into the site. Three injections at fortnightly intervals are usually sufficient, but a lumbosacral support is necessary for three months to make sure that the maximum fibrous tissue reaction has occurred in the treated ligaments.

The injection causes local pain in most cases for two or three days, but the degree of intensity of the reaction varies remarkably, from no pain at all to intense pain. The first dose should therefore be smaller than 1 ml in cases where the threshold of pain is known to be low. The second injection is usually more painful than the first because the ligaments are already somewhat irritable from the first injection. When the response to ethanolamine oleate is good and fibrous tissue is forming well, it will be noticed that there is more resistance to the insertion of the needle and this applies especially on the third occasion.

When the response is slow then a fourth or fifth injection may be desirable. After the last injection an interval of six weeks should be allowed before assessing the full effect of the sclerosis.

Although sometimes the mobility X-rays show an improved stability of the joint, the visual radiological evidence of recovery is usually disappointing even when the clinical result is most satisfactory. There is palpable improvement in tone—i.e. the ligament does not press in so far —and the tenderness diminishes (although during the first two months the tenderness increases).

The explanation, as suggested by Hackett,[60] for the clinical improvement is that the sclerosis results in a firmer attachment of ligament to bone rather than a decrease in the range of movements. Hackett recommends the injection of small pools in different sites in the same ligament and particularly adjacent to the bone where the ligament is attached.

The ligaments which are available for this technique are the supraspinous and interspinous ligaments of 4–5L and 5L–1S and the iliolumbar and sacro-iliac ligaments. Sometimes the sacro-tuberous ligaments will benefit from injection. The technique is applicable to the lower cervical joints also.

The indiscriminate use of sclerosing injections is as bad as the indiscriminate use of corsets, but in the appropriate cases the results are excellent, especially when there is purely ligamentous weakness uncomplicated by disc damage. When hypermobility is secondary to disc damage it is difficult to gauge the effectiveness of sclerosis, but as the posterior longitudinal ligaments and the annulus fibrosus are inaccessible to this method, the results can at best be incomplete. Nevertheless, one of my patients who had recurrent acute episodes with an accompanying scoliosis two or three times a year for five years did not have another acute attack, following the injections, for nine years. He was a farmer who continued to lift hundredweight sacks of corn and remained fully occupied with his heavy work.

In sclerosing the sacro-iliac ligaments 2 ml of ethanolamine oleate is needed at each injection because of the size and area of bony attachment. These ligaments are less sensitive than the supraspinous ligaments of the lower lumbar area in that the painful reaction to the sclerosant is less severe.

Exercises Whether sclerosants are used or not, the tone of the erector spinae muscles needs to be improved. The simplest guide to adequate power—adequate, that is, for average use of the spine—is the ability to extend the spine twenty times for ten seconds with intervals for rest of five seconds. The patient is asked to lie prone, to clasp the hands behind the back and to lift the head and shoulders off the floor so as to arch the spine and contract the erector spinae muscles (*fig. 24*). If power is poor the patient will be unable to do this exercise more than two or three times, and such patients need to increase the number of contractions gradually, say by one a day until they can do twenty ten-second lifts without fatigue. One word of warning here: enthusiastic patients will tend to overdo the extension and nip the spinous processes together and the exercise will cause pain. They may think this harmful and will stop the exercises, therefore they should be instructed to extend to a degree short of causing any pain. If the abdominal and psoas muscles need strengthening ask the patient to lie supine and slowly raise both straight legs together. This exercise should not be advised if the effort causes pain at the lumbo-sacral level.

There are of course a multitude of exercises which are beneficial provided that forced flexion is avoided. But a patient is more likely to carry out one or two simple exercises than a complex series unless this is done under the guidance of a remedial gymnast.

It has been shown[65] that daily exercise is necessary to increase muscle power, and that complete inactivity (as in bed) leads to loss of strength by 7 per cent per day. To increase power in muscle, that muscle must be exercised at the rate of two-thirds its maximal strength until moderate fatigue ensues. Maintenance of power at a certain level can be achieved by exercising at the rate of a third of its maximal strength, but decrease of power occurs if only a fifth of the maximal strength is used.

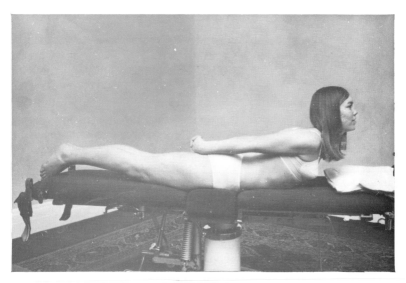

FIG 24 Erector spinae strengthening exercises.

Increased strength is not accompanied by hypertrophy but by increased firmness of tone. In order to achieve hypertrophy (which is not much use except for weight-lifting and advertising!) the muscle must be exercised to the point of considerable fatigue. There is a limit, though, beyond which a muscle must not be forced. If, for example, a muscle is forced beyond tolerable fatigue until it ceases to contract at the maximum of mental effort, the muscle becomes inflamed, swollen, and tender to touch, and subsequent contractions are painful for two or three days.

The importance of *correct sitting posture* cannot be overstressed, because if the patient persists in slumping in a low chair, all the sclerosants and exercises in the world will not produce a lasting response. The car seat, the office chair, and the bed all need attention. It should be stressed that the patient should sit right to the back of the seat and then rest against the back of the chair. If the chair is of poor design a cushion should be placed in the small of the back to maintain a slight amount of lordosis.

The only type of back problem in which a low chair and a slumped position is permitted is that of the patient with a lordosis syndrome (see p. 156) or of the patient with a disc herniation which has caused a lumbar kyphosis and in whom any attempt at straightening leads to increased pain.

The pain of relaxed ligaments is often accentuated in bed because during sleep the muscles relax and the ligaments are stretched. Early morning stiffness and backache usually indicates that the bed is at fault.

129

The ideal design of bed has a solid base and a comfortable mattress resting on top. If the base is springy, a thick board must be placed between the base and the mattress. The mattress can have springs or be made of foam rubber, and it does not need to be hard itself provided that the base is solid.

In general all these points apply even when the discs themselves are damaged or degenerated because it is inevitable that the supporting ligaments will be involved. The cartilage of the disc is insensitive since it has no nerve supply, and therefore the first sign of disc damage is stretching of its supporting ligaments. A herniating disc bulges and stretches the posterior longitudinal ligament. A prolapsed disc has torn the posterior longitudinal ligament. A thin disc leads to approximation of the apophyseal joints and overlapping of facets with consequent strain on those ligaments. A faulty disc therefore always causes ligamentous pain before it causes dura mater pain or nerve-root pain.

The hypermobile patient with elongated and weak ligaments is more vulnerable and is predisposed to disc changes later in life.

The *differential diagnosis of the hypermobile spinal lesion and the unstable stage of disc degeneration* is not easy and in any case the passage of time will blend the two conditions, because hypermobility leads to impaired nutrition and this in turn to degeneration. The degeneration leads to softening of the disc, and already its supporting ligaments are weak because there is little to support the annulus fibrosus, so that herniations become almost inevitable.

Once the simple symptomatology and signs have become complicated, the disc component is playing its own part in the picture. By this is meant that when the symptoms of delayed pain with stretching and weight-bearing and the signs of tenderness and hypermobility, as described at the beginning of this section (p. 119), are complicated by sharp pain which is increased immediately by flexion, the presence of pelvic shifts, muscle guarding, and perhaps nerve-root pain, then the disc, as well as being unstable has herniated.

The weakening of the ligaments is part of the overall degenerative change in discs, so that the common symptom of backache provoked by bending may for a time occur in both syndromes; but the mere fact that this symptom is present does not imply that the disc is degenerating. The condition may not have reached that far. X-rays and mobility tests, as described in the section on disc lesions, help in the differential diagnosis and reference should be made to p. 138 for further guidance.

Hypermobile sacro-iliac lesions are dealt with on p. 184 under the sacro-iliac syndromes.

As already stated hypermobility ensues if an injury tears the ligament badly or if sufficient support is not given to allow full recovery, but other factors can lead to hypermobile painful joints and these need to be considered in management. These factors are:

(*i*) The hypermobile type of person, whose ligaments are already long, is slow to recover from sprains. It is of course difficult to sprain a very flexible joint, but there is an elastic limit to any tissue. If hypermobile ligaments are stretched beyond their limit they do not recover well and they remain sensitive to stretch. They may remain elongated permanently.

(*ii*) When repeated minor sprains affect the same ligament, as in repetitive occupations or sports: several minor sprains in succession can be equivalent in effect to one major sprain.

(*iii*) Positional and mechanical factors may lead to continuous strain of ligaments—e.g. prolonged standing gives rise to pes planus; poliomyelitis of the lower extremity and an unsupported knee produce genu recurvatum; sway posture causes elongation of the femoral ligaments; and a short leg leads to scoliosis and elongation of ligaments on the convexity of the curve.

(*iv*) In pregnancy and childbirth there is a physiological elongation of ligaments, especially in the pelvis, and this is one of the commonest causes of relaxed ligaments.

(*v*) Illness, fatigue, and poor muscle tone lead to relaxed ligaments. Prolonged sitting in bed will elongate the posterior spinal ligaments, and this posture should be avoided. It is better for the patient to get out of bed and sit upright in an adjacent chair rather than half sit in bed. Many chronic backaches date from an operation, an illness, or childbirth where half sitting in bed is allowed or even encouraged by the medical attendant.

The short-leg syndrome This is a subsection of the ligamentous spinal syndrome, which does not necessarily have any hypermobility, but it is of sufficient importance to warrant a section to itself. The subject is also discussed in my *Manual of Osteopathic Technique*, p. 212, but the management of the syndrome needs elaborating.

When a patient presents with a history of backache commencing slowly for no apparent reason, with no history of injury in the past, and with a full range of movements, there is a strong probability that she has a pelvic tilt secondary to an anatomically short leg.

Compensation for a short leg which has occurred during the growing period is usually excellent, and no pain occurs while such compensation is complete. Only when this compensation breaks down do symptoms arise, and this may be at any age from the teens to the sixties.

Compensation, curiously enough, is more complete when the discrepancy between the leg lengths is large rather than small. The patient with $1\frac{1}{2}$ in. of shortening is less likely to develop backache than the patient with $\frac{1}{4}$ in. or $\frac{1}{2}$ in., other things being equal.

The orthopaedic view that it is unnecessary to wear heel or shoe lifts for anything less than 1 in. of shortening is entirely erroneous, and stress should be laid on the importance of lesser discrepancies in the aetiology of backache.

In a series of 100 consecutive cases of backache, 60 per cent were found to have $\frac{1}{4}$ in. or more of femoral discrepancy as compared with 28 per cent of fifty patients who had no backache symptoms.[39]

The compensation for a short leg consists of alteration of position in the sacro-iliac joints, or a tilting of the fifth lumbar vertebra on the sacrum or of 4L on 5L, or the formation of a gradual convexity to the side of the short leg (*fig. 25*). No doubt ligaments themselves become tougher on the side of more mechanical strain, and the musculature must adapt itself to the unequal stresses of walking and standing.

When muscles weaken through reduced physical exercise and increasing age, the ligaments are subject to still more mechanical strain and they give way sufficiently to cause pain. The persistent mechanical strain, even when subliminal as far as pain is concerned, leads to degenerative changes in the strained joints. The discs also degenerate, and at an earlier age than they would if the mechanical strains were symmetrical.

In a similar way, anomalies in the lumbo-sacral area of the spine lead to mechanical stresses and thereby to early symptoms. Absence of bone as in spina bifida occulta puts additional strain on the ligaments. In a series of X-rays of patients suffering from backache, Gillespie[66] has shown that anomalies occur four to five times more commonly than in a similar series of lumbar spine X-rays in patients unaffected by backache. He studied 500 patients with disc lesions and 500 controls. 34 per cent of the disc cases showed congenital lumbo-sacral anomalies compared with 8 per cent of the controls. 16 per cent of the disc cases had transitional vertebrae compared with 4 per cent of the controls.

Management of the short-leg syndrome

In theory the pelvis should be made level as soon as possible, but in practice this is not always wise or practicable. Consideration has to be given to the compensatory mechanisms, the duration of symptoms, and the flexibility of the subject.

Ideally the symmetry of the legs and spine should be checked in children and certainly in teenagers, and if this were done, a great deal of disability later would be prevented. Furthermore, because in this age-group the spinal joints are both flexible and adaptable, the correct

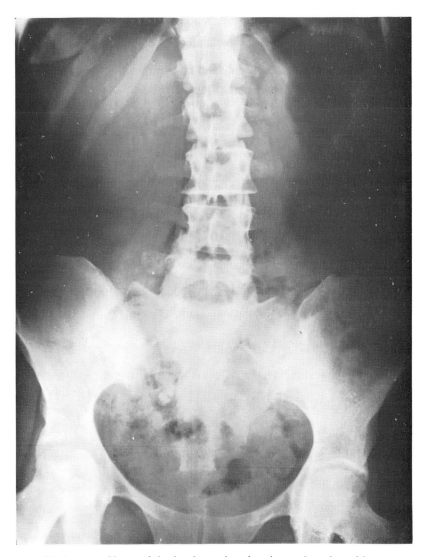

FIG 25 An erect X-ray of the lumbar spine showing a short leg with a convexity to the side of the short leg. This is the usual type of compensation.

amount of raise can be prescribed immediately. The convexity in the lumbar spine will correct fully in such flexible spines, especially if secondary rotation has not occurred. Although we can prescribe full lifts for young people we cannot do this in mature adults because secondary stiffness and degenerative changes have taken place, and any alteration in the base level may lead to symptoms not previously experienced, especially if the change of level is too abrupt.

133

If a young person with symmetrical legs is artificially given a pelvic tilt by, for example, $\frac{1}{2}$ in. raise, the immediate effect on the spine is to create a convexity to the side of the shorter leg. The vertebral bodies rotate to the side of the convexity. As soon as the pelvis is made level again the convexity and the rotation disappear. But in a naturally occurring short leg which has been present for years, the convexity of the lumbar spine, usually to the side of the short leg, creates a relatively fixed rotation of the vertebral bodies to the convexity. Slight rotations are correctible by means of a heel lift, but if the rotation is considerable the heel lift actually increases the rotation even though it reduces the convexity.

In order not to upset the compensating mechanism too quickly the pelvis should be levelled gradually, starting with $\frac{1}{8}$ in. and increasing to $\frac{1}{4}$ in. or more, depending on the amount of original discrepancy. Time must be given (about a month between each increase) for adaptation to take place, and if any rigid joint or joints exist in the spine these should be mobilised.

Symptoms of lower lumbar backache may be superseded by upper lumbar or thoracic backache as adaptation takes place upwards in the spine during the course of the ensuing weeks. It is best to treat these symptoms from below upwards, establishing normality in the lower lumbar region first and working upwards even into the cervical spine. Sometimes occipito-atlantal lesions are secondary to pelvic tilts.

When prescribing heel lifts for primary short legs it is desirable to be guided by erect X-ray films, though a fairly good clinical judgement can be made from palpation of the crests of the ilium and the visual appearance of the curve. Rotation can best be judged by asking the patient to flex forward in the standing position so that one can watch the spine tangentially, looking along it caudally or cranially. The diagnosis of a short leg can usually be made clinically, but it is more satisfactory to take a skiagram in the erect position showing an antero-posterior view of the pelvis and lumbar spine, because even when there is no obvious tilt and no apparent convexity these faults may exist. X-rays of the lumbar spine in the erect position give us double information by showing the effects of posture on spinal mechanics as well as the bony appearances. If any pathological change is seen or suspected in the erect view, then a supine antero-posterior film can later be taken to give more bone detail.

An erect lateral view is helpful mechanically, but owing to the density of the structures and the difficulty in obtaining clear X-rays at the lower lumbo-sacral level, films taken horizontally are needed for bone detail.

Standard views of the lumbar spine are useful for excluding disease, but they are of very little help with mechanical diagnosis. Erect views, oblique views, and mobility films are much more informative, and it is my practice in most back problems to take these views and use only the standard antero-posterior and lateral views when pathological change is suspected and good bone detail is necessary.

The precautions needed when taking erect X-rays are to make sure that the apparatus itself is correctly aligned horizontally and vertically, and to ask the patient to stand symmetrically with the weight equally distributed in both legs. The top of the femoral heads then give an accurate indication of the comparative lengths, and discrepancies can be measured against the lower edge of the X-ray film.

Secondary short legs (i.e. secondary to hip and spinal lesions) are detectible clinically with the patient supine, but this is no criterion as to the true length of the leg, and tape measurements are useless except for gross differences.

If the patient has an acute lesion with asymmetrical muscle spasms, it is better to wait until the temporary distortion has subsided before taking erect X-rays, otherwise a lateral shift of the pelvis and unequal psoas tension can give a false reading of the leg lengths.

Bailey and Beckwith[67] made a study of 545 erect X-rays and found that 45 per cent showed a convexity to the short leg side, 23 per cent showed a straight lumbar spine, and 32 per cent showed a convexity to the side of the longer leg.

When the convexity of the lumbar spine is to the contralateral side of the short leg, the mechanical stresses in the lower lumbar area are even more serious than they are with ipsilateral convexities. The mechanism and cause of such an abnormal response to a short leg is far from clear, but sometimes the degenerative changes at the lumbo-sacral disc are such that internal structural changes could account for the opposing tilt.

When there is a contralateral curve it is doubtful whether heel lifts are ever indicated. In my experience the use of a heel lift for the short leg in these cases merely accentuates the opposing convexity and puts additional strain on the lumbo-sacral joint. The use of a heel lift for the long leg helps in theory to reduce the convexity, but in practice it is not an effective measure and it should only be tried for a short period.

When a heel lift is prescribed, it is important to stress that the patient must wear it consistently. Wearing it one day and not the next merely confuses the picture. If the tilt is permanent, then the heel lift must be worn for the rest of the patient's life, and this must be made clear.

The use of a heel cushion alone is adequate for most men, but in women who wear high heels it is usually necessary to increase the thickness of the sole of the shoe if one cannot persuade the patient to wear low heels instead. With high heels most of the weight of the body is carried forward to be taken by the metatarsal heads, and very little weight is carried by the heels so that any increase in heel height makes little or no difference to the actual length of the legs.

Using a heel cushion inside the shoe is adequate where the discrepancy is only $\frac{1}{4}$ in. but in greater discrepancies the thickness of the leather on the heel itself needs to be altered, and it is often expedient to remove some thickness from the heel of the long leg rather than to increase the height of the heel on the side of the short leg.

3 Acute episodic spinal syndromes

Under this heading is included any acute attack of pain which is of short duration—an acute episode whether it is an isolated one or whether it recurs several times.

The *chief characteristics* of these syndromes are that acute pain is felt in the spine (at any level), and that it lasts for several days and then subsides leaving the patient free from symptoms until the next episode. Muscle guarding is always present and sometimes there is sustained muscle tension.

If the patient has had several such episodes, then it is easy to diagnose this category of syndrome, but if it is the first episode then the acute pain may be a prelude to a number of other syndromes.

There are several types:

1 The *traumatic* type, when obvious trauma anteceded the symptoms and this was sufficiently severe to produce damage to muscle or ligament.
2 The *disc* type when there may well have been a preceeding injury but this was of such a trivial nature that normal tissues would not react in that way.
3 The *muscular* type of acute episode, when muscle pain is the dominant feature and focal points of tenderness can be located in the muscle. Signs of vertebral joint lesions are absent.
4 The *inflammatory* type. The term 'inflammatory' here is used for want of a better term, but some signs of inflammation are evident. This type occurs mainly in the cervical area.
5 A *miscellaneous* group of acute spinal pain syndromes, usually accompanying some pathological process, like gout and herpes (see later syndromes).

The traumatic type of acute spinal episode. This is in fact the beginning of an osteopathic spinal lesion. The injury has usually had some torsional component which has caused damage to the apophyseal joints. It can occur at any age, and it can affect any joint of the spine including the occipito-atlanal and atlanto-axial joints where no discs complicate the picture.

The pain develops immediately after the injury, just as would happen with a sprained ankle. The pain is local, without reference elsewhere, and if bad enough the surrounding muscles will be on guard. The pain is short in duration, rarely lasting more than seven to ten days except when complicated by a subluxation, or when a 'joint bind' or adhesions have formed.

The majority of these spinal joint sprains recover, and even if adhesions and restricted mobility ensue, they become asymptomatic in a week or so.

The treatment of these lesions is described on page 119.

The disc type of acute spinal episode   The characteristic pattern here is that acute pain develops several hours or even days after a moderate strain. In the classical case the patient moves—perhaps to pick up a pencil from the floor, perhaps forwards to turn a tap on in the bath, perhaps to shift a suitcase from a shelf to the floor, or perhaps just sneezes—and then becomes aware that something has moved in the spine. There might momentarily be a sharp pain but it passes off and the person is able to continue her activities. In a few hours the muscles begin to stiffen and to ache. Increasing stiffness becomes apparent especially if the individual sits or lies down and later attempts to move, because the muscles go into spasm with intense cramp-like pain. When severe enough the patient is unable to move without excruciating pain, and may well be obliged to stay in one position for hours for fear of provoking more pain.

The *delay* in the onset of pain is the key point in the history of these cases, and by way of explanation it is reasonable to assume that damage has occurred to an insensitive structure. The only insensitive tissue in the spine is cartilage. Furthermore cartilage is slow to react to injury because it swells only slowly. The histamine reaction to trauma is delayed in cartilage because of the absence of a blood-supply. Not until the swelling stretches adjacent sensitive structures does the pain and protective muscle guarding ensue. The sensitive structures adjacent to the discs are the posterior longitudinal ligaments, the dura mater, and the nerve-roots. The delay after injury may involve two or three hours or two or three days depending presumably on the size of the displacement or in some cases on the gradual oozing of nucleus pulposus through a small defect in the annulus fibrosus, or to the slow swelling of the disc.

Various explanations have been offered by medical writers [68, 69] for the mechanism of disc displacements, such as the tearing of the annulus with displacement of a fragment, or the gradual protrusion of nucleus

pulposus material through a weakened annulus. In clinical practice
the mechanism can only be postulated, but it is helpful to have a working hypothesis. The most useful clinical concept, in my view, is one based
on the degree of protrusion: a small one (called a *herniation*) causes
spinal symptoms only with perhaps some vaguely referred pain, whereas
a larger one (called a *prolapse*) causes predominantly peripheral
symptoms with signs of nerve-root irritation or compression. If the
degree of displacement is in doubt, it is sensible to use the comprehensive term *protrusion*.

Most cases go through the stage of herniation before a full prolapse
occurs. It is postulated that a hernia of the disc is a reversible condition
—merely a bulging which diminishes in the course of time or is helped
back into place by manipulation and/or traction. On the other hand, a
prolapse of the disc is an irreversible condition because the posterior
longitudinal ligament as well as the annulus have been disrupted, and
nuclear or annular material has protruded into the spinal canal.

There may well be several episodes of herniation before a prolapse
ensues. The herniations may last a few days only at first, but subsequent
attacks tend to last longer—say, two or three weeks—and finally a full
prolapse causes reduction in the spinal pain and an increase in the peripheral pain. Whether or not there are abnormal central nervous system
signs depends upon the degree of pressure on the nerve-root.

Many acute episodes of low-back pain are relieved suddenly either
by the patient's own spontaneous movement or with the help of manipulation or traction. Something must have happened to account for the
sudden relief of pain, and repositioning of a herniated fragment of disc
is the probable explanation. Certainly the injury type of acute spinal
episode only recovers gradually because ligaments which have been torn
heal slowly and consequently the pain diminishes slowly. The sudden
release of a 'joint bind' could account in some cases for the rapid relief
following manipulation, but in my view it is possible to distinguish
between mere 'joint bind' and disc herniations by the severity of the
symptoms. A 'joint bind' can give rise to moderate pain but surely
never to the severe pain which accompanies a disc herniation. In
osteopathic practice we are constantly releasing 'joint bind', and
certainly the manipulation does give a sense of release and relief, but
the patient is not in extreme pain and the muscles are not in spasm.

Should intense pain occur instantly after bending, without the delay
mentioned above, it is possible that a prolapse has occurred with its
attendant tearing of the posterior longitudinal ligament but without the
intervening stage of a herniation, and in this event a differential diagnosis problem arises as between a prolapsed disc and the injury type of
acute episode previously described. This is particularly difficult if the

sudden prolapse was a result of some strenuous exertion. Both types have an acute onset. Neither shows any temporary remission of pain, and both may have peripheral pain. The question arises as to whether a ligament only has been torn or whether the torn ligament has allowed the disc to prolapse.

In the first day or two it may be quite impossible to say which of these explanations is the most likely, but the subsequent course of the condition will make it plain, just as at the onset of a febrile illness it may be impossible to make a diagnosis until further symptoms indicate which disease is causing the fever.

The history is of course a great help, for if the patient has had previous acute episodes it is likely to be a prolapse. The type of injury also gives a clue because compression injuries are more likely to cause disc damage whereas torsional strains are more likely to cause damage to ligaments. The age-group most commonly affected by these disc-type episodes is forty to sixty years, because at that age disc material has had time to degenerate. Patients in the younger age-group are more likely to have ligamentous damage only, but one must remember that disc damage can occur in the teens if osteochondrosis is present or if weakness of cartilage is inherited.

Another aid to differential diagnosis is that disc herniations and disc prolapses are invariably accompanied by some deformity of the spinal curve—a kyphosis or scoliosis or pelvic shift—whereas torn ligaments do not give rise to deformity. Even small herniations are accompanied by locking of the two vertebrae in at least one direction. At the height of the attack the intense pain and muscle guarding preclude accurate localisation of the level of the protrusion, but as the spasm subsides the pain and tenderness become less diffuse and the localised blocking of movement becomes palpable. Most locking is obvious from an examination of the general spinal movements and the contour of the lumbar spine, and such locking feels quite different from the restriction of movements resulting from adhesions or 'joint bind'. When applying mobility tests to the area, the blockage gives a positive sensation to the palpating hand, and movement is impossible beyond the limit, not just because of pain but because of hard obstruction.

In the early acute stages, pain is accentuated by any movement and the slightest attempt at examination evokes such pain and spasm that it is wiser not to persist with mobility tests but to rely on palpation alone. Without moving the patient at all it is possible to feel the contour of the spine, the tension of the muscles, and the skin changes. The muscles are virtually *splinting* the vertebral column against any movement. As the pain subsides the splinting may persist, and although the patient will move, only the peripheral joints will be used. Rising from the lying position is effected by turning on to the side and then levering the body up with the arms. The patient uses a similar procedure in order to lie down again. This manner of changing from sitting to lying and vice versa is also adopted by patients suffering from ankylosing spondylitis because of the sheer rigidity of the spinal column, and therefore the differential diagnosis between the recovering stage of a disc protrusion and ankylosing spondylitis needs to be considered. This is especially true with a nervous patient, who through fear of pain continues this spinal splinting long after the pain has subsided.

Another sign in the acute stage of a disc herniation is that because weight-bearing accentuates the pain, the patient tries to reduce the weight on the spine by using the hands to lift or move the body. It is a tell-tale sign when a patient sits with the arms on the sides of a chair trying to support his or her own weight.

If the patient is able to stand or sit, the *tests of compression* and *distraction* help in the diagnosis. The method is to press firmly on the patient's shoulders in the standing position to create an additional compression force on the spine. If pain is increased the test is positive, and this implies that further bulging is occurring. Similarly if the patient's weight is decreased because the operator supports the body under each axilla, lifting the patient gently and vertically, the pain will diminish if a hernia is present.

The *transition from a disc herniation to a disc prolapse* may be gradual but often it is a rapid process. In a herniation, pain is provoked by any movement but especially forward and backward-bending, whereas when the disc prolapses, only forward-bending provokes pain. Side-bending and backward-bending are painless. Pain from a disc herniation is accentuated by coughing and sneezing, but by the time the disc has prolapsed this symptom will have subsided. The compression and distraction tests are positive with a disc hernia and negative with a disc prolapse.

During flexion the erector spinae muscles are on guard against further movement, and the conflict so produced between voluntary flexion and reflex extension may lead to obvious and visible fibrillation of the paravertebral muscles.

With a disc herniation the prone springing test evokes sharp reflex guarding whereas with a prolapse of the disc there may well be pain and muscle tension but no increase of guarding during the springing test.

A disc herniation will block movement—for example, in side-bending to the right when the hernia is bulging to the right, and a sense of hard resistance is felt during the passive mobility test to the right. This sign may persist if a prolapse ensues, but the blockage is less hard and movement is more likely to be limited by pain than by a sense of something solid. In other words, the signs of a disc herniation are more spinal whereas the signs of a prolapse are more neurological.

The size of a disc herniation can be judged by the severity of the symptoms. The size of a disc prolapse can best be gauged by the straight-leg raising test when it affects the fourth lumbar, fifth lumbar, or first sacral roots.

With large prolapses the pressure and the pain may be severe enough to warrant the use of morphia for relief, but in such cases the pain usually lasts only twenty-four to forty-eight hours, and then it is followed by remarkable relief, probably because the nerve ceases to conduct both sensory and motor impulses. Such patients develop considerable motor weakness, numbness, and loss of deep reflexes. Recovery, if it takes place at all, may take six or nine months, and any loss of function which persists after a year is likely to be permanent.

Another type of disc herniation syndrome is peculiar to young adults. In the teens and early twenties the acute episode is followed by de-formity—either a kyphosis or scoliosis—and although the pain subsides quickly the deformity persists for many months, even up to two years. The likely explanation here is that the posterior longitudinal ligament has remained intact while a sizeable disc protrusion has taken place, and that absorption takes a long time. Pronounced distortion in association with little or no pain is confined to this young age-group.

After the severe symptoms have subsided it is easier to judge at which level the disc prolapse has occurred, and it is important to do this so that manipulation, if indicated, can be directed to the correct level. It is as important for the manipulator to judge the level of the protrusion correctly as it is for the surgeon to do so. With accurate manipulative techniques it should be possible to exert the maximum effect at the exact level of the lesion, thereby being more specific and more effective.

For manipulative purposes we are more concerned with the level of the disc which is faulty than with which nerve-root is damaged. The affected nerve-root can usually be determined accurately from a know-ledge of standard anatomy; but, because of the overlap of dermatomes, myotomes, and sclerotomes, because the nerve-roots of the corda equina descend almost vertically and straddle several disc levels, and because the recurrent spinal nerve carries sensory impressions from the posterior longitudinal ligaments above the level of the nerve-root, there may be so much confusion that the surgeon will require a myelogram to make sure of the correct level before operating.

In most instances of nerve-root pain (as distinct from referred pain), pressure on the 3L nerve-root produces pain in the anterior thigh, weakness of the quadriceps muscle, and loss of the knee jerk. Pressure on the 4L nerve-root produces pain in the posterior thigh and medial calf with loss of power in the calf muscles. Pressure on the 5L nerve-root produces pain in the posterior thigh and the lateral calf with loss of power in the extensors of the toes. Pressure on the 1S nerve-root produces posterior thigh and calf pain with loss of the ankle jerk. Pressure on the 2–4S nerve-roots produces peri-anal numbness together with bladder and/or bowel symptoms.

Radiological signs are sometimes helpful in determining the level of the prolapse—for example, gapping of the 4–5L disc space posteriorly strongly suggests a central hernia there. Lateral gapping suggests a prolapse to the wider side. Thinning of the disc is no criterion of the level of the lesion: it merely indicates that the thin disc has undergone some degeneration.

Clinically the level cannot be determined accurately during the acute phase, but as the muscle spasm subsides the springing test becomes more localised, and the tenderness will become better defined. Skin and subcutaneous tissue signs are also helpful at this stage. Flexion mobility tests are of little value in determining the level of a disc protrusion, but blocking which occurs in side-bending or extension can be felt on palpation and this gives an accurate indication of level of the disc protrusion.

Finally, special investigations like epidural and extra-dural injections of procaine give additional help in the differential diagnosis of disc protrusions, but I would refer the reader to other books for details of those techniques.

Treatment of disc herniations In the previous description (p. 138) a clinical distinction was made between a disc herniation and a disc prolapse. This may be considered arbitrary but the syndromes occur so characteristically that differentiation between the two is reasonable. A hernia is considered to be a bulging of the annulus whereas a prolapse implies protrusion through the annulus and perhaps even through the posterior longitudinal ligament. In the light of this hypothesis, the treatment of a herniated disc differs from the treatment of a prolapsed disc because a hernia may be reversible whereas a prolapse is not.

In practice it is often possible to replace a herniated fragment but it is useless to try with a prolapsed fragment. Techniques which will be described to replace a herniated disc can be tried on a prolapsed disc, but they are liable to aggravate the symptoms and will achieve nothing.

The supposition is that in a herniation the bulging disc is prevented from prolapsing by the intact fibres of the posterior longitudinal ligament and outer layers of the annulus, but once these structures give way there is nothing to prevent nuclear material from prolapsing into the spinal canal.

The purpose behind the manipulative treatment of a herniation is to apply forces—mainly of traction and extension—to push the disc material back towards the centre of the disc, whereas the purpose behind the manipulative treatment of a prolapsed disc is to attempt to alter the relative position of the nerve-root and the prolapsed cartilage.

Once abnormal central nervous system signs have made their appearance the implication is that the disc has prolapsed, and any hope of replacing the disc material should be abandoned; but this assumption does not exclude the possibility of repositioning the fragment—i.e. of shifting the nuclear material away from the nerve-root—and the techniques for doing this are described under the section on nerve-root syndromes (p. 171).

The treatment of a disc herniation depends upon the stage to which it has reached, and, as there is a high proportion of spontaneous reso-lution with rest alone, we must apply only treatment which will help the resolution and not hinder it. In all short-term afflictions of the body which can recover spontaneously, claims of success are made for many forms of treatment and false impressions of their effectiveness accrue; but if the rate of recovery is accelerated and no aggravation of symptoms ensues then the treatment is worth while. This applies to the techniques described now.

Tracing the course of the patient's history from the commencement of the acute episode to its resolution, the following treatment is indicated:

At the onset before muscle guarding has set in it is sometimes possible to abort the attack. Unfortunately, at least in the first episode, the patient is unaware of the consequences of the initial symptoms and the sensation of something moving in the spine without significant pain does not prompt the patient to seek advice. After two or three such episodes, the patient recognises the initial sensation, and realises that something can be done during the first few hours, and then it is well worth while applying the vertical adjustive technique described below, provided a practitioner versed in the technique is available. If muscle guarding has already commenced and pain is increasing, little can be achieved by manipulation or traction at this stage, and in my view both are contra-indicated. The same techniques can be tried again after five to seven days of bed rest, because after this interval the muscle guarding has subsided and it is again safe to use traction techniques.

In general there are four types of *traction* (see p. 258, *Manual of Osteopathic Technique*)—sustained, intermittent-sustained, rhythmic, and adjustive. Each has its uses *and* abuses, but adjustive traction only is applicable in the episodic syndromes. The other three methods are contra-indicated because of the risk of increasing the muscle spasm and converting the hernia into a prolapse. With adjustive traction there is an excellent chance of giving rapid relief within the first few hours of the onset and again later on when muscle guarding has subsided; but adjustive traction can be applied at any stage without risk of aggravating the symptoms. The chances of success when muscles are on guard is small, but it is a consolation to know that the technique will not aggravate the condition even if it fails. Torsional techniques are all contra-indicated in this phase of a disc herniation because of the risk of converting the hernia into a prolapse.

Adjustive manual traction In the *lumbar* spine traction techniques can be applied in two ways, the choice depending on whether a kyphosis is present or not. If there is a kyphosis the patient will be unable to extend the lumbar spine, and the first technique is indicated. If there is a scoliosis or pelvic shift and if the patient can be distracted in extension without increasing pain, then the second method is more appropriate.

FIRST METHOD (*fig. 26*)

The operator stands behind the seated patient's back. The patient clasps her hands behind her neck, and the operator's hands pass under the patient's axillae to grasp her forearms. The table or stool should be at the appropriate height so that when the operator straightens up the patient is lifted off the table. The buttocks should be raised 3 or 4 in. and the patient's knees (popliteal areas) should remain resting on the edge of the table. At this point the patient must be persuaded to relax her back so that it remains suspended and automatically slightly flexed. Unless the patient can relax in this position and can feel some measure of relief from this initial distraction, the technique will fail. There is a tendency for the patient to try to extend her knees when lifting her from the table, but this indicates lack of relaxation and must be discouraged.

After the initial stretch the patient should be permitted to return to the sitting position to allow time for her to realise what is being done and what is to be expected so that when next the weight is taken by the operator's arms there will be good co-operation. The operator leans backwards as the patient is raised in order to take some of the weight on his chest and in order to encourage the patient to keep the lumbar spine in flexion. Several preliminary stretches of this nature will help the patient to relax, more particularly if relief is experienced during the pull. The operator must guard against forcing the patient's head forward. The thrust on the patient's forearms is a vertical one so that none of the component of the force is in flexion.

The operator is now ready to use adjustive traction by bouncing up

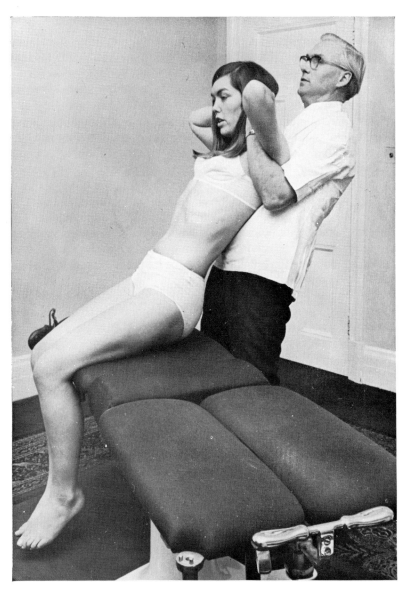

FIG 26 Adjustive manual traction in the sitting position.

and down by flexing and extending his knees An analogous movement
is used when one attempts to shake the bulky contents of a canvas bag
to the bottom of the bag. The operator flexes and extends his knees to
achieve this bouncing movement, counteracting the downward movement
of the torso with the upward movement of his arms. The final adjustive
stretch is achieved by an extra bounce. When successful, the kyphosis

145

disappears and the patient can extend the spine further, straight away. *Strapping* must be applied forthwith to discourage the patient from flexing the spine and re-herniating the disc. The operator should use his whole body as a single unit and should hold the patient firmly so that both operator and patient move up and down synchronously and rhythmically. Unless these details are observed the technique is not likely to succeed. It produces, of course, some strain on the operator's own back, but as his lumbar spine is in extension the risk is small. However, I would hesitate to use this technique on a 250 lb patient!

SECOND METHOD (*fig. 27*)

This technique presupposes that the patient can at least stand up, even though distorted. A preliminary stretch should be made to see if pain is not increased by vertical traction. If pain is increased then the technique will fail and should not be pursued.

The operator stands with his back to the patient. If the patient is short and the operator tall then it is feasible to use this technique without any aid, but if the two are of equal height or if the operator when lifting cannot get the patient's feet right off the ground then the operator will require a platform to stand on. The patient clasps her hands firmly in front and is asked to grip tightly there, while relaxing everywhere else. Standing back to back the operator threads his arms round the front of the patient's arms and takes a firm hold of her loins with the flat of his hands, avoiding digging the fingers in.

The operator's buttocks should be on a level with the patient's lumbar spine to fit into the concavity there. He leans forward and thereby lifts the patient off the floor, taking much of the weight on his own buttocks and some of it with his arms and hands. The patient is now asked to relax by resting her head on the operator's thoracic spine and by letting the legs dangle. This initial distracting force should afford some relief, thereby helping the patient to relax. At least one preliminary stretch is made in order to give the patient a chance of understanding what is being done and of co-operating in the relaxation when the procedure is tried again. The adjustive force is created by bouncing up and down as in the previous technique, and at the moment of fullest relaxation on the part of the patient an extra bounce upwards on the operator's part creates a traction effect on the patient's lumbar spine. The whole thoracic and lumbar areas are involved in the traction, and often separational clicks are felt, but unless the gapping occurs in the lower lumbar region where the disc has herniated, the technique is ineffective. When successful the pelvic shift is seen to be straighter and the patient feels easier straight away.

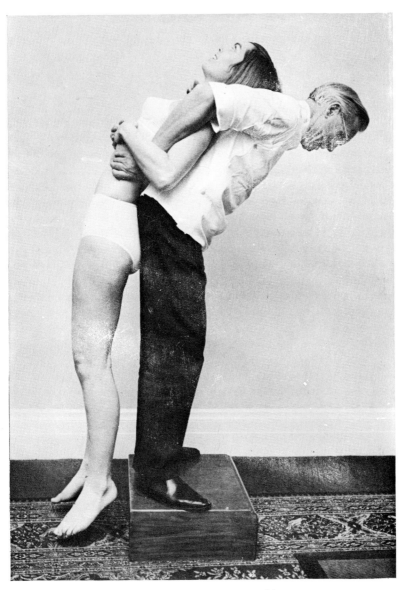

FIG 27 Adjustive manual traction in the erect position.

The type of strapping which ought now to be applied is 2 in. adhesive tape of the non-stretch variety. Two long pieces (about 24 in.) are applied longitudinally, stretching from the scapula down to the sacroiliac areas. The strapping not only provides a degree of support but also serves to remind the patient not to bend (the hairier the patient the greater the reminder!). After attending for this manipulation the patient

147

must be given help in putting on shoes and stockings so that flexion is avoided, otherwise it is a waste of time using the technique. Do not test the patient in flexion to see whether the technique has been successful! *All torsional techniques at this stage are contra-indicated.*

Most patients with a disc herniation in the lumbar spine are obliged to stay in bed because they literally cannot do anything else. In any case it is the best treatment even with those who can manage to stand up. The muscles in spasm can be partially relieved by analgesics and muscle relaxants—e.g. 'Norgesic' tabs. 2 four-hourly. Heat is a comfort and often enables the tension to diminish. The ideal form of heat is a constant temperature source, as with an electric pad. The patient should be nursed on a comfortable mattress resting on a *solid* base. A small pillow placed under the lumbar spine when supine or under the abdomen when prone may give relief, and any position may be adopted which gives most relief. Even sitting may be necessary if a kyphosis has developed and if lying supine accentuates the pain, but such patients can obtain relief when lying horizontally by turning on one or the other side. Micturition and defaecation are problems, and bottles in the bed or a commode adjacent to the bed are necessary. Remember that a bed-pan calls for more agility than a commode! Struggling along corridors and up stairs are absolutely contra-indicated.

Some types of acute episodic back pain are relieved by activity rather than by rest, but these mainly belong to the muscular types of acute syndromes (p. 236). A small disc herniation may produce only moderate guarding which the patient can overcome by alternately contracting and relaxing her muscles as in walking; but, in my view, if the practitioner is sure of the diagnosis and is convinced that a herniation has occurred, then he should prescribe bed rest, even though being in bed temporarily increases pain and stiffness.

The cornerstones of treatment in these acute episodes are bed rest, heat, and analgesics. The majority of patients recover in four or five days. Struggling to work delays recovery and predisposes to further herniations. Massage of the paravertebral muscles gives relief if the patient can first be placed in a position of comfort, but it does little to accelerate recovery. Articulation is contra-indicated because almost any movement provokes muscle guarding.

Once the guarding has subsided enough for the patient to take weight on her feet without increasing the pain, then the adjustive vertical traction technique can be tried, but if unsuccessful it should not be repeated until next day. As the spasm subsides massage and articulation will afford more relief, but no forced movements should be used until all danger of further herniation has gone. In most cases it is wise to wait for two weeks. The full repair of a disc herniation may well take six weeks—i.e. long after the pain has subsided—but this interval should be allowed before any strong specific manipulations are applied.

Specific adjustment is indicated if there is residual restriction of movement after the six-week period has elapsed. Careful and controlled osteopathic techniques are then completely safe. They are in fact essential if residual restrictions persist because immobility implies impaired function and it leads to impaired circulation and thereby to earlier degenerative changes.

There is a tendency to assume, just because the patient is free of pain, that full recovery has occurred and nothing more needs to be done. Both practitioner and patient should direct attention to restoring full movement and muscle power and mechanical perfection to reduce the risk of further attacks, and the patient must be warned that full resumption of heavy lifting is risky within six weeks of a disc herniation.

A programme of graduated muscle exercises (as indicated on p. 128) should be arranged, but the degree of muscle power must be matched with the physical requirements of the patient in occupational and sporting activities. The ideal general exercise to tone up the spinal muscles while avoiding back strain, is swimming, and after recovery from pain all patients should be encouraged to take up swimming regularly. Games which involve jarring and compression of the spine are best avoided. The patient needs to be shown how to use the legs and arms to best advantage to reduce the mechanical strain on the back if lifting a weight is unavoidable. The principle behind this advice is to keep the spine as straight and as vertical as possible while the load is applied, and to distribute the load symmetrically, keeping it as close to the body as possible. The vertebral column will withstand a compression load which is vertically disposed better than a load taken under flexion. The most risky mechanical loads are those in which there is an element of rotation in combination with flexion, as, for example, in transferring a load from one side of the body to the other while the feet remain stationary.

Further attacks can be prevented or at least the risk of further attacks can be reduced by the following methods undertaken between attacks:

1 Correcting the spinal mechanics and posture.
2 Strengthening the spinal muscles by individual and general exercises directed not only to the erector spinae muscles but also to the abdominal muscles.
3 The avoidance of mechanical strains which are known to be excessive for that person.

4 The use of external supports (corsets and belts) if the above methods are insufficient.

5 The use of sclerosants where hypermobility is the problem.

The posture of the patient should be considered under all conditions. In standing, a mid position between lordosis and kyphosis is desirable, and the patient should try to stand 'tall'. Prolonged standing is detrimental for patients suffering from disc lesions. In sitting the emphasis must be on sitting well to the back of the seat, and if necessary a cushion should be placed in the lumbar area to prevent sagging. This is particularly important on long car journeys. The bed should be firm, having a comfortable mattress on a solid base. In bending the spine must be kept as vertical as possible. When making beds or bathing the baby, the mother should kneel for safety. Forced flexion exercises must be avoided.

Strengthening the erector spinae muscles is vital to recovery in most cases, and the progression as suggested on p. 128 will help. In addition good abdominal muscle tone is important, because it has been shown[32] that a sixth of the weight of lifting is carried through the abdomen. If the abdominal muscles are weak, the intra-abdominal pressure cannot be maintained to take some of the load off the spine.

(For thoracic disc protrusions see p. 199. For cervical disc protrusions see p. 210.)

4 Chronic degenerative spinal syndromes

1 Spondylosis affecting the vertebral bodies and intervertebral discs.
2 Osteo-arthritis of the apophyseal joints.

Although spondylosis of the vertebral bodies and osteo-arthritis of the apophyseal joints may occur concurrently in the same patient, and although these are both degenerative in nature, the two conditions are separate diseases in aetiology, in pathology, in symptomatology, and in treatment. There is much confusion between them, both radiologically and clinically; and because osteophytes occur in both, and are the most conspicuous feature on X-rays, the confusion is enhanced.

The following quotations underline the difficulties:

Lumbar spondylosis is essentially osteo-arthritis of the posterior interarticular joints of the lumbar spine.[70]

We have studied spines showing extreme spondylosis deformans and minor arthrosis of the small joints, as well as spines with distinct arthrosis of the small vertebral joints and insignificant marginal outgrowths of the vertebral body edges. There certainly exists some relationship between the two disease entities since both are due to

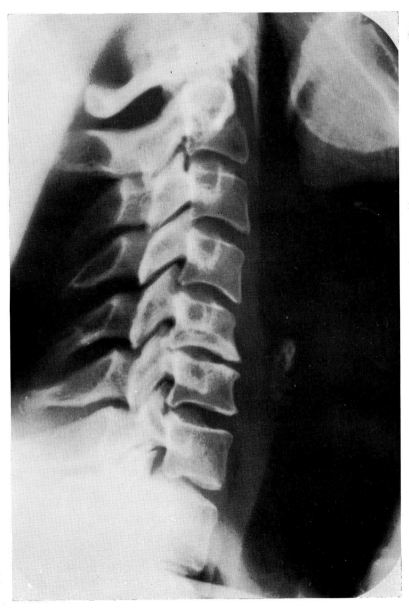

FIG 28 Cervical spondylosis showing isolated degeneration in the 5-6C joint. When one joint only is involved injury is the probable cause. The apophyseal joints are normal.

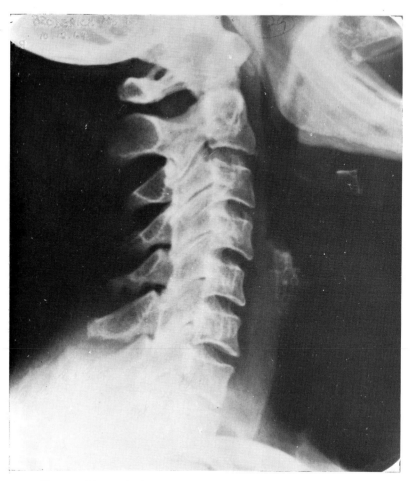

FIGS 29 AND 30 Cervical osteo-arthritis of the apophyseal joints with no evidence of spondylosis between the vertebral bodies.

wear and tear; the vertebrae, however, with their discs, neural arches and small joints are subject to different mechanical stresses and consequently varying degrees of spondylotic changes of the vertebral joints are found, with each change influencing the other.[71]

Disc degeneration and apophyseal arthritis do not always occur at the same level and concentration on the disc lesion may lead to relative neglect of the apophyseal lesions which from a clinical standpoint may be more important.[72]

These statements illustrate the difficulties, but in 1949 Collins[73] pointed out that 'Osteo-arthritis of the diarthrodial posterior intervertebral joints is not necessarily related to the presence of osteophytic out-

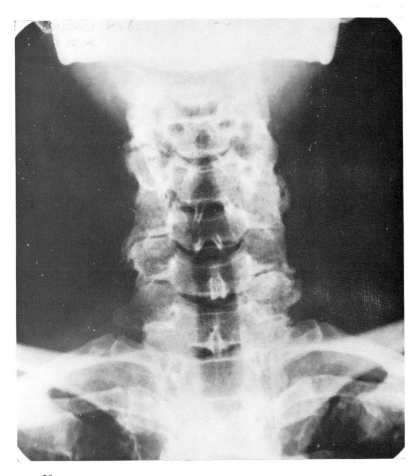

FIG 30

growths on the margin of the vertebral bodies although they are very widely and mistakenly regarded as a manifestation of spinal osteoarthritis'.

The distinction between the two diseases is much clearer in the cervical area of the spine as compared with the thoracic and lumbar areas.

The X-rays shown here (*figs. 28, 29, 30*) have been chosen to illustrate the point that spondylosis can occur without any changes in the apophyseal joints, and that osteo-arthritis can be very obvious without any radiological signs of spondylosis.

In order to help the reader to distinguish between the two states the characteristics of each are tabulated below, but I would also remind the reader that spondylosis is quite different from spondylitis, and therefore these two terms should never be confused. The only type of spondylosis which can be mistaken radiologically for ankylosing spondylitis is the

153

hypertrophic variety of spondylosis deformans, where excessive proliferation of osteophytes leads to complete calcification of the longitudinal ligaments. However, clinically these syndromes are entirely different so that confusion in this sense is unlikely.

The differential points between spondylosis of the vertical bodies, and ostro-arthritis of the apophyseal joints are noted in Table 2.

Treatment of spondylosis Spondylosis may or may not need treatment. Apparently 75 per cent of men and 65 per cent of women over the age of fifty years show radiological evidence of spondylosis,[74] but, a much lower proportion of people have symptoms from the disease. Many merely have occasional stiffness which they often ignore, though the mobility can be increased by manipulation and traction. There are no contra-indications to manipulation except when the disease is complicated by disc protrusions (p. 210). The choice of manipulation depends upon the particular type of restriction present at the time, and the only caution needed is that undue force must be avoided, not only because this is in itself undesirable but because the reaction to trauma, even of mild degree, is excessive. The dictum of 'minimum force consistent with achieving the objective' is particularly important in these cases, especially in the older age-groups. It is a good plan after any specific manipulation to follow the treatment with some intermittent sustained traction to minimise any painful reaction to the manipulation. When the spondylosis is complicated by nerve-root irritation the complication is of more consequence and must be considered first. The treatment should then be directed to reducing the nerve pressure, and this must be given priority.

Treatment of osteo-arthritis of spinal joints In principle the treatment of osteo-arthritis of spinal joints is similar to that in peripheral joints—i.e. improving the circulation by articulatory manipulation and by short-wave diathermy, reducing the friction of adjacent rough surfaces by traction, and minimising trauma by reducing the load upon the joint. In practice the treatment of osteo-arthritis of the lower lumbar joints consists in reducing the lordosis which is present in virtually all cases of osteo-arthritis of the lumbar spine, using articulatory manipulation, avoiding specific adjustments, and applying traction with the lumbar spine slightly flexed; and, if these measures fail, giving short-wave diathermy, protecting with a corset, reducing body weight, and injecting hydrocortisone into the capsules.

Intermittent sustained traction is more effective than sustained traction because the former encourages circulation and the latter strains the ligaments. Traction in the lumbar spine is best performed with the patient prone. A cushion is placed under the pelvis to reduce lordosis and to give an additional separational effect on the apophyseal joints.

TABLE 2

	Spondylosis	O.A. of apophyseal joints
1 Age	30 to 60 years	60 years onwards
2 Sex	Equally affected	Equally affected
3 Frequency	Common	Uncommon
4 Onset	Punctuated by acute episodes	Gradual onset with exacerbations
	Disc herniations are the prelude	Never entirely free of symptoms although quiescent phases occur
	Complete freedom between troublesome phases	
	Course may be asymptomatic	
5 Pain	Local or referred	Predominantly local
	Nerve-root pressure common due to disc protrusions	Compression pain common. Root pressure rare, and if so gradual in onset
6 Stiffness	Temporarily very restricted but no lasting severe restrictions	Increasing though variable with the phases of inflammation
	Stiffness related to muscle guarding	Stiffness after rest which wears off with activity
7 General symptoms	None	None
	Health unimpaired	Health unimpaired
	Erythrocyte sedimentation rate and blood picture normal	Erythrocyte sedimentation rate and blood picture normal
8 Variability of symptoms	Weekly or monthly rather than daily, and related to stresses	Daily and unrelated to any other factors like activity, rest, or weather
9 Pain related to position	Important	Unimportant
10 Aetiology	Injury—years before	Tends to occur in patients who have osteo-arthritis elsewhere
	Poor cartilage inheritance	
	Osteochondrosis	Lordosis in the cervical and lumbar areas predisposes
	Mechancial stresses	
	No osteo-arthritis elsewhere	Minor injuries liable to trigger off an attack
	Anomalies	
11 Pathological changes	Primarily in the disc and adjacent bone of the vertebral bodies	Primarily in the apophyseal joints with osteophytes on edges of facets
	Changes in vertebral body may be splaying, compression, or irregularity	No narrowing of disc spaces
		Vertebral bodies normal
	Apophyseal joints normal, although with some overlapping where discs are narrowed	Loss of articular cartilage and joint space
		Irregularity and sclerosis of facet surfaces
		Pathological changes similar to osteo-arthritis in peripheral joints

155

TABLE 2—*contd.*

	Spondylosis	O.A. of apophyseal joints
12 levels commonly affected	5–7C, mid T, and lower L	2–4C and lower L
13 Signs	Side-bending restriction in the neck	Rotation restriction in the neck
	Movements restricted according to level	Thickening of facet margins palpable and *enlarged*
	No crepitus	Crepitus
14 X-ray appearances	Narrow discs, vertebral body osteophytes, irregular outlines of vertebral bodies and adjacent surfaces	Wide discs, narrowed apophyseal joints with irregularity and sclerosis. Facet osteophytes (best seen in oblique views)
15 Treatment	Good response to manipulation	Poor response to manipulation
	Rhythmic traction appropriate	Relief with traction, especially intermittent sustained traction
	No relief with phenyl butazone etc.	Relief with phenyl butazone
	Short-wave diathermy aggravates when nerve-root pressure is present	Short-wave diathermy gives relief
16 External support	May be desirable in acute phases or to reduce mechanical stresses when unavoidable	Undesirable and only rarely beneficial, because of increased stiffness after wearing support

The traction can be applied manually and the patient can hold on to the top of the table, but this is not the ideal method because it is tiring for the operator, and the patient cannot easily relax her back at the same time as she is gripping the top of the table with her hands. An apparatus like the McManis table is suitable (*fig. 31*), using a chest harness or strap to immobilise the thoracic area. The feet are strapped to the end of the table, a pillow is placed under the pelvis, and the lower leaf of the table is extended and lowered to exert a gentle pull, gradually introduced and gradually reduced for half-minute stretches with five seconds' pause between each stretch.

5 Lordosis syndrome

The characteristic features of this syndrome are:

Lordosis of the lumbar spine.
Backache accentuated by backward-bending and by standing, especially when there is an accompanying enlarged abdomen.
Backache relieved by sitting and forward-bending.

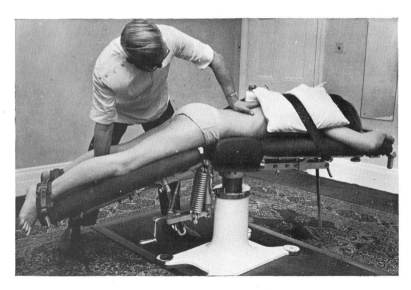

FIG 31 Prone traction technique.

Lying prone accentuates the pain. Relief is obtained by lying on the side with the knees and hips flexed.

Pain may be referred and is usually bilateral, without nerve-root signs unless complicated by a disc prolapse or by spondylolisthesis.

A definition of lordosis is any increase of the lumbo-sacral angle to more than 35°, using the Ferguson method of measuring the lumbo-sacral angle.[75]

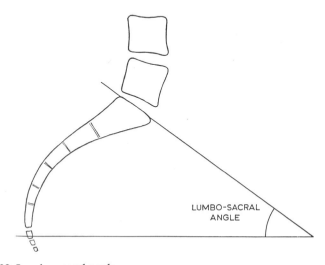

FIG 32 Lumbo-sacral angle.

157

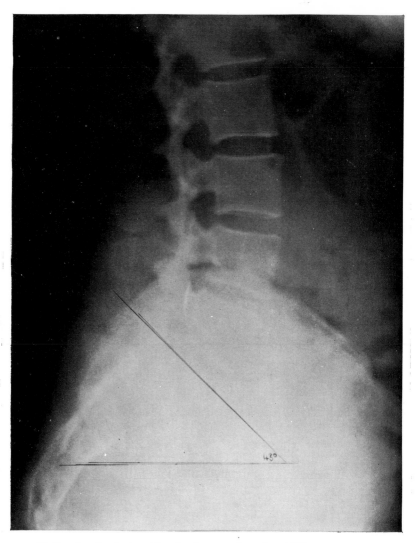

FIG 33 Lumbar lordosis with a lumbo-sacral angle of 43°.

The measurement is only valid if an erect lateral X-ray is taken (*fig. 33*). The superior surface of the sacrum is projected to the horizontal and that angle is measured off.

All the characteristic symptoms are due to the effects of lordosis—i.e. the carrying of more weight posteriorly because of the shift of the central gravity line posteriorly. Consequently more weight is taken by the posterior vertebral arches than is taken by the vertebral bodies and discs. These arches were not designed to carry much weight. (This is in contrast to the cervical spine, where the articular processes and vertebral arches

158

are as thick as the vertebral bodies.) This extra weight carried posteriorly is successively on the spinous processes, the apophyseal joints, the partes interarticulares, and the intervertebral foramina. Indirectly and at a distance from the lumbo-sacral joint there are other disadvantages arising from the lordosis—namely sacro-iliac strain, thoracic kyphosis, and even cervical lordosis. There are visceral effects also from ptosis of the abdominal contents.

Sometimes the lordosis syndrome follows directly from a hyperextension injury.

Disc lesions sometimes complicate the lordosis syndrome. Henderson[76] found that 22 per cent of his cases of spondylolisthesis were complicated by a disc protrusion. He was operating on a series of 216 patients using Gill's method of spinal fusion. However, the lordosis syndromes constitute quite distinct clinical entities, and the lordosis itself does not predispose to disc degeneration until a late stage.

The backache which is due to lordosis is occasioned in the first place by the mechanical apposition of the spinous processes (kissing spines) and by ligamentous strain in the anterior longitudinal ligament. Then if the spines are small, by the apposition of the inferior margin of the lower facets in the partes interarticulares area of the vertebral arch, and finally by degenerative changes in the arch and apophyseal joints. In early cases the ache can be abolished by the infiltration of a local anaesthetic between the spinous processes. In one patient this was all that was necessary to relieve a backache which had persisted for the previous eight years.

The term 'kissing spines' implies too great an approximation of the spinous processes (figs. 34, 35). Apposition can occur even in the erect position, but only when the spines are unusually large. X-rays show sclerosis of adjacent bony surfaces. Sometimes the bone has adapted itself to the shape of the vertebra below, one spinous process showing a convex ridge fitting into a concavity of the adjacent spinous process. Occasionally adjacent spinous processes are oblique so that during extension they come into apposition causing lateral deviation. Much depends upon the size of the spinous processes. When unduly large they may actually prevent the spine from adopting the average amount of lordosis. Such patients are blocked from further extension by this bony apposition and, if this position is sustained, an unpleasant local ache ensues in the lumbar spine. Yet they may be quite comfortable when sitting in a low easy chair. The contrast between this syndrome and the ligamentous strain syndrome (p. 119) is apparent because with the latter patients have more pain when sitting low and the pain is relieved by standing and spinal extension.

If the spinous processes are average or smaller than usual then the

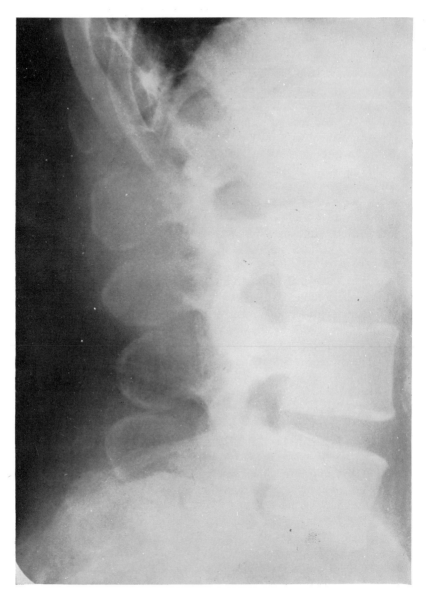

FIGS 34 AND 35 'Kissing' spinous processes. There is sclerosis of the adjacent surfaces of the 3,4 and 5L spinous processes. The adjacent sloping surfaces force slight rotation during backward bending.

lordosis brings the facets into apposition before the spines touch each other. This has two effects, namely, mechanical pressure on the partes interarticulares and stretching of the apophyseal joint capsule due to the overlapping of the facets.

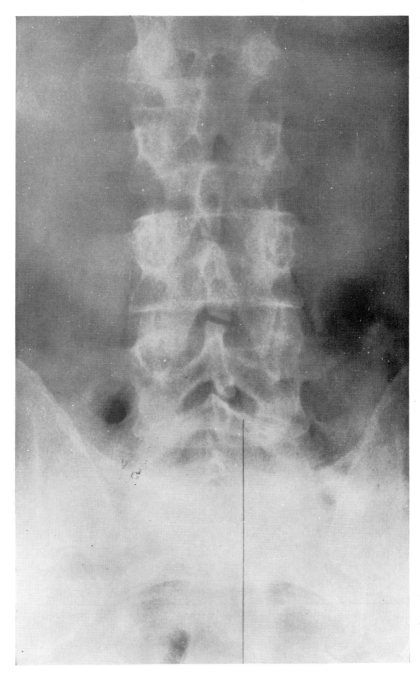

FIG 35

If the condition proceeds still further the chisel-like mechanical action of the lower margins of the inferior articular processes creates a stress fracture of the partes interarticulares. This defect is known as a *spondylolysis* if there is no forward displacement. If the load is too heavy for the fibrous tissue which forms at the partes interarticulares, separation occurs there so that the vertebral body shifts forwards, and this is called a *spondylolisthesis*.

When the partes interarticulares are strong enough to withstand the extra load, sclerosis of the vertebral arch follows, and still later osteo-arthritic changes develop in the apophyseal joints.

The reduced load on the vertebral bodies ought perhaps to decrease the compression of the intervertebral discs; but in fact the shearing strain of the lordosis tends to force the vertebral body forward on the one below, the annulus fibrosus may give way under such strain, and then a disc prolapse is inevitable.

Many lordotic subjects are pain free until the disc prolapses, but this does not imply that lordosis itself does not cause symptoms, otherwise why should correction of posture be enough to relieve such patients of backache? Mere correction of the standing position to reduce the lordosis is in most cases sufficient to achieve this relief of pain. If sclerosis of the vertebral arch is present without spondylolysis, spondylolisthesis, or osteo-arthritis, the backache is dull and local in character and is accentuated in any position involving weight-bearing and extension.

Quite often spondylolysis and spondylolisthesis are asymptomatic apart perhaps from discomfort when arching the spine backwards. Much depends upon the strength and stability of the ligaments. A shearing strain forward is present all the time during standing and walking. I had a patient with a spondylolysis at 3–4L who was a professional ballet dancer for thirty years without symptoms until she was forty-four years old, when presumably the ligaments and muscles began to weaken.

A full radiological assessment of these cases involves two erect views with one lateral and one antero-posterior view to show the influence of weight-bearing, two oblique views to show the apophyseal joints and partes interarticulares, and two mobility views taken laterally to show the effects of full flexion and full extension.

If there is any abnormal forward or backward shifting of the vertebra above on the vertebra below, the spondylolisthesis is *unstable* (*figs. 36, 37*). Such patients require strong lumbo-sacral support until stability has been restored. Manipulation is contra-indicated at the unstable stage, and *forced torsional adjustments are contra-indicated at any stage of spondylolisthesis*.

A defect of the partes interarticulares on one side only, leads to excessive rotation of the vertebral body away from the defective side. All cases in which this deformity is seen in an antero-posterior skiagram should have oblique views to note the state of the partes interarticulares.

Newman[77] described five types of spondylolisthesis. Type I has a congenital defect of the sacral neural arch, with a deficiency of the superior sacral facets, and the partes interarticulares elongate rather than break. Type II shows a defect of the partes interarticulares with or without forward displacement owing to persistent mechanical stress. Type III is traumatic, due to severe hyperextension. Type IV is degenerative, where the whole vertebra (usually 4L) slips forwards on the one below: the partes interarticulares are intact, but the apophyseal joints are osteo-arthritic. Type V is a rare pathological condition secondary to Paget's disease or neoplasia.

In all these cases the intervertebral discs are under stress and they may give way, complicating the picture and reducing the size of the intervertebral foramina still further. The lumbo-sacral foramen is the smallest but it has to carry the largest nerve-root of the sacral plexus and 5L is the most common vertebra to show defects of the partes interarticulares.

If lordosis of any degree leads on to *osteo-arthritis of the apophyseal* joints the clinical picture changes almost imperceptibly at first, but when established the diagnosis can be made both clinically and historically. Osteo-arthritis of the apophyseal joints in the lumbar spine rarely if ever occurs without a concomitant lordosis. There is no doubt that the extra weight-bearing on the facets is a factor in the arthritic changes.

Uncomplicated lordosis causes pain related to position. (Increase of the lordosis increases the pain, and decrease of the lordosis relieves the pain.) When osteo-arthritis supervenes, the pain ceases to have such clear characteristics. The pain can persist in any position, and it is very variable from day to day in an unaccountable fashion. Flexion of the spine only gives partial and temporary relief and stiffness soon develops when the patient remains stationary, as with sitting or lying down.

Management of the lordosis syndrome The treatment of symptoms which are due to lordosis differs from the treatment of most of the other syndromes because the patient is encouraged to sit in a low chair; erector spinae extension exercises are not advocated nor are torsional techniques used except in an articulatory manner. Forcible torsional techniques are risky. In fact it is possible to convert a spondylolysis into a spondylolisthesis by such methods.

When the lordosis is causing pain either in the interspinous ligaments, capsules, or intervertebral foramina, it evokes normal reflex muscle protection, but this unfortunately accentuates the lordosis and so a vicious cycle is established. This is especially so if osteo-arthritic changes have supervened because the forced apposition of roughened articular

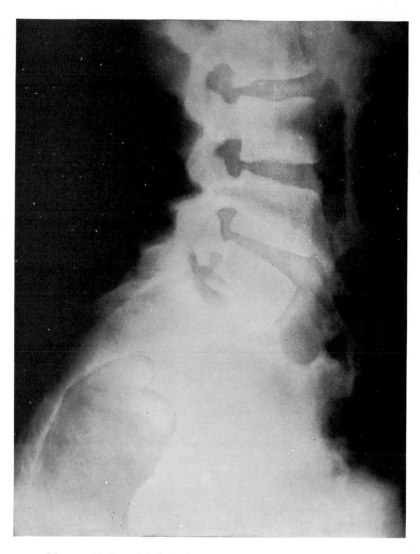

FIGS 36 AND 37 Spondylolisthesis at 5L. The mobility views indicate that there is instability during flexion and extension.

facets accentuates the pain and then the protective muscular tension accentuates the apposition. At all times the opposing facets should be apart. The patient must be taught to flex the pelvis in the standing position and to maintain this position both in sitting and lying. If the patient is unable to do this a firm lumbo-sacral corset should be prescribed, and its reinforced semi-rigid steels should fit the lumbar spine with the pelvis tilted forward—and not backwards. If the usual standing position is adopted for measuring and fitting a corset, the lordosis will

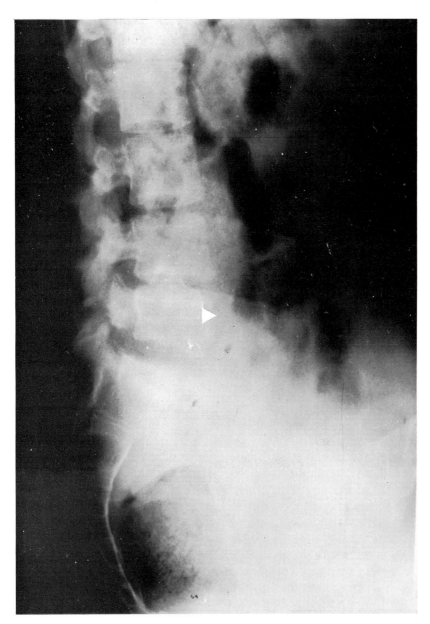

FIG 37

be increased by the corset and it will soon be rejected by the patient because of the increased pain.

Lordosis corrective exercises should be taught to all patients. The posture adopted when standing should be similar to that depicted in *fig. 39.*

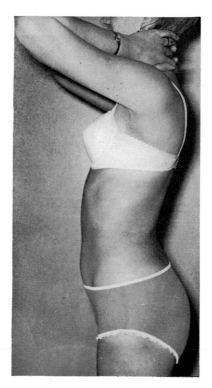

FIG 38 Lordosis.

Sclerosing injections (p. 126) are additionally helpful in unstable spondylolisthesis. The interspinous and supraspinous ligaments at the level of the 'shelf' are the ones to be injected, because these are the ones under most strain.

When nerve-root pressure becomes serious, surgery may be necessary if conservative measures fail.

If a disc prolapse complicates the pattern of symptoms then the treatment needs to be modified, and the first consideration is the degree of pressure on the nerve-roots. If severe enough, surgery may be necessary to relieve the pressure and to stabilise the vertebrae. A bone graft will probably be required.

If surgery is not imperative then conservative measures must take into account the vulnerability of the patient on the grounds of bone weakness as well as disc weakness. These patients with severe symptoms require a polythene type of rigid support, or even a brace, to support the whole spine (e.g. Strange's brace). Manipulations of all kinds, even gentle articulatory treatments, are contra-indicated, not merely because of the risk of accentuating the symptoms but because it can achieve

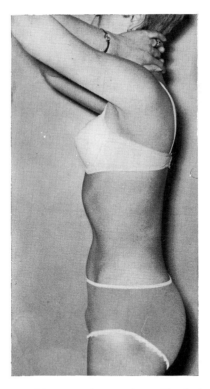

FIG 39 Postural correction of lordosis.

nothing in these difficult circumstances. Rest and immobilisation give the only hope of resolution: it may well take twelve months and even then a corset will be permanently required to reduce the risk of recurrence.

A lumbar disc prolapse can recover well with conservative measures, and the patient can be restored to full activities short of heavy lifting. A patient with a spondylolisthesis may well be rendered symptom free as long as the disc remains intact and the joint stable, but the combination of a disc prolapse with a spondylolisthesis is a permanent risk. Neither the patient nor the practitioner can afford to take liberties with such a spine.

The surgical procedure of choice in these cases is an anterior spinal fusion using the abdominal approach with a bone graft to wedge the vertebral bodies apart sufficiently to obtain normal separation between the bodies and to ensue a reliable arthrodesis. The posterior approach using an Albée-type graft across spinous processes is less effective and often fractures again because of the enormous leverage and shearing strains involved.

167

6 Nerve-root syndromes

When pain originating in a nerve-root is the predominant symptom the patient can be placed in this category. The majority of such patients have had previous symptoms which belong to other syndromes, and they have progressed or retrogressed to this next stage, when spinal pain has diminished or has disappeared altogether, and the limb pain from one or two nerve-roots dominates the clinical picture. All five previous syndromes may lead to nerve-root irritation, pressure, or adhesion formation. It is rare, though possible, for a patient to present with root signs and symptoms without any previous history of spinal symptoms. If this does happen the practitioner should be on his guard lest some less common disease is responsible or the cause is entirely peripheral without any disorder of the spine whatsoever.

Nerve-roots pursue a chequered course from the spinal cord to their exits from the intervertebral foramina, and for details of their anatomy the student must refer to textbooks, but some anatomical facts are worth emphasising because of their mechanical significance.

The posterior and anterior roots in the cervical spine are derived from several bundles before they join together, and the dorsal bundles are more numerous. There are up to fifteen dorsal bundles whereas there are only two to four ventral bundles. The bundles converge together to form a single dorsal or ventral root. They then fuse into a single spinal nerve before dividing again outside the spine. This is significant because if the spinal cord is stretched, mechanical tensions can evoke symptoms if the amount of stretch is beyond the elastic limit of the nerve-root or the individual bundle. The proximal bundles are likely to be stretched first with foraminal compression, but the distal bundles are more likely to be affected by shortening of the spinal column—e.g. when several disc spaces are narrowed. In this event, although the spinal cord remains the same length the shorter spinal column causes relative lengthening, and nerve-roots become kinked when they reach the intervertebral foramina.

The posterior nerve-roots are in direct anatomical relation with the capsules of the apophyseal joints, especially in the cervical area, so that enlargement of these joints and inflammatory exudates can directly affect the sensory fibres which pass into the posterior columns of the cord.

The anterior roots are in direct mechanical relation with the discs (in some cases two discs) as well as with the margin of the vertebral bodies, so that disc protrusions and marginal osteophytes can press on these roots.

The intervertebral foramen not only carries the nerve root but also the spinal artery and vein, the lymphatics, and the recurrent spinal nerve. Reduction in size of the intervertebral foramina by narrowing of the discs or by protrusions and osteophytes can, by mechanical irritation or pressure, set up irritative or inhibitive changes in the conduction of the nerves. In addition, inflammatory exudates can lead to adhesion formation and fibrosis which can effect the conduction of impulses through the nerve-roots.

The relative sizes of the intervertebral foramen and the nerve-root matter. As already mentioned, the fifth lumbar nerve-root is the largest of the sacral plexus and yet its intervertebral foramen is the smallest in the lumbar spine.

In the cervical area where the vertebral artery and vein traverse the foramina of the transverse processes, mechanical irritation of these vessels may further complicate the picture particularly when the vessel walls become inelastic or calcified. Secondary vascular changes can impair the oxygen supply to the nerve-roots and the spinal cord. The spinal artery divides into anterior and posterior branches. The anterior spinal branches supply the grey matter of the cord and the anterior white columns, whereas the posterior spinal branches supply the posterior and lateral white columns of the cord. There is a very rich supply of blood to the sympathetic chain of ganglia which runs down both sides of the spinal column. Consequently disturbances of vasomotor control can affect the blood-supply to the cord, the spinal nerves, and the autonomic nerves.

Another anatomical point is that, although there is very extensive anastomosis of spinal arteries and veins, the veins themselves have no valves and therefore venous drainage must depend largely upon movement and the active venous drainage of the azygos and lumbar veins. Venous congestion may well be a serious consideration in certain mechanical problems of the spine. Farkas[28] made this the cornerstone of his treatment of spinal disorders, using gravity (in different positions) to assist in decongestion of the spinal cord and canal.

Characteristics of the nerve-root syndrome The symptomatology in these syndromes depends upon the level of the lesion and upon whether the nerve is being irritated or compressed. Secondary signs and symptoms arise from the patient attempting to avoid pain.

Mechanical *irritation* of a nerve from intermittent pressure eventually leads to inflammation and swelling of the nerve. This gives rise to *pain and paraesthesiae in the distribution of the nerve.*

Mechanical *pressure* on a nerve when continuous leads to ischaemia of the nerve so that it soon loses its power of conduction. This is expressed clinically as *motor weakness, loss of reflexes, and loss of sensation in the distribution of the nerve.*

Adhesions around nerve-roots are often left behind when inflammatory exudates disperse. The signs of inflammation no longer obtain, and the *pain occurs only when the nerve is stretched*. If the adhesions become dense and 'root sleeve fibrosis' ensues then conduction may be gradually impaired.

The secondary effects of nerve-root irritation or compression arise because the patient either voluntarily or reflexly tries to avoid pain. Scolioses, kyphoses, and pelvic shifts appear in the lumbar area, and torticollis in the cervical area. Tertiary effects develop in muscles and ligaments as a result of these deformities.

A frequent concomitant disturbance of nerve-root syndromes is altered vasomotion and visceromotion in the related autonomic nerves.

When root pain is mechanically produced it is characteristic that changes of spinal position alter the pain, and if there is no inflammation the patient may well be able to adopt a position which is quite free from pain. But once the nerve-root swells and a neuritis is established, the pain is not relieved fully in any position. It occurs day and night, and is worse at night. Heat accentuates the pain peripherally and short-wave diathermy to the spine aggravates the symptoms centrally, presumably by creating more congestion in the intervertebral foramen. Once mechanical irritation sets up inflammatory change, the rate of recovery is reduced, and the pain is sometimes quite prolonged because a vicious cycle is established—the pressure causes the nerve to swell and the swelling increases the pressure. The pain is then perpetuated until the vicious cycle is broken by treatment.

The slow recovery of human nerves after ischaemia has been demonstrated by Barlow and Pochin.[78] After occlusion of the circulation to the human arm by a tourniquet for twenty-five minutes, movement and sensation returned rapidly to normal, but for about ten hours full recovery of the nerve was shown to be incomplete because if a second occlusion was performed within those ten hours, motor and sensory changes developed earlier than with the first occlusion. They contended that slow recovery was an effect of ischaemia from oedema. They found that even if the arterial supply was restored fully, oxygenation of the nerves was delayed by the presence of oedema.

Although the majority of nerve-root syndromes are of mechanical origin, one must never forget that benign and malignant neoplasms can cause root signs and symptoms. In addition other causes of referred limb pain must be excluded before assuming that the problem is mechanical.

The causes of lower extremity pain which are not mechanical are: neoplasms, and diseases of the spinal cord; meningeal irritation from infection, haemorrhage, and injections; post-herpetic neuralgia; osteomyelitis and neoplasms of bone; arthritis of various types affecting the lumbar spine and sacro-iliac and hip joints; visceral disease of the pelvic organs; arterio-sclerosis producing intermittent claudication; local injury and local inflammation in the limb.

Erythromelalgia is a term used for pain in lower extremities together with hyperhidrosis, cutaneous flushing, and cyanosis. The pain is accentuated by heat and is probably due to some disturbance of the vasomotor nerves to the legs. Correction of any lower thoracic and upper lumbar lesions affords some relief in these cases.

Meralgia paraesthetica is a neuritis of the lateral femoral cutaneous nerve. The nerve appears to be irritated mechanically where it passes under the inguinal ligament, and the pain is often relieved by injecting the site with hydrocortisone, but attention to the thoracico-lumbar area of the spine must not be omitted, in case the pain has a central source.

The *anterior tibial syndrome* is due to swelling and tension in the anterior tibial muscles following exercise. The fascia is so tight that the muscles cannot expand and relative ischaemia ensues. It may be severe enough to cause intense pain for several hours after the exercise has ceased. Surgical incision of the fascia relieves this syndrome.

The causes of pain which are not mechanical in the upper extremity are similar to those of the lower extremity, but we must include carcinoma of the lung, angina pectoris, pachymeningitis cervicalis, syphilitic aortitis, cervical adenitis, adhesive capsulitis of the shoulder, amyotrophic neuropathy and irritation of the diaphragm (see Brachial syndromes, p. 203).

Thoracic and upper lumbar nerve-roots may be irritated or compressed just the same as cervical and lower lumbar nerve-roots though less frequently. In the differential diagnosis of all types of anterior chest and abdominal pain, spinal causes should be remembered as a potential factor.

Principles of treatment of any nerve-root lesion

1 Removal of pressure from the nerve.
2 Avoidance of further irritation of the nerve.
3 Treatment of any residual neuritis after pressure has been removed.
4 Treatment of residual muscle weakness.
5 Measures to reduce the risk of recurrence.

1 The removal of pressure from the nerve-root may be the most urgent consideration, but as in all spinal syndromes the time factor is very important. At one stage surgery might be appropriate, yet at another stage it might be contra-indicated even in the same patient.

In the early stage—i.e. in the first forty-eight hours of an acute severe prolapse of a lumbar disc—the signs may be such that an urgent laminectomy should be performed to relieve the pressure. Surgery is indicated when paralysis is severe and complete or when a cauda equina syndrome is present with bladder and bowel symptoms predominating. The majority of cases are less serious and it is safe to wait, even if the pain is intense, before considering surgery. The later indications for surgery are: recurrent incapacitating attacks of pain which are interfering with the patient's livelihood, prolonged intense pain which the patient is unable to tolerate, and persistent pain or deformity (say for more than a year) in spite of all conservative methods of treatment.

The above criteria for surgery exclude over 99 per cent of patients, but if there are obvious indications for surgery the operation should not be delayed otherwise the morale of the patient suffers and recovery is protracted.

The acute spinal phase of a disc prolapse is similar to the treatment of disc herniations (p. 143). Once spinal pain has given way to limb pain, however, the probability is that a fragment of disc has fully prolapsed so that the adjacent torn margins of annulus are in apposition once more and healing is taking place. Then it is useless to try techniques which attempt to replace the disc fragment, and one is concerned to minimise the adverse effects of the displaced fragment. The patient must be kept at rest in the position of least pain. The majority obtain relief when lying in bed on either side or supine with a pillow under the knee of the painful limb, but some patients may even find sitting the least painful position to adopt.

Sustained traction at this stage is often effective. The angle of traction and the weights required can only be gauged by the individual patient. A 'Camp Varco' type of pelvic band is applied with the patient supine. A pulley is attached to the bottom of the bed and the appropriate weights are increased until the patient gets relief. If no relief is obtained or if pain recurs while still on traction, then the traction should be removed as it is achieving nothing and it complicates nursing. The traction should only be sustained for two or three hours at a time, and it is vital to release the weight gradually. Any sudden release may jar the nerve-root and accentuate the symptoms. A form of traction without weights and complicated apparatus is advocated by Masturzo[79] by laying the patient on a sloping slippery surface to 45°. The body is held in check by a thoracic harness so that the body weight acts as its own traction force. Christie[80] has shown that sustained traction for five minutes of 75 lb pull causes an increase of the 4–5L–1S disc spaces by 10–15 per cent, and in practice 60 to 75 lb is needed to effect relief in this acute phase.

Traction and/or bed rest should continue for as long as the pain is decreasing, but if the pain persists after three weeks in bed then an attempt should be made to shift the pressure from the nerve by manipulation provided there are no contra-indications (see p. 279). The technique for altering the relative position of the nerve-root and the prolapsed disc fragment is described on p. 174.

2 The avoidance of further irritation of the nerve may involve the adoption of abnormal postures for a time, but so long as the pain is diminishing, the inconvenience of the temporary deformity is less important than is the avoidance of nerve irritation. The patient may require support by a corset either of the plastic or canvas type. The plaster-of-Paris jackets of yester-year have been supplanted by the semi-rigid lighter polythene corsets which can be removed for washing.

3 Even when the mechanical pressure is relieved the nerve may remain inflamed for a considerable time. These patients are helped with vitamin-B therapy.

4 If muscles have weakened the early application of faradism or interrupted galvanism to those muscles is important for maintenance of tone while the nerve supply is recovering.

5 Measures for minimising the risk of recurrences consist of restoring normal mechanics as far as possible by paying attention to the level of the pelvis, the position of the vertebrae, the power of the muscles, and the posture.

Patients who have large disc prolapses are less prone to recurrences than those with small prolapses. This should be explained to patients, to help them through the many months of recovery.

Nerve-root irritation or compression can occur at any level, but in this section only lumbar levels are considered. Cervical and thoracic nerves are considered under their appropriate sections (p. 199, 210).

Prolapsed lower lumbar disc syndrome Characteristics:

Preceding history of attacks of 'lumbago'.
Lumbar pain followed within hours or days by lower extremity pain.
Abnormal central nervous system signs.
Diminished straight-leg raising test.
Spinal deformity.
Transient vasomotor disturbances in the lower extremities.

The *management* of this syndrome consists of rest, support, and sustained traction as indicated before. Pain may be severe enough to warrant the exhibition of morphine, but usually less powerful analgesics are sufficient. It is important for the patient to obtain sufficient relief to permit sleep, otherwise fatigue aggravates the syndrome.

Manipulation of the spine at this stage is contra-indicated, though relaxation of soft tissues in the lumbar area is comforting; but any treatment applied must only be administered in a position of minimum pain. To apply massage in a position which provokes pain will merely accentuate muscle tension rather than relieve it. Infra-red heat is comforting to the lumbar spine but affords no relief when applied to the limbs, and it may in fact increase the pain. Faradism to the palsied muscles should be started early provided that the patient can be treated in a position of comfort.

As time proceeds the pain should diminish, but if after three weeks of bed rest there is no progress and the straight-leg raising test remains the same, then manipulation is indicated.

Technique of manipulation for a prolapsed lower lumbar disc which is not recovering An anaesthetic, though not always essential, is desirable so that maximum relaxation will facilitate the technique. Thiopentone sodium ('Pentothal') is the ideal anaesthetic because it gives sufficient time for the manipulation, and the recovery phase is gradual enough. Suxamethonium chloride ('Scoline') is undesirable because of delayed muscle pain. Premedication is unnecessary. Methohexitone-sodium ('Brietal') acts too quickly and often produces increased muscle tone before relaxation; the recovery rate also is too rapid. (These remarks do not imply that Brietal is unsuitable for manipulation at other sites.)

The procedure adopted involves manipulating the lumbar spine at the level of the prolapse (see p. 141) and the manœuvre combines torsion plus stretching of the nerve-root, not with the object of reducing the disc prolapse because this is mechanically impossible, but with the idea of shifting the displaced fragment of disc away from the nerve-root. The nerve-root may be riding over the fragment or it may be bound by adhesions as it traverses the intervertebral foramen. Whichever the cause, the technique is the same. If it is merely a question of adhesions then a simple stretching of the nerve might suffice, but if the track of the nerve is being altered by the disc displacement then a torsional movement is needed to alter the position of the disc material.

As soon as relaxation is complete under pentothal anaesthesia the patient is turned on to the side with the painful side down (*fig. 40*). The level of the disc prolapse is located with the fingers. In cases under discussion it will be at 4–5L or at the lumbo-sacral level, and *the method now described appertains to 4–5L with right-sided sciatica.* The only difference between the two levels is that slightly more torsion is required for 5L–1S than for 4–5L.

The patient is placed on the right side, the operator facing the patient, flexing the patient's left knee and hip in order just to gap the

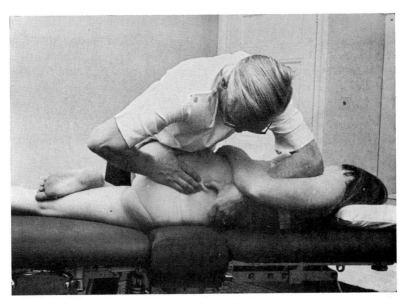

FIG 40 Torsional manipulation of the 4-5th lumbar joint.

4–5L joint very slightly. The left knee is allowed to rest on the table in front of the right thigh, and the patient's left foot is curved over her right knee. This enables the operator to control both lower extremities. More flexion is needed with a lordotic spine, and in this case the patient's left knee is flexed further up to rest in a position which gives sufficient gapping at 4–5L. The posterior aspect of the torso and pelvis should be vertical to the table at this stage.

The next step is to pull on the patient's right arm while maintaining the position of the pelvis as before. The operator must keep his right fingers on the 4–5L joint all the time now, so that while pulling on the patient's right arm to rotate the torso to the left, he feels a sense of tension developing down to the 4–5L level.

The patient is maintained in this position for a moment while the operator alters his own arm positions. The patient's left arm rests on her own left side, and the operator threads his left arm through the space formed by the patient's elbow and her body in such a way as to allow him to rest his left forearm on the patient's left pectoral area. This enables the operator to press backwards on the patient's left shoulder, and it leaves his left hand free to reach the lumbar spine. The operator's right hand is placed over the sacrum, and his index finger remains on the 5L spinous process. In this way an increase in tension can be achieved by pressing the patient's left shoulder backwards and the left side of the pelvis forwards. The patient's left knee must be free to move

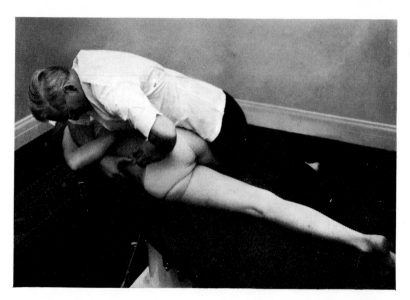

FIG 41 Torsional manipulation of the lumbar spine combined with stretch of the sciatic nerve.

between the operator's two legs. The procedure now is to increase the torsion, more by an increase of the pelvic movement than of the shoulder. At this stage the shoulder should be kept more or less static and the thrust should come from the right hand. In order to achieve this the operator needs to be fully bent over the patient's body, with his right elbow well away from the patient.

It is important for the operator to maintain the position of his right index finger on 5L to make sure that the thrust effects a click at the 4–5L level, and if possible he should also keep his left thumb on 4L. It is easy enough to obtain one or two clicks in the lumbar spine somewhere, but to be effective one must be sure that the 4–5L joint is moved. The clicking sound arises from a separation of the apophyseal joints. This mobilising of the apophyseal joints is part of the procedure to ensure good mobility, and to release any adhesions which might have formed in the 4–5L apophyseal joint on the left.

Now the patient is turned on to the left side (*fig. 41*) so that her painful leg is uppermost, and the operator's objective is twofold—firstly to apply torsional gapping at the 4–5L level, and secondly to stretch the nerve-root. In order to do this concurrently, the same position is adopted as before but the patient's right leg is brought over the side of the table and kept there between the operator's two legs. The operator must arrange his own stance so that his left leg is over the patient's calf posteriorly and his right thigh is in apposition with the patient's

176

right thigh anteriorly in a scissor-like grip which enables the operator to alter the degree of stretch and *maintain full extension of the patient's knee*. The operator is in effect maintaining the patient's right knee straight and flexing her right hip. The degree of flexion is important. If the S.L.R. is 30° with the patient conscious, then the stretching must be at a greater angle than this otherwise nothing will be achieved. About 45° to 50° is correct for that patient. If, on the other hand, the S.L.R. test is 80°, then flexion of the hip must be 90° or more. The patient's straight-leg raising can be controlled well by the operator altering his own leg position. The sequence of this second phase of the technique is to place the patient on her left side, and to flex her right hip and extend her right knee between the operator's legs. At first the operator should be content with 30°, if the patient's S.L.R. test was 30° to start with, and then he should proceed as before applying torsion to the torso by pulling on the patient's left arm and shoulder until tension is again felt at 4–5L. The operator's arm positions are as before and the patient's body position is exactly as before, but now the patient's lower extremity is flexed more, say to 45° or 50°.

The thrust is made as described before but it must be co-ordinated with the extra flexion of the leg. The timing is important. The extra stretch coincides exactly with the thrust. It is by no means easy to arrange, and the correct stance and balance of the operator are vital otherwise it is easy to slip or to miss the correct timing of the stretch and thrust.

The patient is then returned to the resting position while recovering from the anaesthetic. A pillow under the patient's knee is beneficial because having momentarily stretched the nerve it may show increased irritability temporarily, and in any case most sciaticas obtain relief with the knee and hip slightly flexed.

The follow-up care is important too. Immediately after the manipulation some extra analgesic is required, and pethidine may be needed for the next twenty-four hours. Any increase of pain should subside in forty-eight hours, and the patient is then kept in bed for ten to fourteen days according to the severity of the case and according to progress.

If the patient has had chronic sciatica for two, three, or more months, the nerve will be in an irritable condition and even when the procedure is initially successful the nerve will take time to settle. This is why a ten- to fourteen-day period of bed rest is important in ensuring the success of the procedure. It also enables the displaced fragment of disc material to consolidate in its new position. After the bed rest a gradual resumption of activity is permitted. It is not advantageous to rest the patient for more than three weeks. If within three weeks the patient is not vastly better, then further bed rest will not accelerate the recovery and it might delay it because of the weakening effect of prolonged inactivity.

In the period of graduated return to activity the patient should be encouraged to adopt those positions which relieve the pain but those positions which aggravate the pain should be studiously avoided. Most patients are comfortable when standing and lying but not when sitting, though in a few cases the converse may obtain. The point is that one is dealing with an irritable nerve from which all the pressure may not have been relieved by the manipulation. To return to full activity too rapidly may set up inflammatory reactions in the nerve once more. It is important not to have a setback during the recovery phase.

The results of this procedure are excellent, and in an analysis of a series of fifty cases of chronic sciatica (i.e. the sciatic pain had been present for at least two months) which I manipulated under pentothal, 72 per cent showed a significant reduction in pain within two weeks, 24 per cent showed no real change and 4 per cent were temporarily worse. Several patients relapsed later and three went on to laminectomy. No claim is made that the method has a long-term effect and it does not prevent recurrences, but as a short-term measure the relief was real and appreciated by three out of four of the patients. The criterion of significant relief of pain within two weeks of the manipulation under anaesthesia is important and it is a measure of the effectiveness of the procedure. If we had allowed more time for recovery in assessing the effectiveness of the method then the mere passage of time could have accounted for the improvement, but for cases of three, four and five months' duration in whom the pain was persisting unabated—for these cases to get a significant relief of pain in a fortnight justifies the assumption that the method itself was responsible for the relief.

The remaining cases—24 per cent—showed only marginal improvement after a fortnight and the mere passage of time and bed rest could have accounted for the slight improvement. The two cases who suffered more pain after the manipulation were not seriously worse and they had no abnormal nervous system signs—nor did abnormal signs develop following the manipulation under anaesthesia. I did not consider that a 4 per cent risk of aggravation of symptoms was a sufficient criticism of the method to abandon the procedure. I found that the S.L.R. test was a useful guide as to how successful the method was likely to be, but this does not apply to early cases of sciatica.

In acute recent sciaticas a S.L.R. of 10°–20° is no criterion as to the rate and extent of recovery. Many of these recover fully and quickly. But in chronic sciaticas the S.L.R. is a good guide as to the degree of mechanical pressure and irritation of the nerve. All the acute manifestations of the recent disc prolapse have had time to subside and we are left with an essentially mechanical problem. A low angle of the S.L.R. test implies less room for the nerve-root, less opportunity for manœuvre and less chance for the manipulation to relieve the pressure on the nerve-root. A low S.L.R. angle may be due to adhesions alone without direct pressure but in these cases both legs show a reduced angle and the painless straight leg raising evokes a pain on the other side.

In these chronic cases the critical level is 20°–30°. Patients with less than 20° S.L.R. tend to respond poorly to manipulation under anaesthesia. Those with over 30° respond well. Patients who show no abnormal central nervous system signs respond better than those with abnormal central nervous system signs. The numbers showing abnormal central nervous system signs were twenty-three and of these fifteen responded quickly. The others without central nervous system signs were twenty-seven, and twenty-one showed a quick response. That is, 80 per cent of the sign-free cases responded quickly as against 65 per cent of the ones with abnormal signs.

The *contra-indications* to the above technique are the presence of (1) pathological changes other than a disc prolapse, (2) spondylolisthesis or spondylolysis, (3) osteoporosis of the spine, (4) bladder or rectal disturbances indicative of massive displacement involving the cauda equina, (5) a general disease which might render anaesthesia a danger in itself, (6) a S.L.R. of less than 20°. The technique is also contra-indicated, (7) during the first three weeks of the onset of the prolapse.

If the *patient is making progress* after the manipulation and bed rest, then all that is needed is articulatory treatment to the lumbar spine weekly, and later fortnightly to help improve circulation to the spine and as a means of keeping the patient under observation. Torsional techniques are contra-indicated in the phase of recovery. Steps should now be taken to minimise the risk of recurrences (see p. 149).

If, however, *the patient is not responding then further* consideration must be given to the question of surgery or traction or epidural or extradural injections and to the feasibility of a corset to reduce irritation of the nerve-root. Prolonged bed rest is undesirable because it does not accelerate recovery and tends to weaken the general musculature as well as undermining the patient's morale. The patient is better getting about and following her occupation within the limits imposed by the pain and deformity. Activities which accentuate the pain should of course be avoided, especially if pain continues after the activity ceases, because the nerve-root is only being more irritated and inflamed thereby. Many patients are better for walking and standing rather than sitting, and during the first few days after two weeks of bed rest my advice to patients is to adopt vertical or horizontal positions but to avoid half-lying or sitting.

The wearing of a corset at this stage helps in recovery only in a negative sense. The corset reduces the risk of irritation of the nerve and it reminds the patient to take care, thereby reducing the risk of recurrence. In a follow-up series of sciatic cases Dr. J. Barrett (personal communication) found that there was a 25 per cent recurrence rate after large disc prolapses and still more recurrences after small disc prolapses.

Traction at this stage would be of the sustained type because when patients still have nerve-root irritation rhythmic traction tends to aggravate rather than relieve it.

The above description and scheme of management applies to the typical prolapsed lower lumbar disc, but there are syndromes which are not quite typical, and though infrequent these occur often enough to warrant separate descriptions.

1 Management of the prolapsed intervertebral disc involving the third lumbar nerve-root This syndrome differs from fourth and fifth lumbar and first sacral root lesions in several respects:

(*a*) The pain distribution is in the anterior thigh, extending sometimes beyond the knee to the shin but not beyond the ankle.

(*b*) The knee-jerk is diminished or absent.

(*c*) The quadriceps muscle may weaken.

(*d*) The S.L.R. test is 80° or more, but stretching the femoral nerve (Ely's test) by having the patient prone and flexing the knee while the hip remains extended is more painful than on the other side. Comparing the two sides is important because flexion of the knee in this position in any average adult is uncomfortable owing to the quadriceps being stretched to its elastic limit.

(*e*) The sensory loss when present is in the anterior thigh in the third lumbar dermatome.

(*f*) The psoas muscle is often tight, and this keeps the hip flexed or at least prevents much hip extension. It may in fact cause pain and apparent restriction in the hip joint, and it may give rise to a mistaken diagnosis of early arthritis of the hip joint. Lumbar lesions should always be taken into account when considering the differential diagnosis of arthritis and capsulitis of the hip joint.

(*g*) It is rarely necessary to manipulate the 3–4L joint under anaesthesia, and it is safe to manipulate without the reservations which are applicable to 5L–1S (p. 143). Even when specific adjustments at 3–4L are ineffective, I have not found any exacerbation from specific treatment. If the ordinary manipulation at 3–4L is not effective then pentothal should be given, using the standard torsional technique for 3–4L. This should be followed by stretching the femoral nerve with the patient prone as for the Ely's test, i.e. flexing the knee and extending the hip.

(*h*) Careful thought must be given to other pathological causes of 3L nerve-root irritation because the 3–4L intervertebral foramen is very large, and for a disc prolapse to be big enough to cause root pressure implies a much larger displacement than is the case with those which evoke symptoms at the lower two disc levels.

(*i*) Surgery is rarely if ever indicated.

In management, therefore, the response to treatment is usually gratifyingly rapid or disappointingly slow. If abnormal central nervous system signs are present the recovery time is likely to be nine to twelve months rather than three to six months. Permanent disability from third lumbar nerve-root pressure is less likely than at lower levels.

2 Management of disc prolapse with abnormal central nervous system signs and yet no restriction of S.L.R. This occurs, according to Herlin,[21] in cases where the prolapse is very laterally placed. No tension on the root can be achieved by the technique described on p. 174 because the straight-leg raising is 90°, and therefore this is not applicable. However, the standard torsional technique can be applied to both sides quite safely, and this should be tried without an anaesthetic.

3 Prolapsed lumbar disc lesions in young patients The characteristic of these cases is that there is more than average pelvic shift or sciatic scoliosis, yet the pain is not severe and abnormal central nervous system signs are unusual. Furthermore although recovery is protracted in the sense that deformity persists for many months, the patients themselves do not complain of severe pain nor are their activities as severely restricted as would obtain in the forty to fifty age-group.

I do not know the reason, and I have not been able to trace any literature on this point; but one possible explanation is that, even though the disc prolapses, the posterior longitudinal ligament remains intact because it is tougher than the corresponding ligament of an older patient, consequently the prolapsed material cannot protrude far enough to cause root pressure. Another factor may be that all the adjacent ligaments and muscles are more elastic so that adaptation to the deformity is better and therefore less painful.

The management of these cases lies not in giving much treatment but rather in reassuring the patient and her parents that eventual recovery is certain, even though it might take two years. Support with a corset together with strengthening exercises for the erector spinae muscles are indicated, and of course no heavy lifting. A polythene corset may be necessary. At a late stage manipulation under anaesthesia is justified if improvement in the scoliosis ceases.

4 Paralytic type of prolapsed intervertebral disc In this syndrome motor loss is the predominant symptom and sensory changes are minimal. Sometimes there is very severe pain for twenty-four to forty-eight hours and then the pain ceases as dramatically as it came on, but instead of pain there is loss of power and sometimes sensory loss, as if the nerve had given up its capacity to convey pain as well as its capacity to carry motor and sensory impulses.

In these cases the straight-leg raising rest is not impaired and the spinal mobility is not affected, so that spinal treatment does little to influence the recovery. Recovery is the rule, but it may only be partial. Treatment by faradism to maintain muscle tone is all that is needed. Corsets are unnecessary.

5 Central disc prolapse This gives rise to bilateral and symmetrical pain, and the pain may extend to the coccyx (see p. 193). Almost always the pain later becomes unilateral. It may even alternate between the two sides. The probable explanation is that the fragment tracks from the centre to one side or the other, deep to the posterior longitudinal ligament.

If a disc prolapse is unstable, and this is implied if the pain suddenly alters its distribution, great care needs to be taken with treatment in case manipulation or traction or articulation alters the pain for the worse. A polythene type of corset is indicated in these cases for at least three months so that the prolapsed fragment can become stabilised in one site.

The direction in which a sciatic scoliosis deviates depends, according to Armstrong,[81] on whether the prolapsed fragment is medial or lateral to the nerve-root. In right-sided sciatica, if the fragment is medial to the nerve-root, the patient is more comfortable when side-bent to the right, because this creates a concavity to the right, whereas if the fragment is lateral to the nerve-root on the right, the patient is more comfortable when side-bent to the left which creates a concavity to the left. Whether the scoliosis is convex to the painful side or to the painless side, the constant sign is that side-bending to the convexity increases the pain.

6 Cauda equina lesions These are usually due to a massive disc prolapse, and they are characterised not only by wide motor and sensory loss but also by bowel and bladder dysfunction. In describing thirteen cases, Shepherd[82] stated that 'bladder function took the form of difficult micturition or retention of urine; failure of appreciation of the filling of the viscus or loss of urethral sensation, in some cases, stress incontinence. The main bowel disturbance was constipation and in most cases lack of appreciation of rectal distension and loss of anal sensation.

Loss of sexual power occurred in some patients'. The onset of a cauda equina lesion may be gradual or rapid. In most cases there is a previous history of disc protrusions coupled with injury or of lifting strains.

Any disturbance of micturition together with sensory loss in the saddle area should alert the physician to the serious nature of the syndrome, and surgical advice should be sought immediately because any delay in surgical relief of pressure may lead to permanent loss of bladder function and a risk of ascending urinary infection as well as bed sores.

7 Peripheral nerve lesions affecting the lower extremity

Meralgia Paraesthetica This is a peripheral neuropathy of the lateral femoral cutaneous nerve of the thigh. The symptoms are entirely sensory—pain, paraesthesiae, and numbness over the antero-lateral aspect of the thigh and it is due to mechanical irritation of the nerve as it passes under the lateral part of the inguinal ligament. As it takes its origin from the lumbar plexus at 1–2L similar symptoms can accrue from mechanical lesions in the upper lumbar joints and treatment should be directed there first, but if not effective, some hydrocortisone can be injected at the site of emergence of the nerve under the inguinal ligament. The surgical method is to open the channel but this is rarely necessary.

Tarsal tunnel syndrome This is analogous in the foot to the carpal tunnel syndrome in the hand, but it is less common. The tibial nerve is irritated as it passes under the flexor retinaculum just inferior to the medial malleolus. It leads to aching and burning sensations in the foot at night especially after prolonged walking or standing the previous day. It can lead to loss of power in the abductor hallucis muscle. It is treated, as is the carpal tunnel syndrome, by hydrocortisone injections at the site of irritation or by surgical incision of the retinaculum.

Metatarsalgia Pain is felt in the toes when walking and the pain can be elicited by compressing the heads of the metatarsals together. A neuroma is sometimes found when the digital nerve is surgically explored. Treatment, other than surgical, includes the restoration of the foot and body mechanics, and toning up of the intrinsic muscles of the foot by exercises and faradism.

Metatarsalgia can also arise from adhesions, inflammation, and mechanical strains in the metatarso-phalangeal joints. The commonest cause of this is splaying of the metatarsal heads and dropping of the transverse arch. This condition should be treated by manipulation, exercises, faradism, correct footwear, and temporary support with a metatarsal pad.

8 Sacro-iliac syndromes

Pain arising from sacro-iliac joints may stem from mechanical lesions of the pelvis or from diseases of the joints themselves. The latter diseases are ankylosing spondylitis, tuberculosis, gout, osteo-arthritis, and osteitis condensans ilii.

Mechanical lesions may be subluxations and hypermobile strains. Their *characteristic features* are:

Pain in the region of the sacro-iliac joint with referred pain into the posterior thigh, iliac fossa, and buttock.
No central lumbar pain or tenderness.
Pain accentuated by sacral springing tests.
Local tenderness over the posterior sacro-iliac ligaments and the sacro-tuberous ligament on the same side.
Unilateral muscular tension in the erector spinae muscles of the same side.

Occasionally sacro-iliac mechanical lesions are bilateral, one compensating for the other when torsional factors are involved. There is also bilateral sacro-iliac strain secondary to lumbar lordosis.

In establishing the diagnosis of a sacro-iliac lesion we must first exclude disease in the joint and secondly exclude lumbo-sacral lesions before blaming the sacro-iliac joint for the symptoms. In my view only about one in ten of patients who present with pain in the region of the sacro-iliac joint has in fact a sacro-iliac lesion. Most of these patients are suffering from referred pain arising in the lumbar spine. If there are any centrally placed signs or symptoms at all, then the sacro-iliac joint is probably not at fault, even though there is obvious asymmetry in the pelvis. The differential diagnosis between sacro-iliac lesions and lumbar lesions is difficult. It can be just as difficult as, for example, the differential diagnosis between appendicitis and salpingitis.

Movement in the sacro-iliac joints Young[83] has demonstrated radiologically in the later stages of pregnancy that the sacro-iliac joints become increasingly mobile. He shows X-rays which indicate hinge-like and rotary movements. The symphysis pubis increases in width by 4 mm towards the end of pregnancy, and this implies a ginglymus movement at the sacro-iliac joint with corresponding approximation of the posterior superior iliac spines. X-rays taken in the standing position with weight-bearing first on one leg and then on the other leg show an upwards and downwards movement of 2 mm in each direction at the symphysis pubis. This implies a rotatory movement at the sacro-iliac joint. It occurs around the pivot of the concentrated portion of the posterior sacro-iliac ligaments, at the 1–2S level of the sacrum.

I have seen 3 cm of separation at the symphysis pubis in a man aged thirty-five, who fell off a horse. This occurred without any fracture so that the hinge effect at the sacro-iliac joint must have been considerable. Curiously enough he did not complain of sacro-iliac pain, but only of symphysis pain and a sense of weakness of the whole pelvis.

Measurements of sacro-iliac movements can be made clinically by marking the skin with a pencil over an exact part of the posterior superior iliac spine on each side in the standing position, taking care not to move the skin, and then measuring the distance between the posterior superior iliac spines again in the prone position. There is plenty of room for experimental error in these measurements because of the difficulty in finding an exact point on the rounded posterior superior iliac spines and because of the mobility of the overlying skin; but with repeated measurements, keeping the eyes closed while palpating the bony points and lifting the palpating thumb off the skin to make sure that the skin itself is not being moved, I have satisfied myself that there is usually 1–2 mm of movement in the normal young adult, but in view of the difficulty the test is not reliable for clinical assessment. The posterior superior iliac spines approximate when standing and separate when lying prone. This is probably accounted for by the weight of the body pressing the sacrum caudally and anteriorly, and pulling on the posterior sacro-iliac ligaments, so approximating the iliac spines.

The mobility of these joints diminishes with increasing age, particularly in men, and these joints are virtually ankylosed by forty years of age in men and by sixty years in women.

As age advances motion is diminished and later it very frequently disappears completely because of fibrous and bony ankylosis. In men motion begins to disappear about the fourth decade while in women rarely before the fifth decade but more commonly at the end of the fifth.[84]

The small amount of movement at the sacro-iliac joint is of course very difficult to detect. In fact it is impalpable except in late pregnancy. What can be detected, however, is a sense of 'give' in these joints when springing over the sacrum. Sacral springing is the most reliable test for sacro-iliac lesions, whether mechanical or pathological in origin.

Springing the sacrum With the patient prone on a flat table, so that the symphysis pubis is on an unyielding surface, the operator applies the heel of his hand to the apex of the sacrum and springs firmly over it. The arm must be kept straight and the operator should lean well over the patient, so that any yielding of the sacrum can be sensed by the operator's whole arm. To press with a flexing elbow is insufficient and gives false impressions.

While springing over the apex of the sacrum, the other fingers can be used to palpate over the sacro-iliac joint, but the movement there is slight and the movements of skin and muscle are misleading. One can rely only on the sense of 'give' to the springing arm. This is primarily a subjective test, and more significance must be attached to the patient's reply to the question 'Does this cause pain?' than to the objective sensation of movement. If pain is evoked by this test, then the next question is 'Where?' If the pain is at the site of pressure no significance can be attached to it, but if it is felt in the sacro-iliac region this is a positive sign. If the pain is in the lumbar spine then the lumbo-sacral joint is probably at fault. The latter can be confirmed by applying the springing test in the lumbar spine itself (*fig. 7*, p. 53).

Springing of the sacro-iliac ligaments can be achieved with the patient lying supine and flexing her knee and hip fully, then rocking the pelvis by maximum flexion of the hip on the pelvis, or by gapping the sacro-iliac joint using the flexed knee and hip to 90° and then adducting the femur to rock the sacro-iliac joint.

These tests are described on p. 75 of my *Manual of Osteopathic Technique*. The other tests of springing the innominates apart or together using the anterior superior iliac spines for leverage are so rarely positive even in proved sacro-iliac lesions that I attach little importance to them.

Genuine sacro-iliac pain in a young adult, mainly in men, may be due to tuberculosis or ankylosing spondylitis and in the older age-groups to gout or osteo-arthritis. Young women may develop *osteitis condensans ilii* which causes increased sclerosis of the iliac portion of the sacro-iliac joint without true involvement of the joint and without progressing to ankylosing spondylitis. The disease pursues a benign chronic course resolving spontaneously in due course, and all that is needed is some support to the joint in the form of a sacral band.

The characteristic feature of diseases of the sacro-iliac joint is the constancy of the pain which is quite unrelated to position.

Central sacral pain may arise from the lumbar spine but not from the sacro-iliac joints. Low sacral pain is mostly due to disease of the pelvic viscera. Pain and tenderness lateral to the posterior superior iliac spine is never due to sacro-iliac lesions but to muscular changes in the origin of the gluteus maximus. This can be an intrinsic fault in the muscle or it may be secondary to the irritation of the inferior gluteal nerve supply of the gluteus maximus.

Gout of the sacro-iliac joint is discussed on p. 255.

Osteo-arthritis of the sacro-iliac joint is very rare indeed, and although osteophytes are quite often seen they are rarely the cause of symptoms.

Tuberculous sacro-iliitis occurs in adults and commences in the lower pole of one of the joints. Haziness or erosions are seen on the X-ray.

Sacro-iliac strain is provoked mainly by torsional stresses when the pelvis is fixed—for example, transfering a load from one side of the body to the other with the feet stationary. The golf swing is a common cause of sacro-iliac strain, because the sacrum rotates within the relatively fixed innominates. This sort of trauma may lead to over stretching of the ligaments and thereby to a hypermobile joint, or it may subluxate the joint so that the relative position of sacrum and innominates is altered. The commonest type of lesion is a 'posterior innominate' when the upper pole of the sacrum moves forward, and this gives an apparent prominence of the posterior superior iliac spine. Whether a subluxation or a hypermobile strain occurs depends on the convolutions of the opposing surfaces of the innominates and auricular surface of the sacrum. The convolutions can be hitched out of their true position. Sacro-iliac joints which are straight, in the sense that there are few convolutions or very shallow ones, are more vulnerable than are irregular and convoluted joints. It is necessary to take oblique X-rays to determine whether the sacro-iliac joints are convoluted or straight.

The effects of a posterior innominate and of a hypermobile sacro-iliac joint are similar in that the posterior sacro-iliac ligaments are tender to palpation and the sacro-tuberous ligaments are also tender and tense. The tension in the sacro-tuberous ligament is quite easy to feel if the patient will relax the glutei. The ligament passes obliquely downwards and outwards from the sacrum to the ischial tuberosity, and the ligaments on each side should be compared. When the sacrum is tilted forwards superiorly and therefore backwards inferiorly, an undue stretch is occasioned in the sacro-tuberous ligament and this increases its tensions and tenderness.

The 'anterior innominate' can occur, but in most cases this positional fault is asymptomatic.

Another cause of sacro-iliac strain is the repeated manipulation of these joints, especially in the hypermobile type of patient. I have seen many of these cases due to enthusiastic and misguided osteopathic treatment.

Unlike most joints of the body in which we aim at maintaining good mobility because movement is their normal function, we should in the case of the sacro-iliac joints encourage stability and immobility. The only exceptions to this rule are in women of child-bearing age, who need flexible sacro-iliac joints to facilitate labour.

If there is the slightest doubt about the diagnosis of a sacro-iliac lesion, a rectal examination is indicated not only because the sacro-tuberous ligaments and coccyx can be palpated well in that way but because the pelvic viscera can also be examined.

Management of sacro-iliac lesions If there is a positional fault this should be corrected, and if there is a primary short leg this should be compensated for by the appropriate heel cushion. The patient's habitual posture and the type of games she plays must be considered carefully, and advice given to reduce the recurring strain on these joints.

Manipulative techniques to the sacro-iliac joints should be specific and ought not, at least in the first instance, to incorporate lumbar leverage because, however careful the operator, it is well nigh impossible to avoid mechanical stress in the lumbar spine with torsional techniques. Torsional techniques even when directed to the sacro-iliac joint usually cause lumbar apophyseal joint clicks, rather than sacro-iliac joint clicks. If this happens the operator is unable to judge which joint has been responsible for the response to his manipulation. Should the patient recover, the operator cannot be sure that his original diagnosis of a sacro-iliac lesion was correct though both he and the patient may be grateful. If the patient does not respond well, the operator is still in a quandary and is unable to direct his attention to the real fault so that the techniques become pure guesswork. Therefore the techniques which use direct thrusts or leg leverage (figs. 133 and 137, *Manual of Osteopathic Technique*) should be used.

A feature of sacro-iliac lesions which is not apparent in other joints in my experience, is that a number of adjustments need to be given before the joint yields. When using a springing technique with the patient prone and applying pressure with the heels of the hands, one over the apex of the sacrum and the other over the affected posterior superior iliac spine, the operator should spring several times, beginning gently and gradually increasing the pressure. After five or six attempts the joint frequently yields. This may be due to the gradual stretching or fatigue of the ligament or it may be due to some slight alterations of the angle of the thrust.

After adjustment, the sacro-iliac joint should be held with a sacral band (*fig. 42*) or firm strapping, and repeated manipulation should be avoided.

If the ligaments are too weak to hold even with a sacral band, then sclerosing injections of ethanolamine oleate should be given (see p. 126). Usually 2 ml at a time is needed because the ligaments are larger, and in any case they are less sensitive to the needle and to the sclerosant.

Osteitis condensans ilii is included under the heading of sacro-iliac

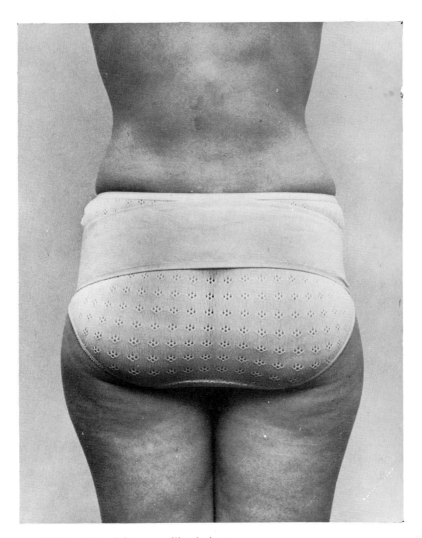

FIG 42 Sacral band for sacro-iliac lesions.

syndromes because it is entirely limited to these joints. It is a radio-logical diagnosis, but patients with this syndrome are usually women (in contrast to the male predominance in ankylosing spondylitis) and they complain of dull bilateral sacro-iliac pain. The X-rays (*fig. 43*) show increased density on the iliac side of the sacro-iliac joints, yet there are no erosions, no haziness of outline, and no ankylosis. The condition is benign and self-limiting. A sacral band may be all that is necessary to relieve the ache. The standard A.P. view is inadequate to distinguish this from sacro-iliitis of ankylosing spondylitis but the oblique views clearly show the difference.

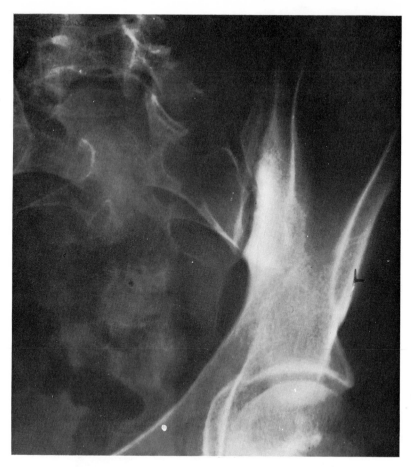

FIG 43 Osteitis condensans ilii. This oblique view shows that the sacrum is free from disease. This male patient had a serum uric acid of 8·1 mgm.

9 Ankylosing spondylitis syndromes

1 Marie-Strumpell and Von Beckterew types.
2 'Stiff-back' syndrome.

The characteristic feature of these cases is excessive rigidity of the spine without much pain.

In the classical picture of ankylosing spondylitis the earliest sign is spinal rigidity, and as the onset may be painless or very gradual the patient may have a 'poker' back before he realises it.

Lack of spinal mobility is a sign rather than a symptom, and patients will rarely seek advice merely because the spine is stiffer than it used to be.

Here a distinction should be made between stiffness and rigidity. Both will cause reduced overall spinal movements, but stiffness implies that the soft tissues are losing elasticity and that the range of movement can gradually even though slowly be increased by stretching, whereas with rigidity there is a solid unyielding quality about the movement.

The spinal rigidity of ankylosing spondylitis should be easily distinguished from the acute stiffness of a disc prolapse. In ankylosing spondylitis there is no muscle guarding or spasm when applying the springing test, though the paravertebral muscles are in a state of continuous contraction. At rest this muscle tension may subside gradually.

The only other disease which has considerable rigidity with moderate pain is the hypertrophic variety of spondylosis deformans, but this occurs in the older age-groups and the enormous osteophytes and altered vertebral shapes easily distinguish the condition radiologically.

The other features of ankylosing spondylitis are that it is a generalised disease with loss of weight, a raised erythrocyte sedimentation rate, anaemia, and sometimes pyrexia; whereas with the stiff back syndrome and osteitis condensans ilii the patient is perfectly well generally.

Ankylosing spondylitis may start in the sacro-iliac joints when it is sometimes confusingly called sacro-iliitis condensans (Marie-Strumpell) or it may start in the cervical spine (Von Beckterew). Both types spread to affect the whole spine. The longitudinal ligaments become calcified, and so do the capsules of the apophyseal joints and the costo-vertebral joints. The calcification is a sequel to arthritis of these joints, and this distinguishes the disease from other forms of arthritis. Although the prognosis is not good and often the condition progresses to a state of flexion deformity of the whole spine, many cases become quiescent before this occurs, leaving the patient with a rigid chest wall and a rigid spine, yet in reasonable comfort. In the active phase of the disease there may be considerable backache and sometimes girdle pain as the intervertebral foramina become smaller. There are phases of exacerbation and remission. Sometimes the hip joints and shoulder joints become arthritic too. The occipito-atlantal and atlanto-axial joints often remain unaffected.

Because of the tendency to natural and spontaneous resolution of the inflammation in the joints, the disease may be limited and may be very mild. This is the probable explanation of the isolated sacro-iliitis condensans cases and the 'stiff-back' syndrome described below. A rigid chest wall may even be the presenting symptom, with the patient complaining about difficulty in taking a deep breath or about aching in the thoracic spine extending forward to the front of the chest. Such patients breath mainly with the diaphragm and have chest expansion of less than an inch.

X-rays of the sacro-iliac joints especially when taken obliquely show haziness of outline, then erosions and finally bony ankylosis. The vertebral bodies show longitudinal calcification, patchy at first and later continuous, leading to the 'bamboo' effect.

The ache of which patients complain in sacro-iliac disease is a persisting dull bilateral pain which is unaffected by position. The pain may radiate downwards to the posterior aspect of the thighs. If a sacral band which circles the pelvis tightly, gives relief this is good confirmatory evidence of sacro-iliac disease because such a small band cannot limit lumbar spinal movements.

The 'stiff-back' syndrome, as mentioned above, may be an atypical form of ankylosing spondylitis, but it is characterised by much stiffness and dull backache without the patient feeling ill, and there are no abnormal radiological signs nor is the erythrocyte sedimentation rate raised.

In osteopathic practice we see a number of patients who fit into this category, and I know of no satisfactory explanation. Their peripheral joints are perfectly flexible and yet it is a struggle to manipulate their unyielding spines. I have tussled with many of them to no avail, but fortunately the symptoms are not severe and they manage their lives without significant restriction of activity.

Stiffness of the spine can of course be a sequel to prolonged inactivity. or the wearing of a plaster-of-Paris jacket or corset. Usually, however, such stiffness is limited to the lumbar spine whereas the 'stiff-back' syndrome affects all areas of the spine.

Management of ankylosing spondylitis Lasting benefit accrues from deep X-ray therapy and temporary relief of pain is best achieved with phenyl butazone, but X-ray treatment is at present in dispute because of the long-term increased risk of leukaemia.

Manipulation of the spine and exercises to maintain mobility both of the spine and rib cage are not contra-indicated except in an acute phase, when rest in bed may be necessary

There is a limit of course to what can be achieved by manipulative techniques, but no adverse effects occur provided excessive force is not used.

The ribs, their costo-vertebral joints, and the thoracic spine need special attention because limited respiration has more adverse effects on general health than does stiffness in the cervical and lumbar areas.

When the disease is quiescent strong articulation should be applied to all areas, and gradually increased mobility can be achieved so long as complete calcification has not occurred. It is also important to maintain shoulder and hip mobility because of the tendency for these joints to be involved, and in any case restricted spinal mobility increases the need for flexible shoulders and hips.

10 Coccygeal syndrome

Coccydynia may be part of a lumbo-sacral syndrome or it may be due to local changes only.

The coccygeal nerves are the terminal nerves of the cauda equina, and they descend centrally with the filum terminale, which helps to tether the spinal cord to the coccyx. These nerves and the filum terminale can be stretched by central disc prolapses from 3L downwards or by the shelf of a spondylolisthesis or by neoplastic causes within the spinal canal. The filum terminale joins the conus medullaris of the spinal cord to the dorsum of the coccyx. It consists mainly of pia mater and contains nervous elements for half its distance. It pierces the dura mater at the level of 2S and receives an investment from it. It pierces the sacral canal and is inserted into the periosteum of the dorsal surface of the coccyx, so that flexion of the coccyx can have a stretching effect on the filum terminale.

In cases where the coccygeal pain derives from above, the pain is poorly defined and there are no localising signs of abnormality when the coccyx is examined. Sitting in these cases does not hurt, but the act of rising from the sitting position will be painful because of the leverage on the lumbar spine. Removal of the cause in the lumbar area will relieve the coccygeal pain without any local treatment to the coccyx itself.

Local causes of coccygeal pain are adhesions which follow injury to the coccyx or the sacro-coccygeal joint. The injury may lead to displacement to either side or to flexion deformity of the coccyx. The displacement may affect one or more of the segments. The site is best examined in the first place with the patient prone so that the lumbar spine, the sacrum, and the coccyx can be palpated symmetrically. It is a useful test to place the palm of the hand over the sacro-coccygeal area with the fingers pointing towards the lumbar spine, and then apply firm pressure against the point of the coccyx. If the coccyx is palpable in the palm of the hand, then it is vulnerable because it has insufficient soft tissue to protect it from external pressure when sitting. Sometimes the coccyx juts out a long way. Such patients find sitting on a hard chair uncomfortable even when there is nothing wrong with the coccyx itself.

If the coccyx is well protected by soft tissue then nothing but a direct blow could damage it, and the mere act of sitting could not cause pain.

Patients in whom the coccydynia is due to adhesions have pain on sitting, especially when seated on a hard chair. The exact site of tenderness should be located, and if the prone position does not give enough space for the examining finger the patient should be turned on to one side so that an examination per rectum can be made, noting the mobility of the sacro-coccygeal joint and the individual segments of the coccyx with the index finger inside and the thumb outside. Palpation of the coccyx is very easy indeed so long as the patient will relax.

The chief movements are flexion-extension, but some lateral and rotatory mobility is possible and is readily detectable during the examination. Any restriction of movement which is at the same time painful, implies adhesion formation, and the opportunity should be taken straight away to manipulate the coccyx in the direction of the restriction to release the adhesions. Soft tears can be felt during this procedure but strong movements are required and it may be quite painful to do. An anaesthetic, however, is only rarely required for very nervous patients.

When there is local tenderness in the terminal segment or in the levator tissues without limitation of coccygeal movement, the cause is some myofascial disorder of indeterminate nature, but which responds well to infiltration with hydrocortisone. These coccydynias have no history of injury and may be of inflammatory nature in view of the quick response to hydrocortisone.

Rarely is a coccydynia of psychogenic origin, but preoccupation mentally with the perineal or rectal functions may focus attention there. *Proctalgia fugax* is a name given to a condition in which spasm of the coccygeus and levator ani muscles takes place for no accountable reason.

A sympathetic hearing, a careful local examination, and an adequate explanation is the most effective method of dealing with these cases; local treatment should be avoided. If the cause is anxiety then local treatment only confirms the patient's suspicions that there is some disease present which has not been disclosed or discovered. On the other hand it is no use ignoring the symptom until and unless the cause can be discovered and the remedy for the anxiety relieved.

Posture when sitting is important not only for the coccyx but for the lumbar spine as well. A slumping posture causes pressure on the coccyx whereas sitting up relieves the pressure. The point to emphasise regarding sitting posture is that the patient should press the buttocks right to the back of the chair before leaning backwards.

11 Thoracic and rib syndromes

Pain in the thoracic spine is a common symptom. The pain may be central or lateral to the vertebral column, and often it radiates round the chest wall. Most of these pains are mechanically produced.

CLINICAL SPINAL SYNDROMES AND THEIR MANAGEMENT   195

Anterior and lateral chest pain, on the other hand, is more likely to be of visceral origin, especially if it is unaccompanied by spinal pain, yet many types of anterior pain are referred from the back so that *spinal causes must be included in the differential diagnosis of all anterior and lateral chest pain.*

In diagnosis our first task is to establish the pathological process, but it is not the purpose of this book to discuss the differential diagnosis of chest diseases or any other diseases for that matter. This manual attempts to take the practitioner to the next stage, that is, the stage of mechanical diagnosis, when pathological causes for the patient's symptoms have been excluded.

Mechanical causes of thoracic and rib pain are:

1 Apophyseal joint lesions
2 Disc lesions
3 Costo-vertebral and costo-chondral lesions
4 Spondylosis.

Simple *apophyseal joint lesions* in the thoracic spine are always of the hypomobile variety because of the small range of normal movements and the limiting effects of the rib cage. They cause pain at their own level, tenderness at the spines and interspinous ligaments, some tenderness over the corresponding transverse processes, some tension of the adjacent paravertebral muscles, and sometimes skin and subcutaneous tissue changes.

The hypomobile type of apophyseal joint lesion is described in the first syndrome of this chapter (p. 114), and most of the discussion there is applicable to the thoracic column. These lesions are common. In fact very few patients, even though they are consulting about cervical or lumbar symptoms, have perfect thoracic spines. The pain is rarely intense because acute traumatic apophyseal joint sprains are rare whereas chronic lesions are common. The lower thoracic joints are the site of acute lesions whereas the upper and middle thoracic joints are the site of chronic lesions. The springing test (p. 53) with the patient prone gives the best information about local restrictions, and if loss of springiness is detected in one or more thoracic joints the more detailed mobility tests should be applied (p. 57, *Manual of Osteopathic Technique*). When loss of mobility is found in a thoracic joint, then the springiness of the adjacent costo-vertebral joints should also be tested in case there are combined vertebral and rib lesions.

Group lesions in the thoracic spine are common. Several vertebrae take part in a kyphosed, lordosed, or scoliosed area.

In addition to mobility tests the standard tests for the skin, subcutaneous tissue, and muscles must be performed (p. 89).

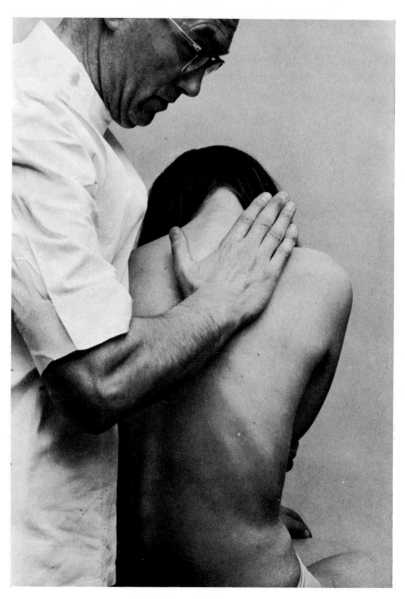

FIG 44 Rib test. Flat of the hands over the angles of the ribs.

A useful *general test for costo-vertebral lesions* apart from the detailed tests (described on p. 65, *Manual of Osteopathic Technique*) is to apply the flat of the hand in the region of the angles of the lower ribs, moving the palm upwards over the angles of successive ribs (*fig. 44*),. The patient should be seated and slightly flexed for this test. An individual lesion

196

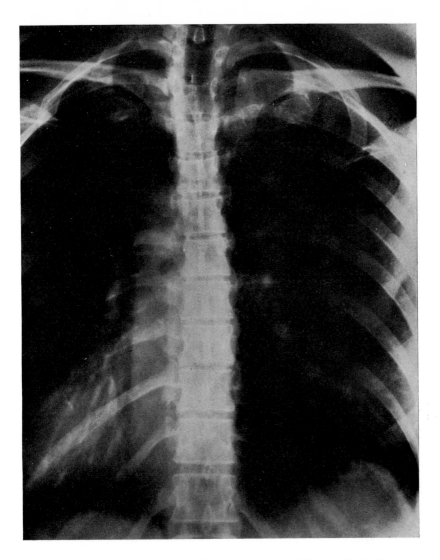

FIG 45 Rib approximations at 4–5 on the right and 6–7–8 on the left.

can be detected by noting undue prominence of the angle of the rib. The prominent rib will be found to be approximated to the rib above. The rib has become relatively fixed to the one above, staying in a position of relative inspiration compared with adjacent ribs (*fig. 45*). The inferior margin of the rib becomes everted slightly owing to the 'bucket-handle' type of movement of ribs during respiration.

Most rib lesions are accompanied by, if not caused by, spasm of the intercostal muscles. A sneeze or a cough with its violent contraction of the whole musculature of the thoracic cage may leave a persistent contraction of one intercostal muscle leading to the approximation of the two ribs. All the intercostal muscles except those between the two implicated ribs relax after the sneeze, but the two ribs involved stay approximated.

The upper of the two ribs may be considered to be in a position of relative expiration and the lower of the two ribs in a position of relative inspiration, but intercostal muscles only actively contract during inspiration and they relax during normal expiration. Forced expiration is a function of the accessory muscles, mainly of the abdominal muscles and the diaphragm. Therefore the net effect of sustained contraction in one intercostal muscle is to elevate the lower rib. An 'inspiratory' type of lesion is thus the only one which can occur from intercostal muscle contraction. These rib lesions with their prominent angles and everted lower edges are therefore the commonest type of rib lesion. The 'expiratory' type of lesion in which the lower rib is held downwards can only occur in the lower ribs—mainly the eleventh and twelfth because of the attachment of the quadratus lumborum to the last rib. The first and second ribs are always inspiratory in type because of the strong attachments of the scalene muscles. These muscles are irritable in brachial-plexus syndromes. They elevate the upper two ribs and diminish the dimensions of the costo-scalene triangle (see p. 214).

The ribs should be palpated from their angles forwards to the sternum, and the inferior edge of the lower rib should be felt and compared with the rib on the other side of the chest. Frequently there is tenderness along the whole intercostal space.

Upper rib lesions cannot be considered in isolation because of their close anatomical links with the cervical spine, the scalene muscles, and Sibson's fascia, and the fact that the pectoral muscles derive their nerve supply from the brachial plexus. Furthermore the rhomboids and levator angulae scapulae muscles are often irritated by lower cervical lesions of various sorts.

Likewise floating ribs cannot be considered except in relation to the lumbar spine because of the attachments of the quadratus lumborum and diaphragm.

Tenderness and tension in the trapezius, rhomboids, and levator scapulae muscles are more likely to be secondary to lower cervical lesions than to upper thoracic ones; but local tenderness in the spinous processes and interspinous ligaments, and reduced mobility in the upper thoracic joints, is evidence of lesions in those upper thoracic joints. These lesions are often unrecognised, yet they can cause symptoms both posteriorly and anteriorly.

Anterior chest pain though often ascribed to heart, lung, and pleural disorders is frequently due to lower cervical mechanical disorders mediating via the pectoral muscles.

Tenderness over the angles of ribs should always lead to palpation of the corresponding interspace between the ribs anteriorly, where unsuspected tenderness can be elicited even though the patient is not complaining of anterior chest pain.

The techniques for manipulation of the thoracic and rib lesions are described on p. 166, *Manual of Osteopathic Technique*. It is easy to obtain separational clicks in the apophyseal joints of the thoracic area, but to be effective the techniques must be accurately localised. Once the lesion has been delineated by mobility tests, the practitioner must not loose his contact with the appropriate spinous or transverse processes while positioning the patient for adjustment, otherwise the effectiveness of the treatment will be reduced. One or two palpable and audible clicks may be quite irrelevant because they may come from adjacent joints. Only a separational click in the restricted joint indicates effective treatment.

Thoracic disc protrusion   Post-mortem studies of the thoracic spine show that protrusions in this area are common even though they are clinically of less significance than are cervical and lumbar disc protrusions.

Thoracic pain, especially when accompanied by girdle pain, which has a sudden onset for no apparent reason and for which no pathological explanation can be found, is probably due to a disc protrusion. The pain may be intense and any movement—even breathing—can be enough to accentuate the pain. Certainly coughing and sneezing accentuate it. The pain of pleurisy is accentuated by breathing, but in these cases breathing is checked at a certain phase of inspiration: the breathing 'catches' and the pain suddenly stops further inspiration. The reverse holds for a disc protrusion because full inspiration, so long as it is smooth and gentle, can be achieved without pain; but when the breathing is hurried or accompanied by thoracic movement then pain is provoked.

A rib lesion as described in the previous section may sometimes be secondary to a thoracic disc protrusion with its referred intercostal pain and intercostal muscle spasm. When the contraction of the intercostal muscles has been sustained long enough the lower rib may remain elevated permanently.

Thoracic disc protrusions are less serious than are cervical and lumbar protrusions because the intervertebral foramina are comparatively larger, so that symptoms are less common. Furthermore each nerve-root has a much smaller distribution compared with those of the brachial and sacral plexuses.

As has been stated in other sections, discs do not herniate or prolapse unless they are weakened by degeneration or by previous injury. The commonest disease to weaken cartilage is osteochondrosis, but this often passes unnoticed because in the majority the symptoms are so slight. However, if wedging of the vertebral bodies in the lower thoracic spine is an indication of old osteochondrosis, then the disease is very common indeed in patients who have disc dysfunction (see p. 240).

The clinical distinction between those patients who have nerve root pressure and those who have none is as useful in the thoracic spine as it is in the lumbar and cervical spines because treatment of the two is different. With the thoracic and milder cases, in which we make an assumption of herniation rather than full prolapse of the disc, the technique of adjustive manual traction should be used.

Adjustive manual traction for thoracic disc herniations is best applied with the patient supine on a table (*fig. 21*, p. 116). The ankles need to be strapped to the two corners at one end of the table. It is inadequate to have assistants to tether the feet because the pull cannot be fully synchronised. The table should have a smooth top, and a blanket should separate the patient from the table-top. The object of this is to allow some sliding on the smooth surface without the patient's skin sticking to the table-top. One small pillow should support the head. The operator sits at the head of the table on a stool of the appropriate height to enable him to grasp the patient's chin and occiput comfortably, and to be able to apply traction with his arms straight and in line with the spine.

The ideal table for this technique is one with a centre pedestal so that the operator can place his feet on the base of the pedestal, and lean back while holding the patient's occiput with the right hand and her chin with his left hand. A firm grip is necessary under the occiput because most of the traction has to be applied there. The left hand applies some traction to the patient's chin, but this hold is mainly used to prevent the head from being flexed too much by the operator's right hand. Two fingers are sufficient on the chin and the other fingers should be loosely resting under the chin, making sure that they are not exerting any pressure on the patient's throat. The operator's left thumb should only rest on her cheek and not exert any pressure there.

The next step is to take up the slack—i.e. to stretch the patient so that the slack in the ankle straps and the sliding of the blanket on the table-top is taken up. The patient should now be encouraged to relax while the method of traction is explained to her.

The operator leans back and gives one or two preliminary tugs so that the patient knows what to expect, and to show that her head will not come off! The traction must be applied in a rhythmic manner, say, at the rate of twice per second. This enables the operator to sense the elasticity of the patient's spine and to regulate the rhythm of the pull to the elastic recoil which is natural to that patient. The small light patient will have a quicker rate compared with the large heavy patient. The operator soon should sense the rate at which he can apply his traction. After perhaps six or seven pulls he should feel the patient relax, and at that moment he should give another stronger pull. Continuous strong traction will not achieve the same effect because the patient cannot relax well. Furthermore a short sharp tug need not be so fierce as a long straight pull.

The patient will experience a sense of relief during the traction, though there may be a painful click at the moment of the final tug. If pain occurs at the start of the pull, then the probability is that there are adhesions tethering the joint at the site of pain. This technique is safe to use in either disc herniations or adhesions, and even if it does not achieve its objective it will do no harm. The decision as to when to apply this technique, bearing in mind the acuteness of the disc herniation, is discussed on p. 117. Similar considerations apply to the thoracic spine. The risk of accentuating the symptoms is much less in the thoracic spine as compared with the cervical and lumbar areas, but I would hesitate to use the technique when considerable muscle guarding is palpable.

When a *disc has prolapsed in the thoracic spine* the above adjustive manual traction will be ineffective. This technique together with other manipulations are contra-indicated until the acute symptoms have subsided. The patient must be rested in the position which hurts least, and supported by strapping to reduce rib movements. Heat and analgesics should be administered. The acute phase subsides more quickly than it does in cervical and lumbar disc prolapses, and the patient should be reasonably comfortable within ten days.

Costo-vertebral, costo-chondral, interchondral, and sternal joint syndromes
Lesions of the costo-vertebral joints have already been described (p. 196).

There are three costo-vertebral joints for each rib. With the exception of the first, the eleventh, and the twelfth ribs, the head of each rib articulates with two adjacent vertebrae and with one transverse process. The movements are small and gliding to enable hinge-like or 'pump-handle' movements and rotatory or 'bucket-handle' movements to occur during respiration. There is an additional movement of the lower ribs consisting of lateral expansion of the rib cage, but this is effected mainly through the elasticity of the ribs themselves.

These costo-vertebral joints become arthritic in ankylosing spondylitis and they seriously limit rib movements. They are also the site of osteo-arthritis in older people, but the frequent appearance on thoracic X-rays of osteophytes at these joints does not imply that the arthritis is clinically active. When actively inflamed, the movements of the lower ribs are painful beyond the quiet respiratory range. The upper and middle costo-vertebral joints are rarely affected by osteo-arthritis.

In scolioses considerable adaptation has to occur in these joints yet little pain arises from them, presumably because the formation of a scoliosis is slow and adaptation has time to take place.

In chest surgery considerable separational force is used to give access between adjacent ribs, and the costo-vertebral joints are severely strained at the time of operation. Some patients have intercostal pain following such surgery, but surprisingly few, and I can only assume that recovery is good because of continuous movement at these small joints from respiration during recovery.

Whenever rib lesions occur as described in the previous section there is inevitably some restriction of movement of the lower of the two ribs at its costo-vertebral joint. However, movements at the costo-vertebral joint are not palpable. The only clincial tests which are helpful in gauging the mobility of the costo-vertebral joints are the ones which test the overall mobility of the ribs. These tests are described on p. 66 of my *Manual of Osteopathic Technique*.

The springing tests for the thoracic vertebrae can be applied laterally over the angles of the ribs, and any sense of resistance there is probably in the costo-vertebral joints. There is usually some local tenderness lateral to the transverse process in the region of the angle of the rib.

The *costo-chondral joints* are often tender in patients who have costo-vertebral restrictions, and both ends of the ribs must be palpated.

These costo-chondral joints are sometimes injured by direct blows. The pain and swelling occurs at the junction of the bone and cartilage, and there may be some displacement between the two. These junctions are about an inch lateral to the lateral margins of the sterum.

The *interchondral* joints are situated between the sixth to tenth ribs anteriorly. Sometimes these junctions are ruptured by injury and the friction can be palpated by holding both the external and internal surfaces at the costal margin moving the cartilages on each other. If one is detached it will click with this test. Patients often become aware of this abnormal movement, and it can become a nuisance especially when sitting or leaning to the same side.

In all these painful sites the corresponding thoracic joints and ribs must be checked mechanically and corrected if faulty.

If no lesions can be detected posteriorly then it is useful to treat the cartilage tenderness with hydrocortisone injections.

Tietze's syndrome is a clinical condition in which one or more of the costal cartilages are painful and swollen. The aetiology of the condition is not known, but it is usually self-limiting and relatively unimportant.

Occasionally the sternal joint between the manubrium and the body of the sternum becomes tender and inflamed. It sometimes clicks during deep respiration.

It is probable that the process of calcification of costal cartilages can be temporarily disturbed to produce local tenderness and pain. The elasticity of the rib cage gradually diminishes as more calcification takes place.

Thoracic spondylosis A description of thoracic spondylosis can be found under the kyphosis syndromes (p. 245). It is characterised by stiffness and a uniform kyphosis. Pain is infrequent, though a dull intermittent backache occurs if its course is prolonged. Interscapular 'fibrositis' is common. There may be a localised scoliosis affecting three or four vertebrae. Group lesions, i.e. several hypomobile lesions together, predispose to spondylosis later. Rib lesions occur secondarily to scoliosis or kyphosis. The symptoms tend to smoulder on for years. Occasionally through some additional mechanical strain acute attacks of pain occur, but the acute symptoms only last for twenty-four to forty-eight hours.

12 Brachial syndromes

The cervical spine is usually considered anatomically and functionally as a unit, but in clinical practice it is convenient to divide the neck into two areas, because the syndromes arising from mechanical faults above the level of 4C differ considerably from those arising below 4C. The brachial plexus derives nerve-roots from 4C to 2T, and therefore it is convenient in the discussion of brachial syndromes to include all mechanical problems which encompass 4C to 2T.

Anatomical considerations It is assumed that the reader of this book has a good knowledge of the anatomy of the area, and it is no part of my task to set down obvious anatomical facts, but certain anatomical and mechanical implications should be stressed before embarking on the separate descriptions of various brachial syndromes which are enumerated below.

The cervical spinal column is remarkable in several respects and I would recommend that the student should have a further look at some cervical vertebrae to confirm the following points.

The column has to protect the spinal cord, which as we know carries almost all the nerves to the rest of the body. Any disease of the cervical column can therefore have a much wider effect than a similar disease in the thoracie and lumbar columns.

The neck has to be mobile and yet it has no supports like the ribs or the pelvis in the other areas.

It has to support the skull as well as withstand considerable leverage when the arms are used powerfully.

It carries its own blood-supply from the vertebral arteries and veins; and, although these vessels are well protected in the transverse processes, the vessels themselves complicate mechanical problems in the region of the intervertebral foramina.

Because of the lack of extraneous supports the vertebrae are designed to support each other. Lateral shearing movement is checked by the upward projecting processes from the vertebral bodies where they form the neuro-central joints of Luschka. Backward shearing movement is checked by the downward projecting processes from the antero-inferior margins of the vertebral bodies, and forward shearing movement is checked by the articular processes. The vertebral arches are of strong compact bone, and the laminae are joined by the strong elastic ligamenta flava. Weight-bearing is shared by the vertebral bodies and the posterior columns made by the articular processes.

The other processes differ from those in other areas of the spine in that the transverse processes are bifid, very short, and virtually impalpable. The articular processes, on the other hand, are large and readily palpable. The spinous processes are bifid and irregular, and they are useless for positional diagnosis. Only the articular processes can be relied on for positional diagnosis. The 7C spine is large and comparable with the thoracic spines. The shorter 6C spine is useful when palpating for levels because this process sinks right away from the palpating finger during backward-bending of the neck.

The transverse processes are grooved in such a way as to form a channel for the emerging spinal nerves. This groove is best seen by looking at the cervical column laterally to see the shape of the intervertebral foramen.

The nerve-roots pursue a chequered course from their source in the spinal cord through to the axilla. Each root has its anterior and posterior components which are covered by dural sleeves. The dorsal root divides into bundles—as many as fifteen bundles—before it enters the cord. The ventral root derives from two or three bundles arising from the antero-lateral aspect of the cord. Some of the posterior bundles lie directly in contact with the anterior part of the capsule of the apophyseal joints. Separate anterior and posterior roots traverse the foramen. The posterior root ganglia are close to the junction of dorsal and ventral roots, and they lie in the groove on the superior surface of the transverse processes beyond the intervertebral foramina.

Mechanical pressure exerted by factors which reduce the size of the intervertebral foramen tends to affect one or other of the roots, but especially the posterior root, and because of this, sensory symptoms predominate over motor symptoms.[85]

The nerve-roots span two discs in the upper cervical region whereas they span only one disc in the lower cervical region as they pass laterally from the cord to the intervertebral foramen. This can influence the distribution of pain from disc prolapses at different levels.

When the length of the cervical column is shortened by thinning of disc spaces, this alters the angle which the nerve-root makes at its exit from the intervertebral foramen. Because the cord remains the same length, the inferior bundles tend to become kinked at their exit.

The scalene muscles are attached to the anterior and posterior tubercles of the transverse processes, but in addition some fibres are attached to the nerve sheaths, so that tension of these scalene muscles can exert a traction effect on the nerve-roots.

The brachial plexus is formed by the 5C–1T nerve-roots. Occasionally it is prefixed to include 4C, and sometimes post-fixed to include 2T, and the roots join together to form the upper, middle, and lower trunks of the plexus, as they descend between the scalene muscles. The scalene muscles are attached inferiorly to the first and second ribs. The triangle formed between the anterior and middle scalene muscles and the first rib is known as the costo-scalene triangle.

Tension of the scalene muscles, which is a common accompaniment of brachial syndromes and can be detected by palpation, further embarrasses the brachial plexus by reducing the size of the costo-scalene triangle not only by pulling on the nerve-roots but also by lateral pressure and by elevation of the first rib. The lower trunk of the brachial plexus has to rise above the rib before it joins the rest of the plexus, so that lesions in the mid-cervical region can irritate the scalene muscles and indirectly influence the lower trunk of the plexus. The tension on the lower trunk is still further increased when congenital cervical ribs are present.

The next mechanical hazard of the brachial plexus is where it lies between the clavicle and the first rib. When these two bones press against each other they impinge first on the brachial vein then on the brachial artery. If space is greatly limited then the plexus can be compressed. These points are discussed under the thoracic outlet syndrome (p. 215).

The vertebral artery and vein traverse the foramina transversario from 6 or 7C to 2C. They lie anterior to the nerve-roots, and they are accompanied by numerous sympathetic nerves. A spinal artery enters each intervertebral foramen and divides into anterior and posterior spinal branches. The arterial supply and venous drainage of the spinal cord is described on p. 169.

The intervertebral foramen is bounded anteriorly by a disc and a joint of Luschka, posteriorly by a capsule of an apophyseal joint, and superiorly and inferiorly by grooves in the pedicles of the vertebrae.

Although 'foramen' is a correct concept, the nerve-roots really transverse a 'tunnel' formed inferiorly and superiorly by the transverse process, posteriorly by the scalenus medius muscle, and anteriorly by the scalenus anticus muscle. This tunnel is perforated transversely by the vertebral artery and vein in a vertical direction.

All these elements have to be considered in the mechanical problems of brachial syndromes.

The foramina and the tunnels can be distorted and diminished by:

Disc protrusions
Osteophytes from the vertebral body margin and neuro-central joints
Osteophytes from the apophyseal joints
Narrowing of the disc space
Tension of the scalene muscles
Swelling of the capsules of the apophyseal joints
Swelling of the nerve-roots
Venous congestion.

Most of these factors operate in the middle age-groups, and the whole picture can be further complicated by loss of elasticity in ligaments, capsules, and blood-vessel walls.

In the young there is plenty of room and everything is elastic and the 'dead' space is filled with fat. There is inherent elasticity in the nerve-roots and the pia and arachnoid, though the dural sheath is inextensible. There is ample flexibility to allow free movement of nerve-roots though the intervertebral foramina during the movements of flexion, extension, side-bending, and rotation.

Extension of the neck can produce direct pressure on the cord by impingement of the ligamentum flavum.[85] This does not matter in the young and when the extension is not maintained for too long, but it can matter a great deal in the elderly when elasticity diminishes and even the normal erect position entails some increase of lordosis. As age advances the thickness of discs throughout the spine reduces, and this increases the kyphosis of the thoracic spine. This throws the head forwards and makes the individual look downwards, but to compensate for this the head is tilted backwards and so the cervical lordosis is increased.

Sudden hyperextension, as in car crashes, can damage the cord even though no bony damage is demonstrable. Quadriplegia has resulted from such injuries without fractures.[86]

Another consideration is that the size of the nerve-root is small compared with the size of the foramen, and considerable bony encroachment may *not* produce any symptoms at all. X-ray appearances can therefore be misleading. Most osteophytes as seen on the X-rays are smaller than in reality because they are capped with chondrophytes. Furthermore the degree of inflammation cannot be judged from X-ray appearances.

Trying to correlate X-ray findings with clinical findings is additionally confused because there can be a lack of correspondence between vertebral and neurological segments, as prefixing and post-fixing of the plexus occurs in 11–12 per cent of patients.[87] The seventh cervical nerve—the largest of them all—passes through the smallest foramen. It makes up the medial cord of the plexus in the majority of anatomical specimens, but it joins the lateral cord in 17 per cent of dissections and the inferior cord in 10 per cent of dissections.

In addition to the anatomical hazards of the brachial plexus, the mere weight of the upper extremities and the breasts has a traction effect on the plexus. Poor posture, the carrying of heavy weights for prolonged periods, and poor muscle tone all contribute as aetiological factors in the mechanics of brachial syndromes.

Acute cervical joint sprains These are characterised by pain and stiffness which develop rapidly after a neck injury. The syndrome is influenced by the severity of the injury, the direction of the force, and the age of the patient. During recovery adhesions may form to reduce mobility.

Severe injuries to the cervical column, like fractures, dislocations, or cord damage, are not considered here because they belong to the field of traumatic orthopaedic surgery; but the damage caused by less severe injuries may go unrecognised merely because the standard X-rays show no bony damage. All such patients should have mobility X-rays taken, and abnormal or hypermobile joints should be treated accordingly. In the hypermobile joint the anterior longitudinal ligament has probably been torn; if not treated properly the injury will give rise to persisting symptoms, and later to considerable degenerative changes in the affected joint.

Torsional injuries can give rise to sprains of the apophyseal joints with or without positional displacement. Sufficient time must be given to allow for recovery before manipulation is used in treatment. If restricted mobility ensues then the appropriate manipulation should be made according to the direction in which restriction persists, and the level at which the sprain has occurred.

The twisting sprain may not be one sharp twist—it can happen, for example, when sleeping in the prone position with the head turned to one side. The sustained twisted position can cause an acute apophyseal joint lesion characterised by pain, swelling, and restricted mobility of the joint itself as well as some overall restriction of neck movements.

'Joint bind' (see p. 82) is common in the cervical spine but it merely gives rise to local stiffness and discomfort rather than to acute pain, and this is easily treated by manipulation.

A true subluxation of the apophyseal joints can occur when the inferior facet of the vertebra above catches on the superior margin of the superior facet of the vertebra below. There is an accompanying kyphosis. This subluxation must be reduced as early as possible. As a rule adjustive manual traction is sufficient without recourse to torsional techniques.

An *inflammatory* type (see p. 136) of apophyseal joint lesion occurs in the cervical spine, particularly at the 2–5C joints. This may be an exacerbation of osteo-arthritis of the apophyseal joint or even a rheumatoid arthritic phenomenon, but an isolated inflammatory lesion can occur for no apparent reason.

The pain is intense and mobility is correspondingly reduced. The range may be limited to a few degrees, because any attempt to move further accentuates the pain and the patient is unwilling to move especially to the affected side whether in rotation or side-bending, though it may well permit some rotation and side-bending to the other side. The patient may prefer to keep her head rotated away from the painful side. Palpation will reveal an acutely sensitive and swollen apophyseal joint. Forward-bending is usually free but backward-bending is considerably limited—i.e. any movement which approximates the facets together provokes severe pain.

The inflammation subsides in two to five days, and the best treatment is heat and rest. Any attempt at manipulation is contra-indicated—in fact, the patient will hardly bear the practitioner to palpate the joint let alone move it. A rubber collar is the best way to provide rest both by day and night.

This syndrome occurs at any age from childhood upwards, though after the age of fifty years the syndrome would suggest a flare up of osteo-arthritis in an apophyseal joint. In this 'inflammatory' syndrome the X-rays show no bony abnormality. I cannot offer any satisfactory explanation, and medical textbooks refer to the syndrome as *acute torticollis*, offering no satisfactory explanation. The condition is not due to an isolated spasm of the sternomastoid muscle, and it bears no relationship to spasmodic torticollis. It would be better described as an acute synovitis of an apophyseal joint, because the swelling is very obvious and at recovery it disappears. It may leave a restricted joint with adhesions, and, if full movements are not restored within say a fortnight, manipulation can be safely carried out as described for the adhesive syndrome. Detailed techniques depend upon the type of restriction and each is described in my *Manual of Osteopathic Technique.*

Such acute apophyseal synovitis is rarely if ever accompanied by nerve-root pressure signs, and the foraminal compression test is negative in the sense that peripheral pain is not provoked by side-bending to the side of pain or by backward-bending. Any movement provokes pain, and the head is held stationary in the position of least pain. When there is referred pain it arises from sustained muscle guarding and is limited to the neck muscles.

Any attempt to apply traction evokes more acute pain and will not be tolerated by the patient. This is in sharp contrast to the case of the patient with a disc prolapse who obtains quick relief from traction.

Hypermobile cervical joints These only occur at the 5–6–7C joints. The subject of hypermobility is discussed in general on p. 119. It may be a sequel to injury or excessive manipulation, or it may occur during a phase of degeneration in a disc.

The condition may be suspected clinically but the diagnosis can only firmly be made by mobility X-rays.

One curious type of hypermobility occurs at 6–7C when, during side-bending, there is excessive rotation. When comparing the two X-ray films, one side-bending to the left and the other to the right, the spinous process of 6C is seen to be well to the left in side-bending to the right, and well to the right in side-bending to the left.

Hypermobile joints should not be manipulated because this only aggravates the pain. A collar may help, but so often the patient has had symptoms for years without the proper diagnosis being established that a collar by itself is insufficient. Then we have to have recourse to sclerosing injections (p. 126).

If there is an accompanying upper thoracic rigidity this area should be manipulated well, taking care over locking techniques to avoid putting any strain on to the hypermobile cervical joint.

Prolonged immobilisation in a cervical collar is undesirable in that it may set up physical and psychological symptoms which are worse than the original ones. The patient may become too nervous to dispense with the collar, and the musculature too weak to sustain the head properly on the neck. It can be extremely difficult to wean such patients away from their collars, especially when pain recurs as soon as they dispense with the support. Six weeks should be the limit for wearing a cervical collar in any condition. If symptoms persist after this length of time, the diagnosis and treatment must be seriously reconsidered.

Immobilisation can lead to adhesion formation, which in turn can cause pain and confuse the issue. Most collars are used on the assumption that the patient has a disc protrusion. The collar gives relief because movement provokes pain. Gradually the symptoms subside and all is thought to be well, but adhesions form and then similar pain occurs with movement. It is not always easy to differentiate pain arising in the first place from the protrusion and later from adhesions. Certainly the patient cannot differentiate them, and the anxiety created by thinking the disc is still 'out' can be a serious problem in management.

Cervical disc protrusions The order of frequency of cervical disc protrusions is 5–6C, 6–7C, and 4–5C. 3–4C and 7C–1T disc protrusions are rare. Mechanically the 5–6–7C joints are the most vulnerable to mechanical strain because of the leverage of the head on the neck and the relative stability of the upper thoracic joints.

Characteristic syndrome—Such patients frequently suffer from episodes of stiff neck and 'fibrositis' of the trapezius and/or interscapular muscles for several years before one of the discs herniates. Then pain is acute, movements are restricted, and referred pain spreads into the sclerotome distribution of the affected level, but not until signs of nerve-root pressure occur can a definite diagnosis of a prolapsed disc be made.

The foraminal compression test and traction tests will help to clarify the diagnosis. When a nerve-root is being irritated or compressed in the lower cervical area, then backward-bending and side-bending to the painful side increases pain and/or paraesthesiae. The distribution of the symptoms indicates the level of the lesion, but the considerations mentioned before make an exact diagnosis of level difficult.

The traction test is the application of a pull on the head at 20°–30° of neck flexion and away from the painful side. If this gives relief of pain or paraesthesiae it is confirmatory evidence of the diagnosis of nerve-root compression in one of the intervertebral foramina.

It should be noted that insufficient traction may not relieve the pain and paraesthesiae. 30–35 lb of pull is usually necessary to give relief, but then if the pull is increased say beyond 40 lb the pain may return.

A frequent accompanying symptom is a sense of neck weakness with the pain, leading to inability of the patient to raise her head off the pillow and a desire to support her head with her hands as she descends into the supine position.

If there has been an injury antecedent to the onset of pain, there is a delay of several hours before the symptoms become acute. This point helps in the differential diagnosis from apophyseal joint lesions.

A rough guide as to the level of the nerve compressed is given below:

5C Pain over the lateral aspect of the shoulder to the arm, and over the pectoral and scapular areas; sometimes loss of power in the deltoid, supraspinatus, and infraspinatus muscles; irritability of the trapezius, levator angulae scapulae, and rhomboid muscles, with normal reflexes.
6C Pain extending further down to the dorsum of the wrist and to the thumb and index finger; paraesthesiae in the same distribution; sluggish biceps jerk.
7C Pain extending from the neck the whole way down the arm and forearm to the index, middle, and ring fingers. The triceps jerk may be sluggish and weakness of grip may develop.
8C The pain extends from the axilla down the medial side of the arm to the ring and little fingers. The triceps jerk may be absent with weakness of the muscle, as well as of the extensors of the wrist and fingers. The first thoracic nerve joins the eighth cervical nerve to form the ulnar nerve, and its distribution is similar.

These distributions are only an approximate guide, and local mobility tests are necessary to define the level of the lesion. A sense of blocking to movement at that level is felt (see p. 96). The side-bending mobility tests, which in effect cause foraminal compression, indicate the level of the lesion once the acute phase has subsided, but in the early stages too much muscle spasm prevents accurate localisation.

Management of cervical disc protrusions If a disc has herniated and there is some prospect of reducing it, then adjustive manual traction should be applied on the earliest possible occasion.

The technique is described on pp. 116, 200. Muscle guarding may prevent the reduction, but guarding is less intense than in the lumbar area and it can often be overcome by some preliminary traction—i.e. intermittent sustained traction.

Specific adjustments involving side-bending and rotation should only be used if the adjustive manual traction technique has failed. Then the side-bending and rotation and thrust should be combined with traction. The thrust must only be used on the painless side, because side-bending to the painful side merely jams the foramina, hurts the patient, and irritates the nerve. This practical point is stressed by Maigne.[88] He called it the 'rule of no pain', and implies that the manipulation should be directed in such a manner as to avoid pain. It is especially applicable in acute disc lesions, but not to other less severe lesions.

Following the reduction of the disc herniation, the neck should be protected from strains by a rubber inflatable collar. The collar should be worn at night also, because of the risk of strain if the pillow is too high or if the head slips off the pillow. The collar prevents sudden and unexpected movements, and thus diminishes the risk of further attacks.

Once the muscle guarding has subsided, the patient will be anxious to remove the collar and this is safe to do, so long as jerky movements (like riding in a car) or vigorous housework are avoided. Care must be exercised in this way for at least six weeks to allow full recovery of the annulus fibrosus and the longitudinal ligaments.

If nerve-root compression or irritation persists in spite of manipulation then the condition should be treated with *intermittent sustained traction*. The method can be applied manually or with the use of a halter. The method is described in the *Manual of Osteopathic Technique*, p. 248. The principle is to use traction with the patient supine and the neck flexed to 30°. An element of side-bending is sometimes an advantage, provided the side-bending is away from the painful side and so long as the pain is better relieved that way rather than by straight traction.

Vertical traction with the patient seated or standing is, in my experience, much less satisfactory. There is more apprehension and therefore less relaxation. The halter tends to create backward-bending which defeats the object of the traction. Vertical traction has no advantage over supine traction to my knowledge. The effective pull is in the order of 35 lb, but it should be applied very slowly, taking several seconds to achieve the full 35 lb. Then the pull should be sustained for say twenty seconds before it is slowly released. Any sudden release is liable to cause an exacerbation of pain. If this happens in spite of care in reducing the pull it at least confirms the diagnosis of foraminal compression pain, and then consideration should be given to applying *continuous traction*.

Continuous cervical traction is indicated only in cases with severe root pains in which intermittent sustained traction is inadequate. When adequate, intermittent traction is far better on two counts—firstly that it can be applied to an out-patient and secondly that it is a more physiological procedure because it enables decongestion to take place. Static traction leads to a slowing-up of circulation in the area and it can cause permanent weakness of the ligaments. Static traction can be applied with a halter attached to weights over a pulley in bed. The neck needs to be kept flexed to 30°, and the weight required depends upon the response, but usually less than 35 lb brings relief because elongation gradually takes place.

Intermittent sustained traction applied as above should be repeated six to eight times and can be applied daily. The less severe cases progress well with alternate days' treatment, and some will make good progress even when traction is applied every third day.

About 90 per cent of patients with acute brachial neuritis due to disc protrusions respond well to this method. However, some are resistent, and these need manipulating followed by more traction. In ideal conditions manipulation should be applied first to remove pressure from the nerve-root and then followed by intermittent sustained traction. This combination gives the quickest response.

Sometimes a collar is needed to prevent the patient from making movements which irritate the nerve-root. The rubber inflatable type is best in most cases because it allows a little mobility which reduces the risk of adhesion formation.

Other physiotherapy measures can be used, infra-red heat is comforting but does not alter the course of the disorder. The position of the head on the pillow is important when resting, and the pillow should provide support in the least painful position—usually about 30° of flexion. Short-wave diathermy is contra-indicated because in practice it is found to accentuate the pain presumably by increasing congestion in the spinal canal and foramina.

Foraminal compression syndrome It is not always possible to be sure of the cause of nerve-root irritation in the cervical spine even though there is a positive foraminal compression sign. The size is diminished by several causes (enumerated on p. 206), but whatever the cause, treatment by intermittent sustained traction is appropriate. Manipulation is sometimes contra-indicated—e.g. if there is active osteo-arthritis of the apophyseal joints, manipulation is liable to increase the inflammation. Manipulation can wait until the inflammation has subsided, and even then manipulation must be used carefully. It is better as a rule just to apply articulatory techniques of mobilisation in osteo-arthritis of the apophyseal joints. Specific adjustments may jar adjacent rough surfaces and increase inflammation.

In all cases of foraminal compression syndrome the patient must be warned not to adopt a position of backward-bending—at least not to stay in such a position because of the risk of accentuating the symptoms. Many acute foraminal compression syndromes have been provoked, for example, by painting the ceiling, star-gazing, or looking up at a cinema screen from the stalls. The cheaper gallery seats are much safer!

On the same basis neck exercises should be avoided, especially backward bending and circumduction.

If in spite of traction and/or manipulation progress is slow, and especially if movements provoke pain, a collar becomes necessary to check the vicious circle of pain causing muscle spasm, causing compression, causing more pressure on the root, causing more pain, causing more swelling, causing more pressure, causing more pain, etc.

Thoracic outlet syndromes Under this heading factors like scalene muscle tension, reduction in the size of the costo-scalene triangle, elevated first ribs, congenital cervical ribs, and costo-clavicular compression can all play their part in the production of pain in the arm, and there may be considerable overlapping of these factors.

Typically there are two syndromes here. A costo-scalene syndrome in which the predominant symptom is pain in the ulnar distribution of the forearm; and a costo-clavicular syndrome in which venous congestion and swelling of the hand, together with paraesthesiae of the whole hand, are the predominant symptoms.

Costo-scalene syndrome

When the brachial plexus has traversed the intervertebral foramen, it may become squeezed by a reduction in the space between the first rib and the scalene muscles. If the costo-scalene triangle is already reduced in dimensions by a congenital cervical rib or a fibrous band situated in place of this rib, then the lower trunk of the brachial plexus has to rise higher and is relatively more easily kinked or compressed.

Ulnar distribution of pain should always arouse suspicion about the costo-scalene triangle, and the first-rib area should be carefully palpated. First-rib lesions may be secondary to positional faults at 1 and 2T, as is seen on this X-ray (*fig. 46*), or the rib may be elevated by tension in the scalene muscles. The nerve-supply to these muscles derive from every level of the cervical spine below 3C, so that any lesion—apophyseal or disc lesion—can irritate these muscles to elevate the first and second ribs and squeeze the triangle.

The management of the costo-scalene syndrome may be similar to the management of these cervical lesions, but specific adjustments of the first and second ribs may be necessary. The techniques for manipulating these ribs is described on p. 175 of my *Manual of Osteopathic Technique.*

If all these measures fail and there is strong evidence that the first rib or a cervical rib is at fault, then surgery to divide the rib is indicated. Sometimes division of the scalene muscle attachment is sufficient to afford relief.

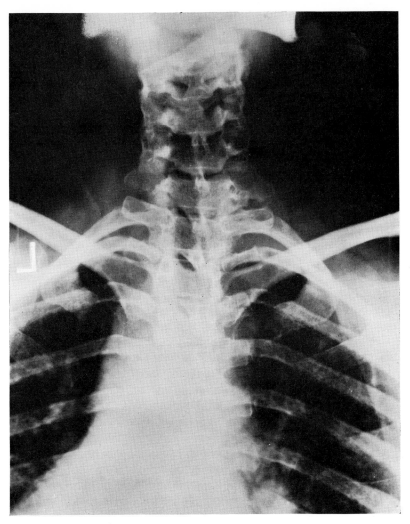

FIG 46 Elevation and approximation of the 1st and 2nd left ribs. Convexity to the left in the upper thoracic spine.

Costo-clavicular compression syndrome

The typical pattern of symptoms in these cases is a feeling of swelling and stiffness in one hand, an increase of numbness, and then tingling. Pain is not a feature.

Compression of the median nerve in the carpal tunnel may accompany it, and there is some overlap of these two syndromes.

The patient may waken in the night with these sensations, or they may come on during the day if the position of sitting is cramped and sustained—for example, these symptoms developed in one patient when at the cinema because the film was exciting and she held the seat tightly for an hour or so!

The simple test to see whether the patient is predisposed to this syndrome is to palpate the radial pulses with the shoulders elevated and then with the shoulders braced down and backwards. If the radial pulse is obliterated in the latter position then the site of the pressure on the artery can only be between the first rib and the clavicle.

If the sign is positive it does not prove that the patient is in fact suffering from a costo-clavicular compression syndrome, but it does indicate a vulnerability. Anterior to the subclavian artery, as it crosses the first rib to be renamed the axillary artery, lies the insertion of the scalenus anticus muscle, and still further forward is the subclavian vein.

Any pressure strong enough to obliterate the artery will certainly obliterate the vein, and while it is rare to observe patients with arterial compression, it is not so rare for venous obstruction to occur from costo-clavicular compression. The swelling of the hand and arm may only be sufficient to cause discomfort—perhaps a ring on one of the fingers is difficult to get off whereas at other times it slips off easily.

If the swelling, discomfort and paraesthesiae, affect the whole of one hand and are unilateral the diagnosis of costo-clavicular compression is more likely. If both hands are involved this diagnosis is less likely (see p. 218). If paraesthesiae affect all the fingers and thumb, the diagnosis is more likely than if only one or two fingers are involved.

Treatment of this syndrome involves exercises to elevate the shoulders. The patient should be instructed not to adopt positions likely to bring on the pressure. She should not carry heavy shopping bags more than for short distances. The whole question of posture should be more than usually checked and corrected. Resting the elbows on the arms of a suitable chair can help the patient to elevate the shoulder girdle without any effort.

Peripheral nerve lesions of the upper extremity When the brachial plexus separates into its cords, divisions, and nerves, it is well protected and surrounded by soft structures in the axilla, but the radial nerve is occasionally compressed as it spirals round the humerus posteriorly. The ulnar nerve also can be irritated or compressed in the groove between the medial epicondyle of the humerus and the olecranon of the ulna. The median nerve is vulnerable to compression as it traverses the carpal tunnel. In addition, the long thoracic nerve and circumflex nerves are sometimes affected mechanically.

Winged scapula

The long thoracic nerve, which arises from 5, 6 and 7C, makes its own way independently of the brachial plexus to the serratus anterior. In some positions it is vulnerable to traction injuries, and as it traverses the scalenus medius muscle it may be irritated by tension in that muscle. Traction of the nerve can cause paralysis of the serratus anterior muscle, the clinical effect of which is winging of the scapula if the arm is abducted or flexed. The best test is to ask the patient to press both hands hard against a wall with the arms at right angles to the body. The paralysed muscle fails to keep the scapula against the chest wall.

Most of these cases recover spontaneously, but it is as well to examine the lower cervical joints with special care and to correct any lesions there.

Deltoid Palsy

The nerve-supply to the deltoid is derived from the axillary nerve with root origin at 5 and 6C. Occasionally this nerve is damaged in fractures and dislocations as the nerve passes round the neck of the humerus.

'Saturday Night' Paralysis

This oddly named syndrome derives from the habit of drunken men falling asleep with an arm hanging over the back of a chair for long enough to cause pressure on the radial nerve as it courses posteriorly round the humerus. The paralysis of the extensors of the wrist and fingers usually recovers quickly and spontaneously, within a few days.

Ulnar Neuritis

The ulnar nerve is relatively superficial at the elbow, and the groove on the posterior aspect of the epicondyle may be shallow and insufficient to afford protection against everyday knocks. Also the nerve may be over-stretched in some of the mechanical lesions of the elbow.

The effect is a neuritis of the ulnar nerve. The nerve is palpable, swollen, and tender. The pain and paraesthesiae affect the ring and little fingers, and any muscle weakness that ensues is to be found in the hypo-thenar muscles and interossei.

Symptoms of this nature may, of course, be due to a costo-scalene syndrome, and if the ulnar nerve is not tender at the elbow then the source must be sought higher up.

Carpal Tunnel Compression Syndrome

The carpal tunnel is relatively small. It carries the flexor tendons of the fingers as well as the median nerve, and it is bounded by bones posteriorly and by the transverse carpal ligament anteriorly. In addition there is a small branch of the anterior interosseus artery passing through the tunnel.

Undue pressure which is frequently repeated, as for example, a char-woman scrubbing floors on hands and knees, is enough to irritate the median nerve and set up a neuritis with its attendant pain and paraes-thesiae in the thumb, index, and middle fingers, and later palsy of the thenar muscles.

The majority of cases, however, are not caused in this way but are due to some disturbance of the water balance in the body, sufficient to cause increased pressure in the hands. This occurs mostly at *night time*, when the patient wakens with the pain and paraesthesiae as described. The pain may radiate into the forearm or even to the arm, and this causes difficulty in diagnosis. Such a pattern of pain can arise from foraminal compression syndromes at the 5–6C level.

Management of this syndrome is by night splintage of the wrist, by hydrocortisone injections into the carpal tunnel, by diuresis to reduce tissue fluid generally, or by surgical incision of the transverse carpal ligament.

All these methods are valid and have their place, but splinting is usually only of temporary value. To some extent it is a useful thera-peutic test, because, if splinting to keep the wrist straight instead of allowing it to extend during the night is enough to relieve the symptoms, this is good evidence that the source of the symptoms is at the wrist.

Hydrocortisone injections are frequently very effective and may be permanently so, presumably because the hydrocortisone has anti-inflammatory properties; but if this fails then surgery should be considered. Even surgery is not always the answer, however, and if symptoms recur afterwards, other factors need to be taken into account. In fact before surgery is decided upon, the mechanical problems in the cervical spine must be investigated and given the appropriate treatment if necessary.

There is still the problem of certain patients—mainly women—who have reached the menopause with its attendant hormonal imbalance and who develop *bilateral* acroparaesthesiae accompanied by swelling of the hands and morning stiffness which wears off when they get up and walk about.[89]

These patients often derive most benefit from diuretics and a reduc-tion of fluid intake. It seems highly probable in such cases that if the tissue fluid imbalance is enough to cause compression at the carpal tunnel then it could also cause compression of nerve-roots in the intervertebral foramina not only in the cervical spine but in the lumbar spine also.

13 Occipital and upper cervical syndromes

For the sake of description the cervical spine has been artificially divided into upper and lower sections. The upper cervical spine, from the occiput to 5C, certainly gives rise to patterns of pain which are quite different from those of the 4C–2T levels, but, of course, there is considerable overlapping and in order not to repeat what has already been described, the student is recommended to read through the section of 'Brachial Syndromes' before reading this section.

The commonest causes of upper cervical pain are hypomobile apophyseal joint lesions (p. 221), nervous tension states (p. 222), '*fibrositis*' of the semispinalis capitis (p. 224), and osteo-arthritis of the apophyseal joints (p. 226).

These syndromes will be described. Each one of them can give rise to referred pain sometimes in the anterior neck, or sometimes in the face, the ear, or the scalp. Any pain in the head and face which cannot be explained on a pathological basis should lead to a closer examination of the cervical spine in case mechanical causes can be discovered to account for the pain.

To complete the picture I have added headache syndromes (p. 227), ear syndromes (p. 230), facial syndromes (p. 232) and eye syndromes (p. 233), emphasising the mechanical factors which operate in some of the unexplained miscellaneous pains of the head and neck.

Before describing the syndromes in detail, the reader is reminded that this area of the spine is complex anatomically, and a revision of the anatomy is well worth while. There is one school of chiropractic which attaches so much importance to the upper cervical area that the occipito-atlantal joint is regarded as the most important joint of the whole spine. Called the 'whole in one' group these chiropractors virtually exclude consideration of the rest of the spine so long as the atlas is in its right place. This of course is carrying specialisation too far, but the very existence of such a group shows that the area is important, and there is no doubt that insufficient attention has been paid to the mechanics of this area by the medical profession.

The upper cervical joints although complicated in many ways are at least *un*complicated by considerations of the intervertebral discs because of course there are no discs at the occipito-atlantal and atlanto-axial joints, and degenerative changes in the discs from 2–4C are rare. Basing my

220

MANUAL OF OSTEOPATHIC PRACTICE

observations on radiological evidence, I have never seen narrowing of
the 2–4C discs in isolation. When disc narrowing occurs at 2–4C
there are always degenerative changes in one or more of the discs
at 4–7C.

In sharp contrast to this observation, it is common to find osteo-
arthritic changes in the upper cervical apophyseal joints and only
rarely in joints below 5C. This observation alone justifies the assumption
that spondylosis at 5–7C is a different entity from osteo-arthritis of the
apophyseal joints at 2–5C (see p. 155).

Applied anatomical points

In addition to the applied anatomical considerations deserving special
mention (p. 203) in the lower cervical area, the following points are
pertinent to mechanical problems of the neck:

Venous drainage from the spinal canal is very rich in the upper cervical
spine. There are four venous plexuses within the spinal canal running
mainly lengthwise, which join with and drain the inside of the skull
from the basilar and occipital plexuses. Many anastomoses occur, drain-
ing the vertebral bodies and joining the longitudinal veins transversely
before they combine together to form the spinal veins which emerge
from the intervertebral foramina as the vertebral veins. In addition to
the plexuses within the spinal canal there are rich venous plexuses on the
posterior vertebral arches subjacent to the multifidus muscles. The
frequent anastomoses of all these precludes any risk of inadequate
venous drainage, but venous congestion and stasis is probably an
important consideration in some of these cervical syndromes.[28]

Regulation of posture is governed largely through the sensory
impressions of the head in space, firstly by the otolith organ of the
vestibule and secondly by afferent proprioceptive impulses from the
neck. 'The receptors for the neck reflexes are probably Pacinian
corpuscles in the ligaments of the cervical vertebral joints particularly
at the occipito-atlantal joint. The afferent impulses pass in the dorsal
roots of 1–3C and come chiefly from the muscles of the back of the
neck.'[90] It is small wonder that disturbances of tone in the suboccipital
muscles can lead to vertigo (p. 230).

The first three cervical nerves not only contribute to the formation of
the cervical plexus, but their posterior primary rami become the greater
occipital nerve, the lesser occipital nerve, and the third occipital nerve
supplying the skin over the posterior half of the scalp, the ear, and the
upper half of the neck as well as motor fibres to the occipitalis muscle
and the semispinalis capitis. The union of the first three posterior rami
is called the posterior cervical plexus. The first cervical nerve, which is

called the suboccipital nerve, supplies the rectus capitis and obliquus capitis muscles. Mechanical faults in the upper cervical joints therefore can have widespread repercussions in the head, scalp, and ears.

The cranial nerves IX to XII emerge from the base of the skull anterior to the anterior arch of the atlas and lie on the longus capitis, rectus capitis anterior, and rectus capitis lateralis muscles. There are direct connecting nerve bundles between these cranial nerves, the cervical plexus, and the sympathetic chain of cervical ganglia which lies anterior to the roots of the transverse processes.

Grey rami communicantes connect the cervical sympathetic ganglia with each cervical nerve.

Abnormal afferent impulses from faulty mechanics in the upper cervical joints can set up an abnormal central excitatory state in the cervical cord and so disturb both the parasympathetic and sympathetic systems (see p. 11). Much osteopathic and chiropractic practice is based on this, but in my view the influence of mechanical faults on the autonomic nervous system is transient except in those patients whose autonomic system is already labile (see p. 14).

After all, if the vagus with its major parasympathetic supply to the viscera of the thorax and abdomen is divided (as in surgical treatment of peptic ulcers) no serious secondary disturbances of the rest of the autonomic system ensue. Furthermore if the sympathetic supply to the head is interrupted as in the Horner's syndrome, no serious disturbances of visceral function ensue apart from the eye signs.

The autonomic nervous system has a remarkable capacity to adjust itself relatively quickly to abnormal impulses so that visceral disorders secondary to mechanical lesions are usually transient and do not lead to pathological changes except when other additional factors are operating (see p. 15).

Hypomobile apophyseal joint lesions Similar characteristics apply in the 2–5C joints to those described at 4C–2T on p. 207, but the occipito-atlantal joint in combination with the atlanto-axial joints have some special features.

When the cervical spine is rotated most of the movement occurs at the atlanto-axial joint, but as the head is turned further rotation occurs progressively further down the neck to the 7C–1T joint. Finally, a few degrees of rotation is possible at the occipito-atlantal joint. (Tests for rotation at this joint are described on p. 46, *Manual of Osteopathic Technique.*) Although this last few degrees of movement is small, it is important for normality at the occipito-atlantal joint.

Flexion-extension is reputedly the chief movement at the occipito-atlantal joint, and about 10° is normal; but surprisingly enough there is an even greater range of flexion-extension at the atlanto-axial joint—namely 15°.

If when testing overall neck movements there is some restriction of rotation, the probability is that the upper cervical joints are at fault. Conversely if side-bending restriction is more obvious, then the lower cervical joints are likely to be at fault.

The techniques for mobilising these joints are described on p. 105, *Manual of Osteopathic Technique.*

A true *subluxation* occurs very infrequently in the upper cervical area (3–5C) in which the facets jam at an angle and the inferior facet of the vertebra above catches at about its centre with the superior edge of the inferior facet of the vertebra below. This may be unilateral or bilateral. The effect of the bilateral subluxation is a kyphosis, and the effect of a unilateral subluxation is a tilt away from the side of the fixation. Adjustive manual traction is the technique best suited to reducing this type of subluxation, but specific adjustments are sometimes necessary also.

In a true subluxation the positional fault is more important than is the mobility fault. That is to say, the position must first be restored by reducing the subluxation otherwise normal mobility will never be restored. The relative merits and significance of position and movement in osteopathic lesions is discussed at length on p. 44.

The atlas is sometimes held in relative flexion on the axis such that the anterior arch of the atlas is low on the odontoid peg and the posterior arch is approximated to the occiput. Similarly the atlas can be held in relative extension on the axis (*fig. 47*) such that the anterior arch of the atlas is high on the odontoid peg and the posterior arch is approximated to 2C. With open-mouth X-rays of the atlas and axis lateral displacements are sometimes seen (*fig. 48*) in which the space, between the odontoid and the lateral mass of the atlas is wider on one side than the other, but this alone is not significant. If there is over-lapping of the facets as well as the altered spacing, then a true lateral shift can be diagnosed. The same applies with the occipito-atlantal joints.

Nervous tension syndromes These are described on p. 62 but as nervous tension expresses itself more frequently in the neck than in other parts of the spine, it is also relevant here. The differential diagnosis between this condition and other causes of neck pain is important not merely because of treatment but because of prognosis.

Neck pain which is due to 'tension' can be relieved by manual treat-

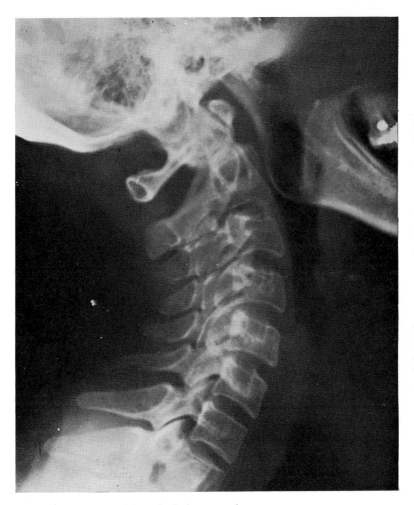

FIG 47 Atlas in a position of relative extension.

ment, but it is only of temporary value because underlying causes are not cured by treating their effects.

The syndrome of nerve pain due to nervous tension is so common that the phrase has even crept into the language. ('Oh! it's enough to give you a pain in the neck.')

Whatever the cause of the nervous tension—whether anxiety or depression, frustration or the general stresses of life—it expresses itself in muscular tension mainly in the semispinalis capitis, splenius capitis, and trapezius muscles. When muscular tension is maintained it produces pain due to the accumulation of metabolites in the muscle. These metabolites can then be a source of irritation which perpetuates the

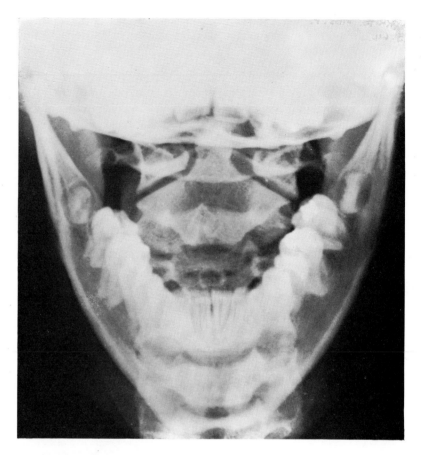

FIG 48 Antero-posterior view of the cervical spine, showing a lateral shift of the atlas on the axis. There is overlapping of the facets as well as asymmetry of the gaps between the odontoid peg and the lateral masses of the atlas.

contraction, thereby establishing a vicious cycle. This constitutes one physical counterpart of psychosomatic disorders.

The muscular component of the psychosomatic disorder can be treated on a physical basis—by massage and heat—but if the nervous tension is not relieved then the somatic part of the psychosomatic disorder may persist and even predominate, thereby misleading the patient and the doctor into believing that the symptoms are physical or mechanical or even pathological.

The *characteristics* of this syndrome are that the patient has difficulty in relaxing, not only in the neck but generally. The patient gives the impression of being 'keyed up', impatient, in a hurry, and anxious to get it over and on to the next thing. These patients often lead an over-stimulated life, have too much to do, and cannot quite catch up with their self-imposed tasks. They have no time to pause and reflect and relax to restore mental and physical equilibrium.

This type of patient may have widespread muscular pains, but often the pains are predominantly in the neck. The tension is diffuse and it affects both sides of the neck, extending from the scapulae to the occiput. The occipitalis muscle is also tight and gives rise to tenderness extending over the scalp from the nuchal line to the vertex of the skull. This tension is best tested for by having the patient lie prone with the head in the mid-line and the nose between two pillows or a slot in the table. The patient, of course, must be generally relaxed. The scalp should then be moved firmly over the occiput. The occipitalis muscle is attached to the lateral part of the superior nuchal line, and it cannot be moved easily but elsewhere the scalp should move freely on the skull.

This prone lying position is also convenient for palpation of the cervical muscles, but it will not indicate all we need to know about the general tension of the neck. Palpation of the semispinalis capitis is best performed with the patient supine, the fingers feeling the tension by rolling the muscles laterally from the mid-line. Palpation of the other posterior cervical muscles is best achieved by using the whole hand to sense the tension. If the tension is of recent origin it is easy to recognise and there are no abnormal physical signs to suggest a physical basis, but when the tension has been maintained for long enough the muscles are not only tender to palpation but hard and 'stringy', and attempts to relax these muscles are unsuccessful. The stiffness of the muscles may even lead to joint stiffness, and then a mechanical basis may be wrongly diagnosed. However, when the tension state has persisted to this extent, those muscles will need physical treatment irrespective of any psychological treatment. In a previously stable individual the psychological help required may not be anything more than common-sense advice—it may be simple advice about how to conduct his or her life. Most of these patients know what they ought to do but they need someone else in authority to instruct them—for example, to stop working at the weekend, or to go to bed earlier, or to cut out alcohol, etc.

Whatever physical treatment is prescribed, no undue emphasis must be placed on it. It is just to help them over their tensions, and it should be gently applied. Any forced or violent treatment is likely to accentuate the physical state, and then the patient will be worse off. Treatment which is soothing and relaxing will assist the patient to resolve her own tension. With this approach, many psychosomatic problems can be solved without deeper psychological aid. Treatment must not go on too long either, because such patients begin to rely on the treatment to give relief rather than to rely on themselves.

Semispinalis capitis 'fibrositis' syndrome The semispinalis capitis muscle is a large mass arising from the transverse processes of 1–6T and the articular processes of 4–6C. Its massive upper extremity is inserted into the occipital bone between the superior and inferior nuchal lines. Overlying this muscle is the thin expansion of the trapezius muscle which is attached to the medial third of the superior nuchal line of the occipital bone.

The *characteristic* of this syndrome is that there is a tight palpable cord in the muscle. Fibres of the trapezius may be included with the semispinalis capitis. The cord is tender and may be the thickness of a finger or pencil. The difference between this syndrome and the previous tension state is that the tension is localised rather than diffuse. The cord, which is found just lateral to the mid-line, may extend distally for two or three inches. The whole muscle is not involved. The pain is local and sometimes referred upwards into the scalp. This state is often chronic and may persist for years; and, athough it only causes discomfort rather than pain, it is a pity that patients should have to put up with it when treatment is usually simple and effective.

Often there is an underlying lesion of the occipito-atlantal joint, but not necessarily so; and in any case at this chronic stage manipulation is of no avail in relaxing the muscle. It needs deep kneading and frictional massage several times. The efficacy of this treatment is enhanced by infiltrating the site with 2 per cent procaine. The injection helps to relax the muscle and to break up fibrous tissue within it.

Osteo-arthritis of the cervical apophyseal joints This is characterised by pain in the posterior triangle of the neck, limitation of movement, and palpably enlarged edges to the articular processes at the affected levels. There may be swelling of the capsules in addition to the hard margins. Sometimes quite large lumps are palpable.

The pain is usually localised but may be referred upwards or forwards or downwards according to the level and distribution of the segmental nerves. Its variability is particularly characteristic, and the pain is unrelated to activity, weather changes, or posture. It may persist for years, and although the condition can become quiescent it rarely becomes completely pain free.

The distinction between osteo-arthritis of the apophyseal joints and spondylosis is discussed on p. 155. These differences are seen in all areas of the spine but are much more clearly defined in the neck.

The differential diagnosis of osteo-arthritis of the apophyseal joints also involves acute cervical joint sprains (see p. 207). In addition it is possible for latent osteo-arthritis suddenly to flare up due to injury, but X-rays will help in diagnosis. The films show irregularity of the joint surfaces and loss of joint space. They show osteophytes either invading the intervertebral foramen or protruding posteriorly. These appearances can be seen in the standard antero-posterior and lateral views, but are better seen with oblique views. The radiologist may miss the diagnosis, especially if only standard views are requested, because the jaw overlaps the 2–3–4C levels and obscures the facets. Many normal necks show a rounded appearance of the facets in the antero-posterior view, but in osteo-arthritis of the apophyseal joints the rounded appearance becomes irregularly enlarged. These points need emphasis because even experienced radiologists frequently miss the diagnosis unless the condition is suggested clinically.

A useful radiological technique to disperse the shadow of the jaw in the antero-posterior view is to persuade the patient to move the jaw during the exposure of the film. The atlanto-axial joints are best seen with the mouth kept open.

The *treatment* of osteo-arthritis of the apophyseal joints consists of gentle articulation, avoiding movements which hurt and using intermittent sustained traction, applied at about 30° of flexion. This should always be done manually at first, to ensure that the patient relaxes well.

If the patient can co-operate and relax, then the traction can be given by halter. The strength of the pull should never be more than 30 lb. Three or four pulls lasting about a minute will be sufficient at first, and as the patient becomes accustomed to the method the pulls can be increased to seven or eight.

If the pain is local and there are no signs of foraminal compression of a nerve-root then short-wave diathermy or micro-wave therapy is indicated, especially when the inflammation is chronically persistent and when traction is not effective.

In the later more severe stages a collar may be needed, but surprisingly few patients require them, and they are better psychologically for not having to wear one.

The reader should remember that ankylosing spondylitis can start in the neck, but the age-group is much younger (p. 190).

Other pathological causes for neck pain, like tuberculosis, secondary carcinoma, and spinal tumours, are not discussed here.

Headache syndromes The causes of headaches are legion, and the reader is referred to other texts for the differential diagnosis of this common symptom.

Intra-cranial causes of headache are not discussed here, nor are headaches which are secondary to generalised disease. Only headaches which are predominantly due to mechanical faults in the cervical spine are now described. Migrainous headaches are *not* due to mechanical faults, but they are often accentuated by such faults and are therefore included.

Bickerstaff[91] is of the opinion that stretching or tension is the basic cause of all headaches, either in the muscles, the vessels, or the dura, and he considers that this is the order of frequency—i.e. that muscular tension is the commonest, blood-vessel stretching the next common, and dural stretching the least common cause.

Of the mechanical types of headache the commonest is that in which there is undue tension in the suboccipital and occipitalis muscles. Instead of the ache being limited to the neck and suboccipital region, it spreads from there up and over the whole of the posterior part of the skull. The headaches and neckaches occur concurrently. They are intermittent. The headache stems from the neck rather than the other way round. It can affect the vertex of the head and even extend to the frontal area, but frontal and vertex headaches which occur in isolation are not usually due to cervical lesions.

The headache is influenced by position and activity—i.e. it can be brought on by certain positions and certain activities—but once present, the headache continues for several hours unless the position or occupation is altered or analgesics are administered.

There are always localised signs in the neck—e.g. stiffness, muscle tension, hypomobile lesions, subluxations. If there are no mechanical signs then some other cause must be sought to explain the headaches.

It is of historical interest that A. T. Still, the founder of osteopathy, noticed that an occipital headache he had when a youth was relieved by resting his head in a sling round the occiput. In his autobiography[92] he describes how this observation started him thinking about mechanical causes of pain.

> One day, when about ten years old, I suffered from a headache. I made a swing of my father's plough-line between two trees; but my head hurt too much to make swinging comfortable, so I let the rope down to about eight inches off the ground, threw the end of a blanket on it, and I lay down on the ground and used the rope for a swinging pillow. Thus I lay stretched on my back, with my neck across the rope. Soon I became easy and went to sleep, got up in a little while with headache gone. As I knew nothing of anatomy at this time, I took no thought of how a rope could stop headache and the sick stomach which accompanied it. After that discovery I roped my neck whenever I felt one of those spells coming on. I followed that treatment for twenty years before the wedge of reason reached my brain, and I could see that I had suspended the action of the great occipital nerves, and given harmony to the flow of the arterial blood to and through the veins, and ease was the effect, as the reader can see.

Even though a high proportion of occipital headaches have a mechanical basis, each patient must be examined medically and the usual causes—e.g. eye strain, sinusitis, digestive disturbances, and neurological and cardio-vascular diseases—must be excluded.

The treatment of occipital headaches depends upon the mechanical diagnosis. Specific adjustments to the affected joint are required. Accuracy of manipulation is as important as the accuracy of the diagnosis. Treatment to the tense muscles by deep massage is indicated in all cases but particularly in those in which the muscular component predominates.

Migraine

Headaches which are migrainous in character—i.e. are unilateral, associated with nausea, vomiting, and a visual aura, and have periodicity—can often be helped by treatment of the cervical spine, not because these headaches are caused by mechanical lesions but because mechanical lesions aggravate the other factors.

Although the ultimate cause of migraine has not been established there are always concomitant vasomotor disturbances within the cranium. During the attack there is an initial contraction of cerebral vessels leading later to a dilatation of those vessels. Mechanical lesions of the upper cervical spine may well aggravate the vasomotor disturbances by their effect on the sympathetic nervous symptom. Migrainous headaches can be influenced therefore by any lesion from 2T upwards, but the commonest lesion is found at the occipito-atlantal joint.

Treatment for migrainous subjects must be carefully applied. Short treatments with emphasis on specific adjustments are more effective than long articulatory and soft-tissue treatments. Patients should be allowed sufficient time between treatments for the effects to be noted, and it is usually unwise to treat them more often than once a week.

Other measures must not be neglected, like the use of drugs, relief of nervous tension, and correction of digestive and menstrual disturbances, but in almost all cases of migraine the frequency and intensity of the headaches can be reduced by correction of the mechanics of the neck without any of these other measures.

Temporal Arteritis

This is a disease of the temporal arteries in the elderly, and it gives rise to unilateral pain in the temporal area of the head. Persistent throbbing headaches with tenderness of the scalp are the chief symptoms. Neck and shoulder pains may occur if other arteries are involved. This disease should not be confused with mechanical conditions which give rise to similar symptoms. The pulsation of the vessels can be felt and the arteries are tender to such an extent that the patient cannot rest the side of her head on the pillow. The erythrocyte sedimentation rate is raised.

An indirect vascular factor can arise from tension in the cervical muscles because the venous drainage of the head can be impeded by such tension and it gives rise to a *congestive type of headache*. This is a diffuse heavy headache, pulsating in character. When the retinal veins are observed ophthalmoscopically these vessels are seen to be fuller and darker than average. In these cases other causes of increased intra-cranial pressure must be excluded, and if no obvious cause can be ascertained the patient should be given the benefit of the doubt and the neck treated expectantly. If the headaches are relieved by treatment then mechanical causes must have been responsible.

Post-concussional headaches are frequently not due to brain damage, but to the unsuspected neck damage which occurred at the time of the accident. The cervical spine should be examined carefully after head injuries even though the symptoms do not direct attention to the neck. If headaches persist after two weeks in cases in which no serious cerebral damage has occurred, there is a strong probability that they are of cervical origin.

Ear syndromes Pain, tinnitus, and vertigo are all symptoms referable to the ear, and they can all occur without overt evidence of disease. (Deafness has always an organic basis and is not considered here as part of a cervical syndrome.)

As with headaches due to mechanical causes in the cervical spine, it is possible for patients to suffer pain referred to the ear from the neck via the lesser occipital nerve and the greater auricular nerve. When pain in the ear cannot be explained on a pathological basis then the cervical spine should be examined, not because of these nerves only but because the tympanic plexus which supplies the tympanum, the eustachian tube, and the mastoid air cells derives its nerves from the sympathetic chain of the internal carotid plexus and in turn from the cervical and upper thoracic sympathetic nerves.

Tinnitus only rarely responds to mechanical treatment of the neck and therefore is unlikely to be related to mechanical factors, but *vertigo* is frequently related and many cases respond well to appropriate mechanical treatment.

The theoretical basis for this claim is not clear, but balance is a complex mechanism depending not only on the semi-circular canals but also upon proprioceptor messages from musculo-skeletal structures and upon intact cerebellar tracts to the vestibular apparatus in the mid brain.

The upper cervical joints provide receptors for the tonic neck reflexes which affect balance, so that any abnormal afferent impulses from these joints, their capsules, and the muscles which move them, can give rise to vertigo.

These upper cervical joints are a frequent site for adhesions, subluxations, and osteo-arthritic changes, but they are rarely involved in spondylosis which affects the lower cervical intervertebral joints.

In any discussion on the subject of vertigo there is room for widely diverging views because there are vascular, labyrinthine, and ocular causes as well as vertebrogenic causes. Some of these overlap—for example, arterio-sclerosis of the vertebral artery occurs in the same age-group as osteo-arthritis of the 2–4C apophyseal joints, so that any aetiological classification is difficult and may be influenced by the bias of the observer.

There are, however, two common types of vertigo—one in which sudden alteration of position causes vertigo and the other in which a sustained position will provoke it. The former is more likely to be vascular in origin because the rate of change in position is too rapid for the blood-supply to adapt itself. The latter is more likely to be verte-brogenic because the direction of sustained position sufficient to produce the vertigo is usually the direction in which there is some limitation of movement. Trying to move the neck in this direction sets up such a bombardment of afferent impulses from the upper cervical joints that the vestibular apparatus is temporarily disturbed.

This latter type of vertigo was described well by Ryan and Cope,[93] who made a plaster cast to hold the patient's head and neck firmly in relation to each other. Tipping the patient then did not reproduce the vertigo, whereas without the cast the neck movements immediately provoked an attack of vertigo.

These mechanical causes manifest themselves quite differently from Ménière's syndrome, in which there are paroxysms of vertigo and multiple attacks with long spells of freedom, which are unrelated to mere position of the neck or torso.

In some cases the vertigo has been precipitated by traction of the neck and in other cases the vertigo has been relieved by traction. This would appear to be inconsistent, but much depends upon the manner of the traction and the nature of the mechanical fault. If adhesions are present in the upper cervical joints and these are stretched, then this merely accentuates the abnormal afferent impulses. These adhesions need release by specific adjustive manipulation so that the joints can move freely again and then the vertigo will subside. If, on the other hand, there are osteophytes invading the intervertebral foramina and irritating the upper cervical nerves, then gently applied traction will open the foramina and so reduce the abnormal afferent discharge.

The type of traction best suited to this case is intermittent sustained traction horizontally applied with the neck flexed to 30°. The traction is slowly induced and slowly released; it lasts not more than thirty seconds and not more than 30 lb pull is applied.

The technique is described in more detail in my *Manual of Osteopathic Technique*, p. 249.

Facial syndromes The nerve-supply to the face is sensory through the trigeminal nerve and motor through the facial nerve. There is a communicating twig between these nerves—the zygomatic branch of the seventh with the maxillary branch of the fifth forming the infra-orbital plexus—and there is considerable overlapping of skin distribution by the great auricular nerve and nervus cutaneus colli from the second and third cervical nerves.

Clinically it is an observed fact that facial pain can occur secondarily to cervical spondylosis. It is just possible, because the central nuclei of the trigeminal nerve extend well down in the spinal cord as far as 3C, that mechanical faults can reflexly influence these nuclei to create an increased central excitatory state, and thereby reduce the threshold of painful stimuli.

Any facial pain which is not due to sinusitis, dental sepsis, mandibular joint lesions, or other organic cause may be arising from upper cervical lesions, and these lesions warrant treatment on an empirical and clinical basis, even though the modus operandi of the facial pain is not fully documented.

Paroxysmal facial neuralgia

This is an acute facial pain which comes on in waves of great intensity and may be provoked by the slightest stimulus—e.g. eating, talking, chewing, or washing. This condition is not in my experience related to mechanical causes and treatment of the neck does not relieve it.

Facial palsy

The aetiology of facial palsy is often obscure. It frequently follows exposure to cold which can lead to swelling of the nerve in the facial canal just above the stylomastoid foramen. Sometimes mechanical faults are invoked as the cause, but in my experience it is rare to find mechanical lesions in association with Bell's palsy, and mechanical treatment does not materially influence the course of recovery.

Similarly *chronic facial spasm* is not related to mechanical causes and mechanical treatment affords no relief.

Campbell and Lloyd[94] studied forty cases of facial pain which was unlike paroxysmal facial neuralgia. The patients were in the forty to fifty years age-group, 60 per cent women and 40 per cent men. Nearly all of them had pain in the orbit and eye, as well as in the occiput and neck, and the pain was not provoked by talking, eating, washing, etc. Many had flushing of the side of the face during an attack, with sweating, lacrimation, nasal congestion, and pupillary changes. There was occasional ptosis, and a Horner's syndrome was present in one patient.

Forty per cent noticed that movements of the neck either increased or decreased the pain. Usually flexion increased and extension decreased the pain. Twenty-five per cent of these had had previous neck injuries. On examining these patients they found that alteration of the position of the neck, and particularly immobilisation of it, not only relieved the pain but also caused the sweating of the face to stop and the pupillary changes to be reversed.

These cases strongly suggest a close link with the cervical spine and the cervical sympathetic chain of ganglia, and such cases frequently respond to the appropriate specific manipulation of the neck.

Eye syndromes It is not unusual for patients who are having osteopathic treatment to declare that their eyesight seems better. This has been quite spontaneous in many of my patients. I do not claim any special experience of eye problems and no claim is made that osteopathic treatment influences eye pathology, yet it is quite feasible that correction of cervical mechanics and improvement of cervical spondylosis could improve the nerve- and blood-supply to the eyes via the cervical sympathetics.

Klippel-Feil syndrome

This condition, consisting of a short neck, tilted head, and stiff neck was described in 1912. It is really an extensive disturbance of development in which such anomalies, as hemivertebrae, synostoses, and cervical ribs occur. The treatment of it must take into account the degree of deformity and the compensatory hypermobility. There is no point in manipulating a synostosis, and where hypermobile joints complicate the picture we must be particularly careful once the specific manipulations are used which may be needed to free the restricted joints.

14 Cervical myelopathy

This disease is now an established clinical entity, and it is so frequently associated with cervical spondylosis that the condition warrants a section in this manual. In spite of the association of the two conditions relatively few cases of cervical spondylosis become complicated by cervical myelopathy.

Trevor Hughes[95] stated that in a prospective necropsy series of 200 consecutive adults he found fifteen cases with myelopathy and six cases with radiculopathy due to cervical spondylosis.

Brain[68] stated that cervical myelopathy was the commonest disease of the spinal cord after middle life. It may mimic motor neurone disease, disseminated sclerosis, subacute combined degeneration, and also extra medullary and intramedullary tumours. Even syringomyelia may be simulated.

Cook[86] showed that the spinal cord could be damaged by direct injury through the cervical spine. Even quadriplegia occurred with hyperextension injuries without bony damage. The mechanism is that during hyperextension the ligamentum flavum projects well forward into the spinal canal and this can damage the spinal cord. Myelograms have shown that hyperextension can block the flow of fluid into the spinal canal. Apart from injury, the cord can be pressed upon by osteo-phytes projecting posteriorly from the vertebral body margins. Thick bars form which are sufficient to cause direct pressure on the anterior columns of the cord. Trevor Hughes[95] considers that narrowing of the antero-posterior diameter of the spinal canal is the most important aetiological factor.

Another factor which probably accounts for some of these myelo-pathies is that the vertebral artery can be grossly distorted by osteo-arthritis of the apophyseal joints and venous congestion can accrue from blocking the vertebral veins.

Kremer[96] describes a syndrome which he calls 'drop attacks' in which the patient suffers from vertigo, weakness of the limbs, and falling to the ground. He attributes the symptoms to temporary insufficiency of the blood-supply to the vertebro-basilar system and points out that these symptoms can be provoked or exacerbated by movements of the neck, especially where there is spondylosis and distortion of the vertebral artery.

It is well known in other parts of the body that pressure on an artery can provoke spasm even if the artery is divested of its nerve-supply. Furthermore micro-traumata of the vessel walls can have a cumulative irritating effect on the sympathetics which course along the vessel walls. Such vascular spasm could lead to ischaemia in the spinal cord and in turn to degenerative changes in both the white and grey columns.

Thus almost any of the diseases of the nervous system (apart from those affecting the brain and cranial nerves) can be mimicked by cervical myelopathy. In fact cervical myelopathy should figure in the differential diagnosis of almost all of the neurological diseases.

The treatment of cervical myelopathy depends upon the causal mechanism. If the symptoms are slight and cervical movements do not immediately provoke paraesthesiae, then gentle manipulation is safe; but if there is considerable spondylosis and if symptoms are brought on by adopting certain positions, then it is unwise to manipulate or even to exercise the neck except within a short compass. These patients require a collar—preferably one which allows a small range of movement. In some cases continuous traction of 5–10 lb will relieve the symptoms. Roberts[97] treated a series of cases of cervical myelopathy with collar immobilisation and found that a third of them showed improvement, a third showed no change, and a third deteriorated.

Once degenerative changes have started in the spinal cord and chromatolysis has occurred in the neurones of the cord, those neurones do not recover or regenerate. Full recovery is not feasible, though deterioration may be halted.

The vital question is whether mobilising the neck helps the circulation to the spinal cord or hinders it. The question is not easily answered except in those cases where the distortion from spondylosis is considerable, and where the changes in the vessels are already well advanced. If the diagnosis is made early mobilising treatment can improve the blood-supply.

One of the most significant neurological signs is paraesthesiae in the legs or torso when the neck is at its limit of movement in any direction but especially in flexion or under traction. This sign means that the cord is tethered and the spinal movements are mechanically irritating the cord.

The mobilising treatment must be gently applied, taking into account the loss of elasticity in all the tissues, ligaments, vessels, and nerves. The progress of treatment must depend upon the improvement of physical signs and symptoms. At the slightest sign of deterioration, mobilisation must cease and be replaced by immobilisation.

Although osteopathic bias is towards restoring normality, there is a limit to what can be achieved and we must recognise the limit. If the pathological changes have advanced thus far our objects must change: we must just help to minimise their ill effects rather than attempt the impossible.

Amyotrophic neuropathy This disease of obscure origin may be related to cervical myelopathy and occur in conjunction with spondylosis. The

R

patient is suddenly affected by widespread paralysis of one upper extremity, and the muscles are too diffusely affected for the explanation to have a nerve-root basis.

The course of the disease is not unlike poliomyelitis in so far as the paralysis is rapid in onset and slow to recover. There are no constitutional symptoms, and the patients are in the middle age-group. Recovery is usually complete and full in about a year.

Treatment should be directed to mobilising the cervical spine and improving the blood-supply to the cord. The muscles need help with electrical treatment to maintain tone while their nerve-supply recovers. What power there is should be conserved, and exercises should only be pursued to the point of slight fatigue.

Neuralgic amyotrophy This is similar to amyotrophic neuropathy but it involves peripheral nerves only. There may be considerable pain for several days followed by loss of power—e.g. in the serratus magnus from the long thoracic nerve, in the deltoid from the circumflex nerve, or in the spinati from the suprascapular nerve. There is no obvious cause and many show no obvious cervical lesions to account for the attacks.[98]

However, the level of origin of the nerve-supply should be treated by articulatory techniques and specific adjustments where indicated.

15 Soft-tissue spinal syndromes

In this context 'soft' tissues include muscles, tendons, fascia, fat, and areolar tissue. Many changes in these tissues are subservient to the changes in the 'hard' tissues of bone, ligaments, capsules, and cartilage, and they are relatively unimportant *per se*, but it would be a mistake to dismiss the soft tissues out of hand. The study of collagen has advanced recently and these studies have focussed attention on diseases of connective tissues.

The division between 'soft' and 'hard' here is purely a convenient convention, and it has more significance clinically than histologically or pathologically.

The clinical syndromes which appertain to these soft tissues are, again for convenience, divided into (a) muscle syndromes, and (b) connective-tissue syndromes.

Soft-tissue lesions occur all over the body, and the spinal soft tissues cannot be considered in isolation; but I am deliberately limiting my observations to those soft-tissue syndromes which are expressed predominantly in the spine.

Muscle syndromes 'Fibrositis' is a term which has fallen into disrepute because, although there is such a clinical entity, the term is misleading since no evidence of inflammation can be seen in any fibres. Unfortunately no other term has been adopted to cover this clinical syndrome.

'Fibrositis' is characterised by tight and tender muscle bands within the substance of the muscle. Pain in a muscle is no criterion of 'fibrositis' because pain from deeper structures is often segmentally expressed in the corresponding myotome, but if pain is *accompanied* by palpable small muscle bands which can be rolled under the palpating fingers, which are tender to pressure, and which can be obliterated by infiltrating with procaine, then we have all the characteristics of 'fibrositis'. If this 'fibrositis' occurs in an isolated site it is always secondary to another cause, but if it occurs in several unrelated sites then a generalised cause must be considered.

'There is a form of myalgia arising in muscles supplied by an irritated root, which simulates so-called 'fibrositis' both clinically and in its response to local injections of procaine, and is responsible for a variable and sometimes considerable total of the patient's discomfort. Electromyographic studies show that tender spots in the muscles are as a rule the seat of a localised increased irritability and a continuous discharge of action potentials which last as long as the needle remains in the muscle.'[36]

When palpating muscle (see p. 50) we should note its quality of tone and record abnormal tension, isolated tight bands, or guarding with provocation, and we should also test its power. Finally we should notice if contracting the muscle isometrically causes pain or not.

Poor tone and weakness go together, and the mechanical inferences of this are usually obvious. Abnormal sustained diffuse tension in muscle implies a protective reflex state, and the underlying cause of this must be established. *Guarding* of muscle implies a reflex contraction when some deeper structure is moved. It is accompanied by pain and in examination of the spine it is best evoked and tested for by the 'springing' test (p. 53). Guarding is always an important physical sign and testing for it must never be omitted from the examination of the spine. *Localised muscle bands* are best elicited by palpating the muscle transversely (p. 99). The erector spinae muscles should be palpated in this way from the occiput to the sacrum in all spinal syndromes. These tight bands can occur at any level. The semispinalis capitis site has already been described in detail (p. 226). Other common sites besides the erector spinae muscles are the trapezius, rhomboids, spinati, quadratus lumborum, and glutei.

If the 'fibrositis' is isolated the faulty mechanical cause must be corrected, and usually the muscle pain subsides with this correction. However, if the muscle changes have become chronic, persisting say for many weeks, then the fibres become very hard: sometimes even infiltration with a local anaesthetic is insufficient to relax the fibres, presumably owing to fibrosis of the muscle. In these cases, correction of the primary joint fault is insufficient to cure the 'fibrositis'. It will persist and will need treatment in its own right. The most effective treatment is frictional massage with or without the help of local anaesthesia. Another method is to apply 'inhibition' to the muscle. In osteopathic parlance inhibition is a term used for the application of continuous pressure over a muscle with the object of relaxing it. It was thought that continuous pressure maintained for a minute or so 'inhibited' the afferent impulses within the muscle from reaching the spine, thereby reducing abnormal afferent stimuli and thus quietening down the central excitatory state created by the lesion (p. 11). The 'inhibition' was considered to have the opposite effect to 'stimulation' of the muscle, when frictional massage was applied to 'stimulate' more afferent impulses and thereby increase the central excitatory state.

This explanation is illogical because sustained pressure over a muscle causes its own afferent pressure impulses to reach the cord. They may be different from the afferent impulses of the contracted muscle, but the probability is that the pressure merely adds to the total of the afferent discharge from the periphery to the centre. Yet, whatever the theoretical explanation is, inhibition has a useful clinical application. There is no doubt that sustained pressure over a contracted muscle will (if the contraction is not too severe) gradually relax that muscle so that the pain will subside. The sustained digital pressure is likely to bring about a temporary ischaemia of the muscle at the site of pressure. There is also a reactive hyperaemia due to the liberation of histamine which follows any minor damage to tissue. This hyperaemia sweeps away the metabolites of sustained contraction, and the muscles can then relax once more.

Sustained contraction of muscle causes a local accumulation of metabolites in that muscle. These substances irritate the muscle and maintain the contraction, so establishing a vicious cycle. The pressure ischaemia followed by a reactive hyperaemia breaks into the vicious cycle and normality is restored. Although this explanation is difficult to prove, there is clinically at least a skin hyperaemia following the pressure, and a palpable reduction in the tension of the muscle. This explanation of 'inhibition' seems more likely than the supposed reduction in afferent impulses.

Any method which improves the blood-supply to the muscle will have the desired effect—massage, externally applied heat, or counter-irritants. However, unless the source of the muscle's irritability is treated the benefit of these methods will be but temporary.

When 'fibrositis' is generalised it may be due to toxins from influenza and other fevers, septic foci as in tonsillitis and dental sepsis, or gastro-intestinal disturbances. Raised uric-acid levels in the blood render muscles irritable, as in the so-called gouty rheumatism. Climatic variations particularly the combination of cold and damp and changes of barometric pressure can accentuate muscular pain, though there must be some predisposing factor as well. The application of cold to the surface of the skin causes contraction of those muscles which lie immediately subjacent to the cold skin. This may well account for some lumbago attacks. Even visceral disturbances follow exposure to cold—the diarrhoea and colic which follows the exposure of the abdomen in a hot climate to the cold draught of a fan, the congestion of the lungs and even pneumonia following the exposure of the chest to cold, or the constriction of the vessels in the throat from getting cold wet feet.

These are all examples of somatico-visceral reflex disturbances. They are temporarily disturbing the viscera, just as spinal lesions can temporarily disturb their related viscera.

Connective-tissue syndromes The collagen diseases do not particularly affect the spine: they more usually affect the limbs. But panniculitis, which is a disorder of fatty tissue, frequently affects the back. Panniculitis is best detected by rolling the skin to include the areolar and fatty tissues which lie superficial to the deep fascia. The roll of fat is tense and tender, and there is difficulty in 'picking up' the roll. The skin puckers and gives the *peau d'orange* effect. This is due to shortening or tethering of connecting fibres between the skin and deep fascia. The fat is harder and denser than normal. The commonest sites for panniculitis are over the upper medial condyle of the tibia, over the glutei, and over the deltoids, but the soft tissues overlying the paravertebral muscles and the spinous processes are also commonly affected. The skin-rolling test (p. 90) is sometimes a guide to the level of an osteopathic lesion, but if there is generalised tenderness this is more likely to be due to panniculitis than to the lesions. The 'dowager's hump' of the cervico-thoracic area is an example of panniculitis there. It can be present with or without a cervico-thoracic kyphosis of the spine.

The *treatment* of panniculitis consists of dieting to reduce weight and keeping fluid intake low, together with strong massage of the tender fat using petrissage, tapotement, and cupping. All these methods should be used strongly to make an impression and to soften the panniculus of fat.

Nodular panniculitis differs from the above in that small nodules of fat, varying in size from that of a currant to a walnut, lie encapsulated between the deep and superficial fascia. The commonest site is in the gluteal area and crest of the ilium. Sometimes the nodules are tender and this occurs especially if they are recently swollen. They can be treated by deep frictions and petrissage, but they are more effectively dispersed by infiltrating them with a local anaesthetic and then hammering them hard with the fist. While infiltrating the nodule the needle can be used to puncture holes in the capsule and this facilitates the escape of fat when the nodule is hammered.

It is of course a mistake to assume that just because a nodule or an area of panniculitis is tender that the tenderness is due to the nodule. The tenderness may well be due to some deeper structural fault. If in doubt then by all means treat the panniculitis. If it fails to respond then the tenderness is certainly from another source.

16 Osteochondrosis syndromes

The characteristic feature of this disease is a *kyphosis*. There may or may not be any pain but there is always reduced mobility in the affected area of the spine. The kyphosis affects several vertebrae.

The disease may be active or quiescent. It becomes active in the early teens, but once established the kyphosis persists for the rest of the patient's life, even when symptoms subside completely. Mild cases may pass quite unnoticed and the occasional backache in the young may be dismissed as unimportant. An observant parent may notice the child becoming 'round-shouldered', and in spite of entreaties to stand up better he or she soon lapses and finds difficulty in sustaining a good posture.

The common area involved is the thoraco-lumbar (10T to 2L) (*fig. 49*) but any thoracic or lumbar level can be affected. It always affects more than one vertebra and the intervertebral discs between are damaged.

No satisfactory cause has been established, but the condition is not inflammatory; rather is it a disorder of growth, the first changes occurring in the cartilaginous rings at the anterior margins of the vertebral bodies.

Scheuermann[99] was the first to describe the condition. He noticed that the vertebral bodies became wedge-shaped and that their adjacent surfaces were irregular.

I am convinced that it is a generalised disease of the whole spine because, although the lower thoracic vertebrae are obviously affected more than the rest of the spine, such patients are predisposed to disc

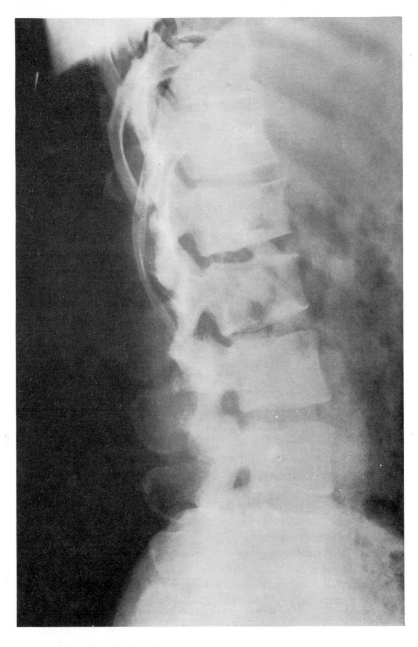

FIG 49 Osteochondrosis of the thoracic spine with several Schmorl's nodes.

degenerative changes in the lumbar and cervical areas more often than other subjects who do not show any wedging of the lower thoracic area. Furthermore the age of onset of disc protrusions is earlier in old osteochondrosis cases than in cases not showing a thoraco-lumbar kyphosis.

The disease is not merely an epiphysitis of the cartilaginous rings because the majority of cases also show Schmorl's nodes on X-rays. Schmorl demonstrated that cracks occur in the cartilaginous plates which separate the nucleus pulposus from the vertebral body, and that nuclear material squeezes through into the vertebral bodies.[100] This leads to irregular calcification and irregular superior and inferior surfaces of the vertebral bodies as well as to the wedging mentioned before.

The disease therefore involves the cartilaginous plates as well as the epiphyseal rings. Because the quality of the cartilage is poor and it cannot stand the weight of the body, compression occurs mainly in the front of the vertebral bodies. The normal nutrition of the discs is impaired and blood vessels invade the nucleus pulposus, leading to fibrosis and loss of mobility. The shock-absorbing qualities of the discs are lost and the spaces grow thinner more quickly than occurs in normal spines.

If the poor quality of cartilage is generalised, as I suspect, then the lower C and lower L discs will be affected by mechanical stresses at an earlier age than with other subjects.

This is in fact borne out in practice, because although the active phase of osteochondrosis ceases when growth ceases at the age of twenty years and symptoms subside, there is only a short five or ten years' freedom from symptoms before the spine becomes painful again.

Curiously enough the lower thoracic and upper lumbar kyphosis remains quiescent in most cases, but because of this rigid group, more mechanical stress occurs above and below. Compensating hypermobility develops in the compensating lordosis, the ligaments protest, to give rise to ligamentous backache, and in due course the discs degenerate more and protrusions ensue.

The differential diagnosis of kyphosis includes osteochondrosis at any age. Other causes in the young are tuberculosis, ankylosing spondylitis, and postural kyphosis from weak musculature. In the older age-group kyphosis may be due to osteoporosis, spondylosis, or neoplasm, but these conditions are discussed in the next section.

The history helps in the differential diagnosis. In osteochondrosis the onset is always insidious, the symptoms never severe, the patient is not ill, and the condition rarely interferes with her life apart from fatigue and backache after strenuous exertion. With *tuberculosis* of the spine the onset is also gradual and symptoms may not be severe, yet the child is ill, and the springing test of the spine evokes sharp guarding. The kyphosis is angular and the X-ray show rarefaction and collapse of two adjacent vertebrae with uniform narrowing of the disc space between. There are no Schmorl's nodes or irregularity in the adjacent surfaces, and there is no reactive sclerosis as in osteochondrosis. *Ankylosing spondylitis* starts in the sacro-iliac joints, and it leads to a long kyphosis of the thoracic spine. The picture is of such generalised stiffness that the diagnosis is usually obvious clinically as well as radiologically. There is a *postural type of* kyphosis due to debility and weak muscles or polio-myelitis, but this kyphosis is correctible, there is no rigidity and the X-rays show no deformity.

Treatment of osteochondrosis Bearing in mind that this disease is mild and persistent, the growing child will need supervising for several years. It is as well to have serial X-rays taken at six-monthly intervals to observe the changes.

The majority of cases can be treated with gentle mobilisation in the form of articulatory techniques mainly and occasional specific adjustments so long as no undue force is used. There is no contra-indication to manipulation, but obviously excessive force is undesirable. In spite of treatment, however, the joints will remain more restricted in range than will normal joints.

The backache can usually be relieved in this way. Strengthening exercises involving extension of the spine are desirable on two counts— they improve muscle tone and they minimise the deformity. Swimming is therefore the best exercise. Jarring games and gymnastics must be avoided, and heavy lifting is taboo.

Without painting too gloomy a picture, the true state should be explained to the patient and the parents, emphasising the point that excessive activity and weight-bearing may cause further deformity of the spine. The youth should be advised against taking up any occupation in which he will be expected to do heavy lifting.

Although kyphosis is the salient feature of the disease, a scoliosis may also develop because of unequal ossification of one or more vertebrae. These lateral curves should be corrected as far as possible, and if a short leg is present it is especially important to use the appropriate heel lift to balance the pelvis.

The treatment of late, quiescent, or old osteochondrosis is directed at minimising its deleterious effects—namely, rigidity in the group affected —and coping with the compensatory hypermobility or lordosis, both in the cervical and lumbar areas.

Any attempt to restore *full* mobility to the kyphosis is doomed to failure, but this does not mean we should not try to achieve as good mobility as possible. In fact, if moderate force only is used and an increased range is obtained, then the extra load on adjacent areas will be eased. This reduces the risk of hypermobility symptoms. Once symptoms of hypermobility have developed, these need our special attention (p. 126) because even if we attempt to restore mobility in the adjacent hypomobile section, the hypermobile joints will continue to protest.

Most old osteochondrosis areas are asymptomatic, and unless symptoms develop they are best left alone. I have sometimes been astonished on radiological examination at the hypertrophic osteophytosis associated with old osteochondrosis which is without significant symptoms.

17 Kyphosis syndromes in the adult

A kyphosis may persist into adult life from an osteochondrosis in youth, as pointed out in the previous section. The differential diagnosis of kyphosis in the young is discussed there also, but in this section we are dealing with those kyphoses which develop de novo, after the age of forty years.

The causes are:

1 Thoracic spondylosis
2 Osteoporosis
3 Pathological fractures
4 Paget's disease
5 Tuberculosis (p. 260)

If a kyphosis is mobile it is painless, and it is probably a physiological response to other mechanical considerations—for example, a lumbar lordosis, an ankylosed hip, anterior poliomyelitis, or habitually poor posture either sitting or standing.

All other kyphoses are accompanied by rigidity in the affected area because there is some underlying pathological process. This may be quiescent and painless, as with old osteochondrosis, spondylosis, early osteoporosis, and Paget's disease, but at any stage these diseases together with the others listed above can become painful as well as rigid.

Most spinal kyphoses affect the thoracic spine, but a straightening of the anterior curves of the cervical and lumbar spines should be considered as a kyphosis. If there is an actual reversal of these cervical and lumbar curves then there is a true kyphosis in those areas.

The triad of kyphosis, pain, and rigidity in the spine is always serious, and we must never make the assumption that the cause is mechanical even though disc protrusions are the commonest cause of this triad. We must in practice assume the worst and prove that the cause is not pathological before concluding that the mechanics of the spine are faulty—i.e. *a rigid and painful kyphosis must be considered pathological until proved otherwise.*

Thoracic spondylosis (fig. 50) leads to a long uniform kyphosis because of the narrowing of the disc spaces and because the loss of disc substance tends (when uncomplicated by protrusions) to occur in the weight-bearing part of the disc. In the thorax the centre of gravity passes anterior to the spine so that more weight is carried anteriorly than posteriorly, and the discs narrow anteriorly and become wedge-shaped. The sequelae of this are an increase of the posterior curvature and an overall loss of height. As age advances these changes occur to a greater or lesser extent in all people. Postural habits may accentuate the trend or they may reduce it. Even mental attitudes can influence the shape— e.g. 'being bowed down by grief' or 'being upright and sprightly even into old age'.

As the degeneration proceeds the discs not only become narrowed and wedge-shaped, but the margins of the vertebrae throw out osteophytes. These occur mainly anteriorly because of extra weight-bearing there, and when the osteophytes impinge against each other they cause pain. A spinal brace with shoulder straps which effectively checks more flexion also reduces the pain. Such pain is deeply placed, poorly localised, and either posterior or anterior in the chest wall.

The *management* of early thoracic spondylosis consists of manipulating the area in extension rather than in flexion (for technique see p. 150, *Manual of Osteopathic Technique*). Articulatory techniques must also be used to improve extension. Erector spinae strengthening exercises and attention to posture are important. Specific adjustive traction (p. 116) is applicable in almost all cases whether a disc protrusion is suspect or not. Sustained traction is of little use in this area, nor is there much application here for intermittent sustained traction. Breathing exercises and swimming help to extend the thoracic spine and are both helpful. The costo-vertebral joints take part in the stiffening process and articulatory techniques to mobilise these joints are indicated, especially when the chest expansion is poor.

Osteoporosis of the spine leads to kyphosis where the vertebral bodies become compressed, but even before this the vertebrae become sensitive and in an active osteoporosis the signs and symptoms are very characteristic, as described below.

The clinical features of osteoporosis of the spine are:
Thoracic kyphosis—angular or uniform
Lumbar lordosis
Weight-bearing increases pain: the patient prefers to support her spine by taking some weight through her arms

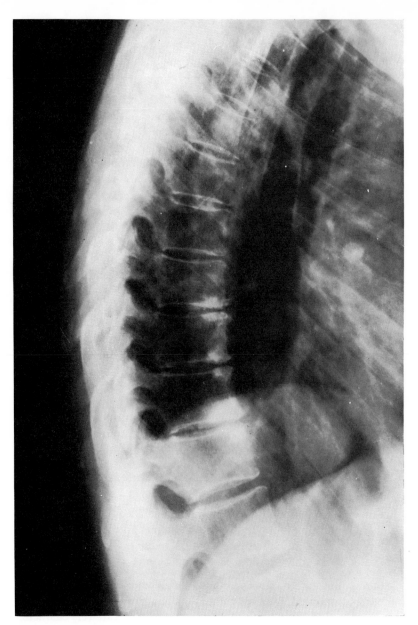

FIG 50 Thoracic spondylosis with sclerosed osteophytes anteriorly at 8–11T.

Compression of the spine increases pain
Distraction of the spine relieves pain
The springing test evokes a reflex guarding response and is worst at
the most porotic area or at the site of a compression fracture

The patient moves with great care to avoid jarring, but when careful she can move slowly without pain

Movement is accompanied by grunting which implies a catching of the breath, and the patient is reluctant to lie prone because of increased pain in the process of getting there

Slow breathing is possible but when respiration is quick the breath is arrested by pain

The pain may be girdle in type, especially when a vertebra has collapsed

In osteoporosis the unfailing sign is guarding with the springing test. The muscle guarding is widely spread, unlike that in a disc protrusion which settles down in a few days and becomes quite well localised to the level of the protrusion. The whole of the thoracic and lumbar spine can be involved, but the commonest site for this positive springing sign is in the lower thoracic area. A positive springing test is always significant and must never be omitted as part of the general examination of the spine. It implies spinal disease or an internal derangement of a disc.

The *aetiology* of osteoporosis is not fully established, but contributing factors are increasing age, loss of ovarian secretions, deficiencies of vitamin D calcium and protein, disuse and rest, steroid therapy, hyperparathyroid and hyperthyroid activity.

The age of onset in the commonest type of osteoporosis is earlier in women than in men, and four times as common because the menopause disturbs the calcium metabolism, the effect of which is to increase the loss of calcium via the renal tract, yet the serum-calcium level remains normal. The loss from the kidneys is made good in the blood by depleting the bones of their calcium. Osteoporosis ensues in the whole skeleton, but the spine is more vulnerable in that the vertebral bodies become sensitive to weight-bearing and jarring long before compression fractures are evident radiologically. Peripheral bones take part in the porosis, but they do not become sensitive. However, peripheral bones and vertebrae are more likely to fracture than are normal bones. Cancellous bone is depleted before compact bone, so that on X-rays the contrast between the bodies of the vertebrae and their compact-bone outline assumes greater definition than with normal bones. The outline looks as if it has been 'pencilled' in by the radiographer (*fig. 51*). The trabeculae become more widespread and thinner. The discs become 'ballooned' uniformly (cf. postcentral disc expansion, p. 250), and the bodies of the vertebrae become bi-concave. If additional compression has occurred then the vertebra becomes wedge-shaped, or the superior or inferior surfaces crack and become angulated, or the line becomes

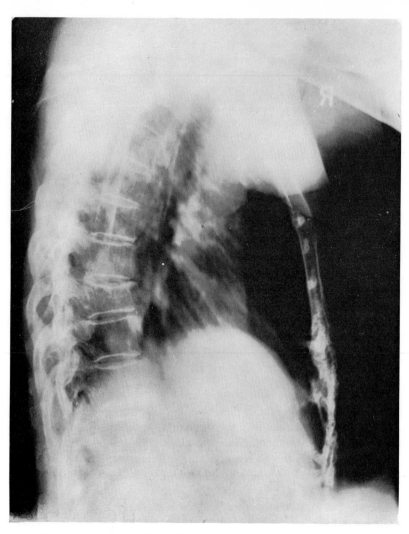

FIG 51 Osteoporosis showing collapse of 8T and 'pencilling' of the outlines of the vertebral bodies. The costal cartilages are excessively calcified. This frequently goes with bony decalcification.

discontinuous. Often several vertebrae become wedge-shaped. If one only is involved then the kyphosis is small and angular, but if several are involved then the kyphosis is rounder and longer.

There are two other radiological appearances which although not directly attributable to osteoporosis, nevertheless indicate the vertebral body's reaction to increased pressure of either body-weight or intra-disc pressure. These are reinforcing lines of calcification (*fig. 52*) and post-central disc expansion (*figs. 53, 54*). The latter is often seen in the lower

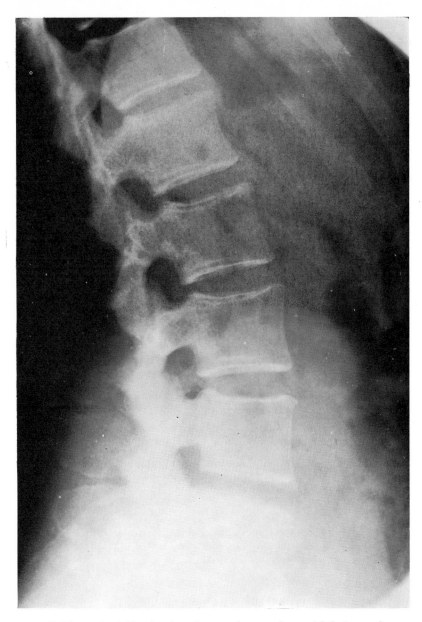

FIG 52 Lines of calcification just deep to the superior and inferior surfaces of the vertebral bodies are probably indicative of the vertebral response to increased intra-disc pressure.

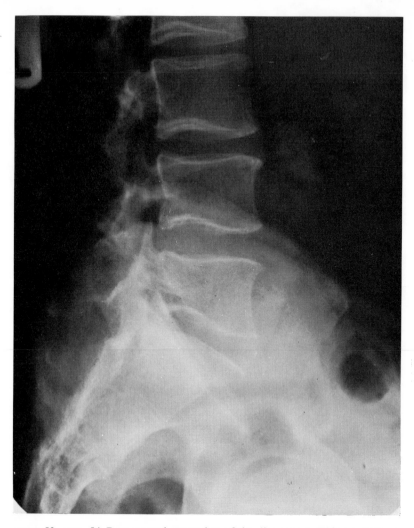

FIGS 53 AND 54 Post-central expansion of the disc spaces. This appearance is usually associated with a 'cupid's bow' effect on the inferior surfaces of the lower vertebrae, in this case 2L to 5L.

lumbar discs and occasionally in the thoracic discs. The corresponding antero-posterior radiological appearance is the 'cupid's bow' effect on the lower surfaces of the lumbar vertebrae. The fourth and fifth lumbar disc spaces are the most commonly involved.

The differences between osteoporosis and osteomalacia in adults is that with the latter the bones become soft rather than brittle, and become mis-shapen rather than fractured. Osteomalacia, which is a disease definitely due to vitamin D deficiency, leads to loss of calcium

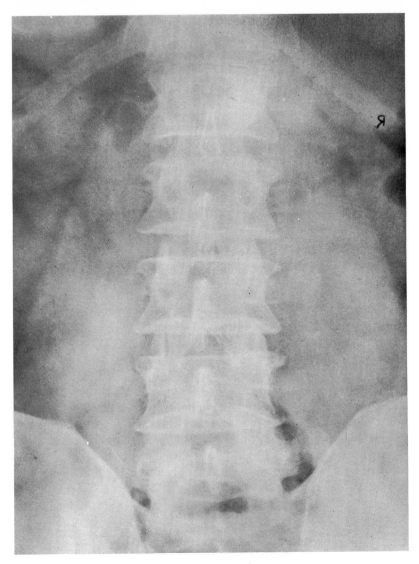

FIG 54

from the bone but the bone cells remain, whereas with osteoporosis both calcium and bone cells diminish. Osteomalacia is fortunately rare whereas osteoporosis is common in the elderly.

When a *fracture* occurs in an existing osteoporosis the injury may be trivial, such as a simple fall or even lifting a light weight. The patient realises something serious has happened to the spine, and is immediately aware of pain which soon increases in intensity. If vomiting and shock follow a trivial spinal injury this should immediately arouse suspicion of a pathological fracture.

251

The signs are an angular type of kyphosis (a gibbus). The gibbus may be small and pass unnoticed. The paravertebral muscles are in tension, and guarding is evoked by the springing test. The symptoms and signs are not always severe, and unless the physician is alert to this syndrome the patient may suffer unnecessarily because of delay in the diagnosis.

Pathological fractures also occur in other diseases of the spine. These are referred to on p. 262.

The treatment of osteoporosis is chemical and not mechanical. All manipulations are contra-indicated. Vitamin D 5,000 units daily and a calcium preparation like Calcium Gluconate 600 mg t.d.s., together with an anabolic steroid (e.g. 'Dianabol' 5 mg daily) must be taken for three months. In many cases the pain will subside within a month and the spine will accept weight-bearing without pain, but it is unwise to assume that full repair has taken place for three months. The springing test is invaluable in assessing progress because while porosis is clinically active, the springing test is positive. This guide to progress and the help it gives in deciding about further medication is much more reliable than X-ray examination, because exactly comparable X-rays are almost impossible to achieve even if the exact exposure is used each time. This is because the mains voltage and the chemicals can both vary, and time factors in developing the films vary with every patient.

The use of spinal support in osteoporosis may be a difficult decision because osteoporosis is accentuated by inactivity and immobilisation yet some vertebrae are so friable that a support is necessary to check further collapse of more vertebrae. A spinal brace with shoulder slings should be as light as possible to minimise the extra load on the spine.

Medication should be kept up longer than seems clinically necessary because of the risk of relapse. The patient must be encouraged to take a full diet rich in calcium, protein, and mineral salts. Fluorine has recently been found to reduce the incidence of senile osteoporosis.

Paget's disease causes a generalised kyphosis of the spine if several vertebrae are involved, but occasionally an isolated vertebra is affected by the disease. No treatment seems effective. There is increased density of bone, the trabeculae are thicker and coarse, and the body of the vertebra becomes flattened vertically and widened transversely (see also p. 264).

18 Scoliosis syndromes

In severe structural scolioses, whether of congential or idiopathic origin, or secondary to poliomyelitis, pulmonary disease, etc., osteopathic treatment by manipulation is no more effective than are other orthodox procedures in restoring the shape of the spine, but some of the effects can be minimised by treatment. Small localised scolioses can sometimes be corrected by manipulation. Minor long scolioses secondary to a short leg, a pelvic tilt, postural balance, or occupational habits can be materially straightened by the appropriate manipulation, and anciliary methods of heel lifts, corsets, exercises, and correction of posture (*figs. 55, 56*).

When a scoliosis is forming the vertebral bodies sometimes rotate into the concavity of the curve and during flexion the curve straightens out, but at a later stage the vertebral bodies rotate away from weight-bearing into the convexity of the curve to produce a pronounced 'high side' on the convexity of the curve. Once this has happened morphological changes must have taken place in the discs, ligaments, muscles, and vertebral bodies so that the curve is irreversible and correction is impossible.

Those scolioses which are due to intense muscle spasm, as in disc protrusions, are temporary in most cases, and treatment directed to curing the disc displacement will eventually resolve the scoliosis. No more need be said about this type of scoliosis as the management is secondary in importance to the disc, and the reader is referred to the appropriate sections in this book (p. 142).

A localised scoliosis affecting say five or six vertebrae is frequently due to the hypomobile type of spinal lesion (p. 114). If a tilt has occurred then compensation for the tilt is automatic to restore equilibrium in the opposite direction, but the compensation may involve several vertebrae. Occasionally the tilt to the opposite side is excessive, and a curve is found opposite to what is expected. These cases are difficult to explain, but it is probable that there is considerable internal derangement in the architecture of the disc at the site of the tilt.

Another common cause of a localised scoliosis is osteochondrosis (see p. 243) because of the distorted shape of the discs and vertebral bodies.

Correction of long scolioses which are secondary to a short leg is usually possible especially in the young before structural changes have become permanent. If such changes have occurred or if there are additional lesions which reduce mobility, then correcting the curve from below may be incomplete or attempts at correction may bring on more symptoms at higher levels in the spine.

When using heel lifts to restore the pelvic levels, the process must proceed slowly: in an adult the heel lift should increase by only $\frac{1}{8}$ in. at monthly intervals. The immobile joints will require manipulation to facilitate the new orientation of the spinal contours, and it is policy to

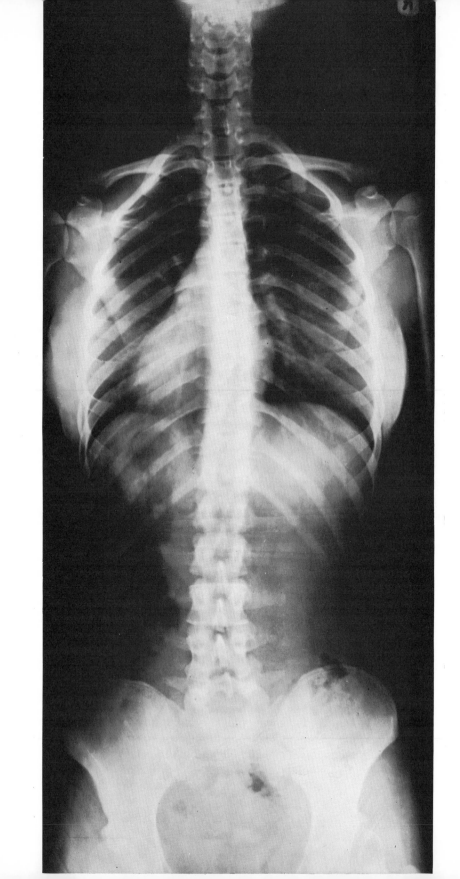

work from below upwards. Sometimes the patient, when first seen, has pain in the lower lumbar spine which is soon relieved by the heel lift but is replaced with a pain in the thoraco-lumbar area. This in turn recovers to give rise to a pain in the thoracic or cervical area. These reactions arise only in patients whose spinal joints are not fully mobile.

Young patients should have the full heel lift almost straight away, and the sooner the better.

It is rarely necessary or desirable for adults to wear the full heel correction. If a patient has $\frac{1}{2}$ in. of shortening, then $\frac{1}{4}$ or $\frac{1}{8}$ in. may be sufficient to relieve all the symptoms. It is a matter of relieving abnormal ligamentous tensions without upsetting the compensatory mechanisms too much(for further discussion of the 'short-leg' syndrome see p. 132).

With an established scoliosis the patients may be perfectly happy and symptom-free, but like other patients they can strain their backs and have pain in the usual manner. In such cases, however, if the patient has not been seen before, the practitioner may not be sure how much of the curvature to attribute to the recent injury and how much to attribute to the previous state. Our task should be directed to relieving the new symptoms and to trying to restore the status quo of the spine.

In most scolioses there are asymmetrical muscular tensions which give rise to symptoms, and these 'soft tissue' conditions need treatment even though the curvature cannot be effectively straightened.

Many scolioses are comfortable for years, but as age advances the mechanical strains become too great and the supporting soft tissues give way under the strain so that deformity increases. In these cases, if the muscular power and ligamentous state cannot be improved, then a suitable corset or brace may become necessary.

In severe scolioses there may be adverse effects upon the heart and lungs. The lungs are smaller and deformed. Resistance to blood flow is increased, and this may eventually lead to pulmonary hypertension and right ventricular heart failure. In the late stages there may be dyspnoea even at rest.[101]

19 Spinal gout syndromes

Classical gout is well known and is accompanied by a raised serum uric-acid level in the blood, but a rise does not necessarily produce typical gouty arthritis. This metabolic disorder can express itself in many tissues or in various sites, one of which is the spine.

Spinal gout can be so acute that the symptoms mimic those of a

FIG 55 Scoliosis secondary to a short left leg.

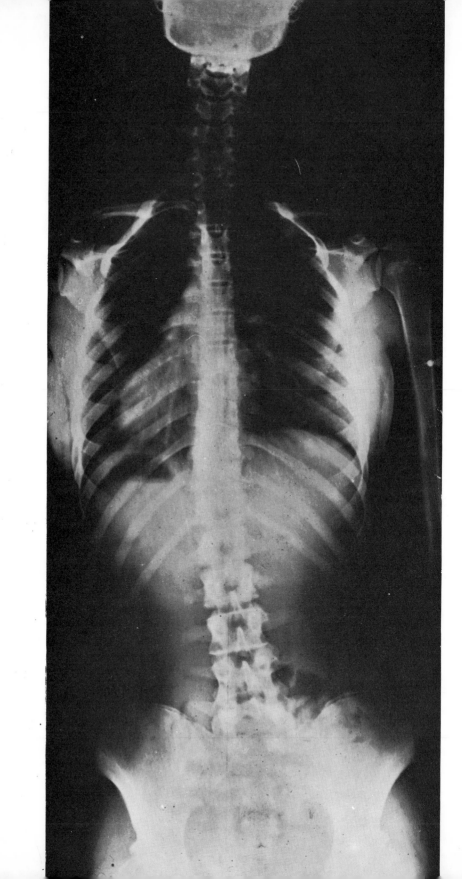

prolapsed intervertebral disc. What is more confusing is that occasionally a patient, who has a genuine disc prolapse and also a raised serum uric-acid, has such irritable muscles that the muscle guarding, which accompanies his or her disc displacement, is so intense that it seems to be out of all proportion with the other signs.

The onset of the disease is abrupt and sharp. Classically it occurs in an apparently healthy male who is awakened at night with severe local pain in one joint, like the big toe, wrist, elbow, or knee, but the sacro-iliac and other spinal joints may also be the site of pain. Typically there is a slight pyrexia, and in a few hours the peripheral joint becomes red, swollen, hot, and tender. There is marked limitation of joint movements because of pain. Effusions form and inflammatory oedema is very widespread. There may be lymphangitis, and the condition may be confused with an infected joint or a cellulitis. In the spine the inflammation is too deep to be superficially apparent, but the protective muscle guarding is intense and the limitation of movement is virtually complete. The symptoms may subside in a few days and then clear up completely to leave a normal joint or a normal spine, with no residual signs whatever. This can be surprising, but in reality it should be a help in diagnosis because other forms of arthritis tend to smoulder on between exacerbations. The attacks increase in frequency and may affect several joints. This leads to residual pain, stiffness, and deformity in peripheral joints. In established cases tophi form in the ear, nose, olecranon, prepatella bursa, and tendons of fingers, toes, wrists, ankles, or heels. Even tennis elbow can be a manifestation of gout. It is worth remembering this, especially if the pattern of the tennis elbow is not typical or is bilateral, or if other joints and soft tissues are involved from time to time.

In addition to the arthritic form of gout, there is a muscular form, 'gouty rheumatism' for want of a better term. The gouty rheumatism expresses itself clinically in three ways:

1 A vague muscle ache which tends to come and go, affecting different areas at different times.
2 Excessive muscular pain following minor muscular effort. The average person experiences pain and stiffness after unaccustomed exercise. These patients either have pain and stiffness after relatively minor muscular exertion or the ache persists for a disproportionate length of time.
3 Excessive irritability of muscle when reflexly provoked.

FIG 56 Comparison of scoliosis after the wearing of a heel lift together with articulatory treatment.

A severe form of this latter occurs in the paravertebral muscles of the spine. Such patients move with care because any rapid movement sets up muscular spasm with so much pain that it checks further movement, and yet if they move slowly the spasm can be avoided. These patients are often diagnosed as having prolapsed intervertebral discs, but they show no abnormal neurological signs, and X-rays of the spine show no bony changes or disc narrowing. The care with which such patients move is surprising: it makes one wonder at first if they are exaggerating their symptoms deliberately. After taking time, for example, to lie prone on the examination table, the patient can relax again and may be quite comfortable, and yet spinal mobility and springing tests provoke muscle guarding straight away. Excessive reflex reactions of this sort make one wonder again if the patient is neurotic; but after giving such patients uricosuric drugs and seeing them again within a few days moving freely and with all the signs gone, one can then no longer attach any psychological label to the patient. One such patient, when turning or altering his position, used his arms to minimise the use of his spinal muscles, sweated while moving and went red in the face, and his arms trembled with the apparent effort.

Gout is a disorder of metabolism characterised by an excess of uric-acid in the blood, the deposition of sodium biurate in articular and periarticular tissues, and recurring attacks of acute pain. It is an inherited or constitutional condition, but it may occur secondarily to polycythaemia, chronic leukaemia, and pernicious anaemia in which there is excessive breakdown of nucleic acid.

Studies with radioactive isotopes on gouty subjects show that there is an increase in the freely diffusible uric-acid in the blood and body fluids. The total normal pool of uric-acid in the body is 0·7–1·4 g, whereas in gouty subjects the total may rise to 4 g or more. The highest recorded total was 31 g. The most useful clinical test is the estimation of the serum uric-acid level in the blood. Its normal range is from 2 to 5 mg per cent, though this depends to some extent upon which laboratory test is used. Any estimation over 5 mg per cent is suspect, but one must remember that the level varies from day to day. In addition the mere level of uric-acid in the blood is not the only factor in the deposition of sodium biurate in the tissues because, in the secondary gouts, deposits are rare even though the serum levels rise much higher than in primary gout.

Uric-acid is a metabolic end-product of protein which forms from the breakdown of nucleic acid in the body. It also forms from glycine in gouty subjects.

In most animals—at least the carnivorous ones—uric-acid is further oxidised and excreted as allantoin. It is a curious thing, and an argument in favour of vegetarianism, that the anthropoid ape and man do not have this ability to change uric-acid into allantoin. Allantoin is 200 times more water-soluble than is uric-acid. In birds and reptiles this is a physiological necessity because most of their nitrogenous wastes are eliminated as uric-acid and not as urea. The vegetarian argument is that if we were intended to be carnivorous and eat much animal protein we should be provided with the enzyme—uricase—for converting uric-acid into allantoin.

About a third of the uric-acid eliminated by the kidneys from the body is endogenous in origin, and about two-thirds of it is exogenous. From this knowledge it is clear that we can make an appreciable difference to the level of serum uric-acid by decreasing the protein intake in the diet.

Exactly where the metabolic fault lies in the gouty subject has not been satisfactorily worked out. It may lie in the ingestion of too much protein, and many gouty rheumatic subjects come into this category. These cases can obviously be treated effectively by dietetic means. It is noteworthy that alcohol as such does not play a significant aetiological role, but red wines appear to precipitate acute attacks of pain. Other factors may be that too much uric-acid is formed endogenously or that conditions in the local tissues themselves may be more suitable for precipitation.

It is significant that the pains of gout are worse at night, when the circulation slows down and when precipitations can more readily occur. The crystals tend to form in cartilage and periarticular tissues, and the severity of pain is explained on the grounds that the crystals prick into the sensitive periosteum setting up acute inflammatory reactions. The reaction to crystal formation must be considerable because in an established case X-rays show erosion of the ends of the bone—the so-called 'punched-out' appearance.

When a patient with spinal pain complains that it is worse in the early hours of the morning, it is worth having the serum uric-acid estimated whatever the rest of the symptoms are.

Williams[102] has pointed out that osteophyte formation in the vertebral column is more prevalant in patients with a raised serum uric-acid than in those with a normal level:

A comparative statistical series was collected from patients between the ages of 45 and 60. Efforts were made to eliminate all cases whose serum uric-acid determination might be altered by disease or medication. One hundred patients were chosen whose X-rays of the spine showed extensive osteophyte formations which could not be explained on a basis of abnormal skeletal stress or toxic factors. Of this series, 67 were men and 33 were women.

The average uric-acid reading was 7·4 mg per 100 ml of blood serum for the men and 6·2 mg for the women.

A control series of 100 patients of the same age-group was chosen from X-rays of the spine which showed no osteo-arthritis or moderate osteo-arthritic changes secondary to a mechanical alteration which was apparent. This series consisted of 35 men and 65 women. The average serum uric-acid determination was found to be 4·7 mg per 100 ml in the men and 3·8 mg in the women.

Osteophyte formation occurs as a sequel to the protrusion of disc material as is shown by Schmorl and Junghans. Does this justify a linkage between disc degeneration and disorders of purine metabolism?

In the management of acute spinal gout the acute phase must be treated with drugs in the usual way—colchicine, phenylbutazone, allopurinol—and no local treatment other than complete rest should be used; but the management of chronic gout, whether affecting the spinal joints or soft tissues, should either be dietetic or allopathic, or a combination of both. The dietetic advice should not merely be to restrict the protein and acid-forming food intake but also to increase the alkalising foods—i.e. the vegetables and salad content of the diet.

20 Osteitis spinal syndromes

The vertebral column is not often the site of infective inflammatory disease, but tuberculous osteitis can occur and staphylococcyal osteomyelitis sometimes develops there.

Tuberculous osteitis can occur at any age but is more frequent in early adult life. There is a gradual onset of pain, usually in the lower thoracic spine, and the individual will prefer not to engage in vigorous activity in the early stages, without necessarily being able to explain why. As weeks pass the pain becomes apparent and is worse with jerky movements. General symptoms develop and the patient becomes ill with lassitude, anorexia, loss of weight, and mild pyrexia. Then a kyphosis and perhaps an abscess develops, but these symptoms appear late. What is required is an early diagnosis.

The early signs are the ones which need emphasis. Rigidity and muscle guarding are the key-signs, and the springing test (p. 53) is vital. If this test were used in all spinal examinations, and if suspicions were aroused in the physician's mind in every patient who had a positive muscle-guarding reaction to the springing test, very few pathological disorders of the spine would escape early detection.

All patients with the positive springing test should be X-rayed to exclude pathological changes before assuming a mechanical diagnosis.

The earliest X-ray finding is haziness of the trabeculae. The haziness may be due to the patient moving while the X-ray was being taken, but in that case the whole film is hazy. If one or two vertebrae look hazy and all the others are normal, this should arouse suspicion. Usually two vertebrae are involved and the bodies become rarefied; they soften and become wedge-shaped. The disc between thins but does not become fully absorbed. Tuberculosis can affect the cervical spine, the lumbar spine, and the sacro-iliac joints. In the cervical and lumbar areas rigidity, pain, and muscle guarding are the chief effects. In the sacro-iliac joints the springing and gapping tests again are invaluable for presumptive diagnosis, but the final diagnosis can only be established by radiological examination. A localised bulging of the paravertebral shadow strongly suggests a cold abscess. These occur at the site of the disease and only later track down fascial planes.

The differential diagnosis of tuberculous osteitis of the spine involves consideration of other diseases:

(a) *Calvé's disease* is a rare destructive disease of a vertebra said to be due to an eosinophilic granuloma. It affects children of five to ten years of age. The bone becomes rarefied and may collapse to produce a kyphosis with pain and deformity, but the adjacent disc spaces are normal. With sufficient rest these children's spines recover well.

(b) *Osteochondrosis* affects several vertebrae, and irregularity of shape rather than haziness of outline, is characteristic radiologically.

(c) *Malignant disease* may affect two adjacent vertebrae, but this is very rare to start with. There is localised rarefaction but no haziness of trabeculae in the adjacent normal bone of the same vertebra.

(d) *Osteoporosis* may lead to angular kyphosis, but all the vertebrae are involved in the rarefaction, not just two as in tuberculosis.

(e) *Staphylococcal osteomyelitis* of the vertebral bodies. This is a more acute disease with pyrexia, severe pain, and intense muscle guarding. It can commence slowly and then reliance must be placed on finding a raised sedimentation rate, leucocytosis, and afternoon raised temperatures.

(f) *Sacro-iliac diseases* are bilateral (p. 186), but tuberculous sacro-iliitis is unilateral at its commencement. Considerable destruction is usually apparent by the time a diagnosis is established. It starts in the lower pole of the sacro-iliac joint.

21 Neoplastic syndromes

The characteristic feature of a neoplasm of the spine is that it produces almost constant symptoms, and once pain begins it remains continuous irrespective of position or of movement. Little relief is obtained from the usual analgesics. Eighty per cent of cases present with pain—i.e. root pain—and dull central backache. This may be worse at night and relieved by activity. Backache which persists and fails to respond to rest should arouse suspicion.

The reader must refer to other texts for detailed accounts of neoplasms of bone and nerve tissue; but, because of the relative frequency and importance of the subject and because all practitioners who deal with the spinal column will sooner or later have patients suffering from neoplasms, the most significant aspects of this problem are set down.

Secondary malignant deposits in bone are the commonest cause of pain in this context. They usually derive from primary growths in the breast, prostate, and lung, and more rarely from the colon, stomach, bladder, thyroid, kidney, and uterus.

The lumbar spine is the commonest site, but occasionally the thoracic and cervical vertebrae are affected, as is the pelvis. In the first instance only one vertebra is involved but later more vertebrae may be affected. The intervertebral discs act as a temporary barrier to spread between one vertebra and the next. The majority of secondaries are *osteolytic* and show in X-rays as an area of rarefaction without any reactive sclerosis. Sometimes the bone looks as if it has disappeared. Adjacent bone is normal in appearance, and the growth is circumscribed though not well defined. Soon the body of the vertebra becomes too soft to support the tissues, and wedging—with a kyphosis—develops. At that stage pain is present even if it had not been present before, and it may be severe. Some secondary bone deposits, especially from a primary prostatic carcinoma, are *osteosclerotic* and show increased density on the X-ray. This density is patchy, especially if it affects the pelvis.

Constant pain unrelieved by any position is a significant warning that something *serious* is wrong with the patient. It is true to say that psychogenic pain is constant, unrelieved by analgesics and unaltered by position, but the psychopathic personality embroiders the pain with exaggerated phraseology.

Blood tests are helpful. The erythrocyte sedimentation rate is raised. In prostatic carcinoma the serum acid-phosphatase is raised above the normal level of 3 units per cent. In Paget's disease the serum alkaline-phosphate level is raised above the normal of 13 units per cent.

Once a kyphosis has developed, the spinal movements are painful and the springing test evokes the characteristic reflex guarding of the paravertebral muscles. By this time referred pain and signs of root irritation have usually started. If the disease progresses, paraplegia develops and the cord is affected. The kyphosis and the radiological wedging of the vertebral bodies have to be differentiated from those which occur in osteoporosis, but with osteoporosis a group of vertebrae is porotic and may show ballooning of the discs leading to the appearances of the fish-tail vertebrae that are characteristic. The wedging of secondary deposits can be lateral, but this is unusual in osteoporosis.

After the pathological fracture has occurred some attempt at repair takes place, and sometimes the vertebra becomes sclerosed with callus; but the diagnosis is usually established before this stage has been reached.

Multiple myelomatosis affects the spinal column in middle-aged people. It affects more than one vertebra at the outset; and, if it is not diagnosed earlier from its generalised symptoms of anaemia and pyrexia, it may commence suddenly with signs of vertebral collapse. Before this the symptoms are vague and diagnosis is difficult. Multiple punched-out areas of rarefaction occur in other bones besides the vertebrae, and the Bence-Jones protein found in the urine is pathognomonic. This is easily tested by heating some urine in a test-tube; precipitation of Bence-Jones protein occurs at 50°C and then it redissolves again with higher temperatures.

Once the spinal column is involved the pain becomes intense, and high dosages of morphia may become imperative. I regret to this day when I was a house surgeon allowing a patient to suffer needlessly because I thought I ought to limit the dose to the standard 15 mg.

A *haemangioma* is a benign tumour of blood-vessels, and it occasionally affects the vessels in the body of a vertebra. I have never seen one which caused symptoms, and they have only been diagnosed radiologically. They show as long streaky lines in the vertebral bodies. No treatment is needed, but the patient should be X-rayed from time to time to note any changes.

Intraspinal neoplasms cause backache and root pain. They are mainly benign tumours of the nerve sheaths and meninges rather than spinal cord tumours.[103] They slowly expand to block the spinal canal, at first causing intermittent pain and later continuous pain unaffected by position or movement.

X-rays may show pressure erosion of the posterior aspect of the vertebral bodies. Lumbar puncture demonstrates a spinal block and myelography is important to delineate the tumour. Gautier-Smith[104] emphasises that the early manifestations of lumbo-sacral neurofibroma cannot be distinguished clinically from those of prolapsed discs and, as they are benign, surgical removal is usually very satisfactory.

Summary of warnings in the history and the signs and symptoms which point to serious pathological processes.

1 A patient who presents with backache, having a history of malignancy during the previous two years, must be assumed to have secondary malignant deposits in the spine until this is proved otherwise, even though the onset is mild and the signs and X-rays are negative. Usually such patients have a raised erythrocyte sedimentation rate.

2 When the onset of back pain is late in life, without any previous history of back symptoms, the patient is more likely to have osteoporosis or secondary deposits than some simple mechanical fault.

3 When there is serious loss of spinal function, or shock, or vomiting after trivial spinal injury or strain, the patient is likely to have a pathological fracture of the spine.

4 Intense pain which requires morphia for more than forty-eight hours may indicate serious disease.

5 Severe pain, deformity, and muscle spasm in areas of the spine other than the lower cervical and lower lumbar should arouse suspicion of disease.

6 Constitutional signs which accompany back pain like pyrexia, loss of weight, malaise, and excessive weakness suggest disease.

7 Loss of power which is too widespread to be accountable by a single nerve-root lesion suggests neurological disease.

8 Loss of sphincter control is never due to simple mechanical causes.

9 Continuous pain unrelated to posture is unlikely to be mechanical in origin.

10 A normal erythrocyte sedimentation rate does not exclude disease entirely.

22 Miscellaneous diseases involving the spine

Paget's disease
Morquio's disease
Brucellosis
Alkaptonuria

Paget's disease can affect the spine and pelvis as well as the skull, femora, and tibiae. It is not serious, and for our purpose here, its recognition is what is important. Occasionally the widening of a vertebra causes distortion and persistent nerve-root pressure symptoms.

The classical later stage of the disease can be diagnosed from the enlargement of the head, the heavy stooping posture, and the bowing of the femora forward and the tibiae laterally; but the cases which cause some difficulty in diagnosis are those where there is a dull vague backache unaffected by position or movement. In these cases the diagnosis can only be made radiologically. The affected vertebrae have large coarse tràbeculae, and there is increased density with splaying and flattening. One isolated vertebra can be involved or several. The disease often affects the sacrum or the innominates. No manual treatment is effective, and usually analgesics are sufficient to relieve the pain.

Morquio's disease is a rare disorder of bone formation. It is a chondro-osteodystrophy affecting mainly the thoracic vertebrae. It leads to stunted growth, kyphosis, and restricted hip movements which make walking difficult. The epiphyses show irregular ossification, and the vertebral bodies are narrowed and wedge-shaped, with scalloped anterior surfaces. Although treatment of this condition cannot influence the shape of the vertebral column, articulatory and soft-tissue treatment can give some relief from backache. An increased range of movements can be expected from treating children while they are growing.

Brucellosis, now fortunately rare, can lead to advanced degenerative changes, especially in the lumbar spine. It should be suspected in patients who have lived in infected areas of the globe, and in whom spondylosis is more evident than that which would occur spontaneously. The treatment is similar to that for the usual form of spondylosis.

Alkaptonuria is a rare metabolic disease of amino acids, which affects the cartilages of the body rendering them brittle and friable. The discs become thin and calcified irregularly. The spine becomes rigid—not unlike an ankylosing spondylitis clinically, but the X-rays show no changes in the sacro-iliac joints and the ligaments are not calcified. The symptoms are not severe and the condition is best left alone.

There are other diseases which can afflict the spinal column, such as Cushing's syndrome, acromegaly, thyrotoxicosis, typhoid fever, syphilis, actinomycosis, hydatid disease, leukaemia, Hodgkin's disease, chordoma, sarcoma, aneurysmal bone cyst, and osteoid osteoma, but the spinal problem in these diseases is merely of secondary importance, and they are mentioned here only for completeness. The reader must look elsewhere for an account of these diseases.

23 Visceral backache syndromes

Visceral disease expresses itself in manifold ways, and when pain is a feature, it is usually felt anteriorly in the chest or abdomen. Because of this most medical examinations are made with the patient lying supine. During my medical student days I never saw a patient turned over to lie prone for a detailed examination of the spine, except in the ortho-paedic wards. This is a pity, because even if the patient does not com-plain of backache among other symptoms, the visceral disease often leads to paravertebral muscle tension and tenderness in the spinal seg-ments related to the nerve-supply of the viscus. Mackenzie[105] pointed this out in 1925.

However, backache may be the presenting feature of some visceral diseases, and those who specialise in spinal problems must constantly bear this in mind. A general examination should never be omitted, even in patients whose symptoms are obviously of spinal origin.

In general, visceral backache is *characterised* by a diffuse dull con-tinuous ache which is unrelated to posture. The local signs in the spine are not well defined, but the paravertebral muscles are sometimes tense and tender at the level of the nerve-supply of the viscus. There are no articular signs of muscle guarding, blocked movements, or sharp pain on particular movements.

The pelvic viscera can cause dull continuous mid-sacral backache. Gastro-intestinal pain may be felt in the upper lumbar spine. Renal pain may be felt in the loins, and cardiac or pulmonary pain can be felt in the mid-thoracic spine.

A list of diseases known to cause back pain includes: cardiac infarct, pneumothorax, carcinoma of the oesophagus, peptic ulceration, pancreatitis and carcinoma of the pancreas, retro-caecal appendicitis, pyelitis, polycystic kidney disease, gall-bladder disease, enlargement of the liver, neoplasms of the bowel, chronic salpingo-oöphoritis, pelvic endometriosis, coitus interruptus and other sexual disturbances, and uterine diseases—i.e. fibroids, carcinoma, cervical erosions, large gravid impacted uterus, and dysmenorrhoea.

It goes without saying that visceral backache must be treated by tackling the source, but it must be remembered that when long estab-lished reflexes have created muscle and joint changes these may persist even after the primary source of symptoms has been eradicated. The residual muscle tension and joint restrictions in the spine may well need local treatment even when the pyelitis or cholecystitis has subsided.

Gynaecological backache Backache which accompanies the menstrual periods is common, and if it never occurs at other times the cause is likely to be gynaecological. However, backache which is merely accent-uated by the menstrual cycle, and which occurs at other times as well, has usually a mechanical or structural cause.

Gynaecological backache is not well localised and the pain is felt lower than that of structural backache. The patient points vaguely to the centre of the sacrum. The pain is diffuse, and there are no localising signs of tenderness or impaired mobility.

Uterine displacements rarely cause backache except when accompanied by adhesions which limit the movement of the uterus or when associated with prolapse of the uterus, so that when palpating bimanually our concern should be more to determine the mobility than to determine the shape. Prolapse of the uterus and vaginal walls can only be effectively palpated with the patient in the standing position, asking her to bear down during the examination.

When the uterus is tethered by adhesions the organ should be moved firmly by the palpating finger to try and elicit pain. If backache is so provoked, this is strong evidence of a gynaecological cause.

When a prolapse is present, wearing a pessary is a useful diagnostic treatment because, if the backache is relieved, then again the gynaecological cause is established.

Stretching of the sacro-uterine ligaments either by prolapse or by tightening with posterior parametritis has a pulling effect on the anterior sacral nerves which gives rise to backache.

Unsatisfactory sexual intercourse, as with coitus interruptus and incomplete orgasm, can lead to backache which is psychogenic in origin. Backache which occurs on the day following intercourse is more likely to be due to lumbo-sacral ligamentous strain than to a gynaecological abnormality.

Backache which follows childbirth can be due to relaxed ligaments or disc lesions, and sacro-iliac strains are common. These are dealt with in the appropriate sections of this book.

Backache which develops during pregnancy may be ligamentous or discal in origin, but it is more likely to be due to lordosis.

24 Psychogenic spinal syndromes

A distinction should be drawn between psychogenic disorders in which backache is a feature and those cases of backache due to mechanical faults in which excessive anxiety exaggerates the whole picture.

Backache may be one of the symptoms of major mental disease, such as depression, psychosis, schizophrenia, and severe neurosis.

When backache is due to mental disease, the back should not be treated, otherwise these symptoms will be accentuated, and management will become more difficult; but one must not forget that mentally deranged patients can also suffer injury to their spines.

Psychogenic causes should be suspect when the spinal symptoms are out of proportion to the physical signs; when tenderness is excessive and widespread; when the physical signs are inconsistent with each other; when full movements are present and there are no signs of the ligamentous strain syndrome; when there is a history that all treatments have made the patient worse; when there is no relief from any analgesic; when new symptoms take the place of old ones; when other symptoms, like fatigue, palpitation, or headaches are also present; when symptoms are bizarre in character; when the patient keeps consulting one doctor after another; when the symptoms are described in exaggerated terms; or when severe and serious symptoms are described with an accompanying smile!

When we examine patients who are psychologically disturbed we find moist hands, poor handshake, rapid pulse, tension and inability to relax, brisk reflexes, and exaggerated, delayed, or anticipated responses to tests, with altered responses when the patient's attention is distracted to some other part of the body.

Sometimes patients come along with symptoms which are due to mechanical faults previously unrecognised by several doctors. These patients are liable to use exaggerated phrases with the object of drawing sufficient attention to ensure that the doctor does not dismiss these symptoms as of no consequence. When such patients with genuine physical pain realise that the new doctor understands and believes in their pain, the mental relief is as great as the physical. The stage is then set for genuine help and physical treatment. Such patients then cease to exaggerate and begin to use normal phraseology to describe their symptoms and their response to treatment.

Some of the most grateful patients are those in whom anxiety has led them to believe that they are suffering from serious disease, yet in whom a simple mechanical fault has been explained and clearly demonstrated and then cured by the appropriate mechanical treatment. Their relief from symptoms is all the greater because the anxiety has also been relieved.

It is sometimes justifiable to allow patients to retain a physical symptom which is an expression of their psychological problem because it is a good excuse for their inadequacy, but a physician should not agree with and lend his support to an excuse for the patient to avoid duties which she should perform for others.

We should never create psychological symptoms by any treatment. This may be done unwittingly, but I have come across patients who have what I call a 'positional neurosis'. They come in complaining that this bone or that one is out of place or that their pelvis is displaced, and that 'so and so has manipulated my bones, but the bones keep coming out of place as soon as they are manipulated back'. It is not easy always to convince such patients that their bones do not go in and out of place.

I fear that some practitioners keep patients on treatment for months or even years on this pretext, but I cannot deprecate this mismanagement too strongly.

When simple common sense, sympathetic attitudes, and demonstrated reassurance fail to cure psychogenic backache then it is time to call in the psychiatrist.

4

THE ART OF OSTEOPATHY

Fine art is that in which the hand,
the head and the heart of man go together.
The Two Paths JOHN RUSKIN

The practice of osteopathy is an art based on knowledge. Perfection in any art demands constant practice and painstaking attention to detail. The artist needs to be single-minded and purposeful in his pursuit of perfection, and he needs to be temperamentally attuned to his subject at an early age. It is sometimes said that great artists are born not made. This is only half a truth. Such people may be naturally gifted in a particular direction, but the greatest quality required is the ability to work hard and long, to absorb as much knowledge as possible from every available source, and then to mould that knowledge with original ideas and interpretations.

The basic knowledge is anatomy—living dynamic anatomy—not just dissection anatomy. This in turn implies knowledge of physiology because functional anatomy is alive; it is the living structure of the body. But even before the student can study anatomy and physiology he must have had a sound general education, including the subjects of biology, chemistry, physics, and mechanics.

Medical anatomy tends to be 'dead' anatomy because it is taught from the dissection room. It is also geared to the needs of the surgeons of the future.

Medical physiology tends to be based in the first instance on animal physiology; the student spends too much time in my view on animal experiments and not sufficient time on their application to human physiology in the study of his own and his fellow student's muscles, joints, gastric juices, etc.

The two subjects of anatomy and physiology need to be integrated, and anatomy needs to be equated with living structures at the earliest possible moment. The skeleton should not merely be studied as dry bones. The bones should be visualised on the living normal subject. A femur should have all its shapes described and its muscle attachments demonstrated, but then the student should feel his own femoral condyles, the adductor tubercle, the greater trochanter, and the sciatic notch. He should palpate the biceps femoris and feel resisted contractions in it, learning to locate all structures in the living normal subject.

While on the topic of the femur, the student should learn about the arterial supply, the histology, the activity of the marrow, and the interrelationship of the bone, calcium metabolism, the liver and spleen, and so on.

If these subjects could be taught without artificial watertight compartments the student would learn to appreciate the normal, and later on would be in a better position to recognise the abnormal. I have taught medical graduates who have never before palpated the mastoid process let alone the transverse process of the atlas.

How many students who successfully pass their anatomy and physiology examinations could locate the articular processes in the cervical spine? Yet these structures are superficial and obvious to palpation. How many preclinical students could feel a muscle and say whether it was in good tone or not? How many have studied the functional capacity of their own heart and lungs?

Living applied anatomy and physiology in the normal subject should be the basis of the osteopathic students' training. After that he can learn about the abnormal, the faulty mechanics, and the diseased conditions of patients at a clinical level.

Of course it is possible to miss out these basic studies and merely apply treatment. There have been successful bonesetters who have learned a few tricks, becoming expert technicians in a limited sphere, but this is not applying osteopathy in its full sense. Furthermore there is considerable risk in just applying a treatment without first making a diagnosis.

The physiotherapist's training does not dwell on aetiology and diagnosis but rather on techniques and treatment, leaving the diagnostic side to the qualified medical practitioner. The physiotherapist is a technician who learns a series of treatments and applies these under guidance, and this is quite in order.

An osteopath may have a training in techniques alone and can become quite adept, but without the basic knowledge of aetiology, pathology, and diagnosis he will make many mistakes.

Equally a medical graduate who has had no training in osteopathy can learn a few manipulations and, with his basic diagnostic knowledge, he may avoid too many errors; but without mechanical knowledge— without studying vertebral mechanics, physiological movements, mobility tests, and so forth—he too will make errors, and the value of manipulation will be discredited.

The ideal osteopath is one who has studied the basic subjects and become competent in all preclinical subjects, who has acquired the essential medical knowledge in all its aspects, and who has then specialised in the study of body mechanics, mechanical diagnosis, and mechanical treatment.

Such a graduate—one who has graduated into mature adulthood, who has studied Life itself, and who has a compelling urge to help his fellow man—can then apply his knowledge so that it becomes an art. Art is involved in this work because we have not infinite knowledge about the structure of the body and how it becomes faulty. Furthermore, mechanical problems are rarely the only ones which patients suffer. They may need help with their anxieties as well as with their backache. They may need advice about their work, hobbies, and posture as well as about their sciatica.

If the character of the osteopath is sound, his motives are genuine, and his knowledge is wide, he can then inspire confidence. These qualities are even more important than the skill of manipulation.

The art of osteopathy can be compared with the art of playing a musical instrument. The practitioner is the artist, and the instrument is the human body. The musician can learn to play intricate melodies after he has painstakingly learned to play the scales and arpeggios. The pianist must develop his muscle power for the fortissimo passages and delicacy of touch for the pianissimo passages. So too must the osteopath learn the basic theme of normality before he can learn the variations on the original theme. He must learn the techniques of palpation, massage, and articulation before he goes on to acquire the skill of specific adjustments.

One advantage the musician has over the osteopath is that he can rely on his instrument. Unfortunately the human body is so variable an instrument that it is often impossible 'to play the same tune on any two spines'. The player has to adapt his technique to the instrument he is playing, and he must be able to attune his own personality to that of the patient. In a busy practice he may have to adjust himself from, say, an enthusiastic golfer coming about his annoying elbow, to a deeply anxious patient worried about cancer, or to the impatient business man who wants his neck 'clicked' into place between board meetings. Such adaption requires a flexibility of mind as well of muscles on the part of the practitioner.

Osteopathic practice is, in the main, 'office' practice. The patients attend by appointment. The rooms should be attractive and clean, and the facilities for dressing and undressing adequate. It is a waste of time for the patient to dress and undress in the consulting room, and patients need a while to adjust themselves to their new surroundings. Most patients are worried, and the door should be opened to them with a smile of welcome and reassurance. A short wait of a few minutes is ideal so that they can recover breath after rushing in to be on time for the appointment. The osteopath needs pleasant competent staff to create a friendly atmosphere right at the onset. The consultation itself should be unhurried, and ample time should be given to history taking and examination. If X-rays are needed the ideal arrangement is to have facilities on the spot or at least nearby, and without undue delay so that the diagnosis can be confirmed early and advice given even if treatment cannot be started straight away. The majority of patients should be X-rayed not merely because it helps with diagnosis but because the fact of taking an X-ray completes the examination and has a reassuring effect on the anxious patient.

Before examining the patient the practitioner should wash and warm his hands not only for cleanliness but because cold hands are unfriendly and they set up muscle tensions which were not there before. If the operator has taken trouble to arrange everything well in advance, and has established a good initial rapport, the patient may tolerate his cold hands but this will be a shock, both physical and mental. The hands are the vehicle by which the operator communicates confidence and assurance, and if they are cold they are a poor vehicle. The hands must be firm and searching but not hard or prodding. They speak for themselves, and patients sense their communication more easily even than the spoken word.

The art of osteopathy should be directed to help the patient recover from his or her disability. It is the application of principles, rules, and precepts, modified by experience, which creates harmony within the body of the patient. It is in this sense that it is creative. No tangible end-product is produced; but creating a happy comfortable person out of a depressed, hopeless, and pain racked patient is creative work in the the finest sense. Attaining such objectives gives the practitioner his greatest sense of achievement. This is the culmination of his years of study and hard work. The satisfaction from such achievement is beyond any other reward, but other reward there should be—financial reward for advice and treatment given. This serves not only the livelihood of the practitioner but is a mode of thanks on the part of the patients. It is a measure of sacrifice in their recovery, and while fees should not be excessive they should be commensurate with the status, the effort, and the training of the practitioner.

The confidence of the practitioner in himself and his own ability increases with age and experience and with the successes he obtains. Thus confidence is enhanced by a series of successes, and dashed to the ground by a failure when success was expected.

The osteopath should always remain humble in the realisation that, even when the patient recovers well and fully, he—the osteopath—has merely been instrumental in helping Nature to restore normality. Were it not for this law of Nature which is constantly operating, our efforts would look poor indeed. Many of us accept praise and reward from patients when the true recovery is due to Nature herself. There is no harm in the patient being appreciative, but the osteopath in turn must appreciate Nature's healing forces. He should be glad and humble, recognising that he is merely removing some mechanical obstruction to the natural recovery of the patient.

If the osteopath adopts a cock-sure and over-confident attitude, he will surely suffer the 'fate of Icarus' many times. Failures are salutary lessons; but when, from knowledge and experience, the osteopath can be confident of success in a particular case, this confidence can and should be imparted to the patient. Many patients need the reassurance of a confident manner, but it is unwise to predict 'cures'. It is better to be continuously optimistic about the outcome, and as the treatments continue and some initial improvement takes place, then both practitioner and patient can rightly add to their confidence in recovery.

Arrogance and conceit, pomposity and affectation are not the qualities which lead to success in osteopathic practice. But modesty and sincerity, sympathy and dedication are the qualities which will evoke the greatest response and thereby the greatest success in this work.

The osteopath should learn from every patient. He should learn more from his failures than from his successes. We osteopaths have such a powerful agent in our hands that successes are to be expected and some patients respond when we least expect it, but we should observe the changes which have occurred and seek a satisfactory explanation for the recovery. When a patient is getting better it is so easy to relax the attention, and neglect the details, and just give some haphazard treatment, leaving Nature and time to resolve the rest of the patient's symptoms. An attempt should always be made to note and palpate the changes which have occurred to see if they tally with the recovery.

Many of the lesions we find are small in themselves, and there is a great temptation to 'find' lesions to account for the patient's symptoms and then, as soon as the patient recovers, to cease to take an interest in the mechanics. It is important to have firm criteria in mechanical diagnosis because it is very easy to be misled—and in fact to mislead oneself —into believing that such and such a lesion is present. We should be as objective as possible, always searching for physical signs which are independent of subjective sensations.

This sort of make-belief happens in other spheres of medicine. It is easy to imagine heart murmurs, for example, and to try to fit them in with the clinical picture; but then what about the murmur which is obvious and yet the patient has perfect functional capacity? Equally so, once the patient's chest is asymptomatic, it is understandable to dismiss the odd rales and rhonchi as unimportant.

We attach more importance to signs which fit in with our concept of what is wrong with the patient. We would all like a simple explanation. Other signs and symptoms which do not fit in with the diagnosis tend to be discounted, and although this is humanly understandable it may lead us into errors of diagnosis. Ideally we should try to remain detached and certainly to avoid getting emotionally involved with our patients: what I mean is that when a patient is getting better we must not just 'preen our feathers' because we are being praised, but rather retain a scientific searching attitude and ask ourselves why has she got better and whether this experience can be of help with other patients.

We should ever be conscious of the fact that the patient may have recovered in any case. We must not even rule out of our detached approach the possibility that the patient has recovered in spite of the treatment, and that the treatment might have aggravated the symptoms or delayed the recovery. This is what I mean by being humble.

It is not easy to remain detached in our appraisal of successes, and the only type of case in which we can be absolutely sure that our intervention has helped is that in which symptoms had become chronic and unremitting, and then quite suddenly recovery follows straight after treatment.

It is also natural to search for some explanation other than the treatment given when the patient's symptoms are aggravated, but the practitioner should be prepared to accept blame if the sequence strongly suggests that the treatment was at fault. He should learn from these sequelae, and avoid making the same mistake again. It is common in all branches of medicine to turn a blind eye to our failures and to take pride in our successes.

A reasonable detached view must be maintained, and a single bad experience over a method of treatment must not lead us into discarding the treatment for ever and for every other patient.

Certain orthopaedic surgeons condemn manipulation in capsulitis of the shoulder in every case because in some they found that the symptoms were accentuated. Consequently many of their patients continue to be incapacitated for long periods unnecessarily. If a form of treatment is effective in some cases and not in others it is our duty to try to find out in which category our patient belongs. With experience it is possible to tell which patients are likely to respond well and which will not.

The student of osteopathy, as with any other subject, has to accept what he is taught, but he should receive it with an open mind. There is room for differences of opinion and differences of approach in most subjects, but especially so in osteopathy. The student is at first quite unable to sift the wheat from the chaff, and only his own experience will enable him to do this at a later stage. He can observe the teacher's methods, however, and he can usually judge whether the teacher is good or not, whether he is just repeating parrot-fashion what he himself has learned, or whether he has been thoughtful and observant and is speaking from experience.

The student should try to learn from everything he does, but he must not base an opinion on one or two observations alone. He must not just learn a set of movements and apply them rigidly to all patients. It is very easy to allow oneself to adopt a stereotyped routine, but this is fatal to art, and the student should always be willing to try out other methods and approaches.

It is disconcerting to change one's habits or mode of thought and to find that the new method is no better or is worse than the old. Then we must go back to the older method, but the experience has been worth gaining. ' . . . to thine own self be true, and it must follow, as the night the day, thou canst not then be false to any man.'*

When patients seek advice from osteopaths they do so because there is something wrong and the condition has failed to recover spontaneously or the medical advice they have had has not helped so that symptoms persist.

The patient goes to a particular practitioner because she has been recommended to do so. Consequently before she arrives she has probably satisfied herself that he is a competent person to entrust with her problem. The patient has already some idea of what to expect, and she has already been favourably impressed by the reputation of the practitioner and by her own reception as she enters the rooms. She is full of hope, she is nervous, and she is worried about meeting a stranger, about what she will be told, and about the prognosis. She will be uncertain of what the treatment will be and its outcome. It is the duty of the physician to assuage these fears, and to explain in simple non-technical language just what is wrong with the patient, to give a reasonable explanation of why things went wrong, and to show that the treatment proposed is reasonable and one which, based on past experience, has been effective with other patients.

In these ways the physician is establishing a good rapport with the patient. Gone are the days when the doctor just listened to the symptoms then made his examination and prescribed a medicine or left instructions for treatment to be carried out. When two people meet—the patient and the doctor—the doctor must be in charge yet must not dominate merely by force of personality. Adequate explanations must be given so

*Hamlet, William Shakespeare.

that the patient complies with the doctor's advice by persuasion and reasoning rather than by force. Much better co-operation will be achieved in this way. A friendly feeling and mutual trust must be established. Not only must the patient trust in the doctor's advice but the doctor must trust the patient to carry out his advice. The interplay between the character of the patient and the character of the doctor operates at all times, and the response to treatment is in large measure a response to this interplay. The interplay of personalities is felt in a physical plane much more between osteopath and patient as compared with allopathic physician and patient because there is much more physical contact. Physical resistance to osteopathic treatment spoils any chance of success, and the ability of the osteopath to achieve relaxation on the part of the patient is a measure of the successful rapport between the two.

The patient is ready to relax if confidence is established. A good deal of confidence can be instilled before touching the patient, but this is only fully achieved when the osteopath places his hands on the patient.

In spite of overt willingness to accept the treatment, the patient may unwittingly resist one's efforts. It may only be necessary to ask for relaxation for it to be given wholeheartedly and without reservation, but if the patient is not willing enough it suggests either that pain is preventing relaxation or that there is a deeper fear which has not been overcome. When a patient is not relaxing, one's first question should be 'Am I hurting you?', rather than just instructing the patient to relax. With the best will and the fullest co-operation, she will be unable to relax if the condition or the manœuvre is causing pain. That is why an anaesthetic is sometimes necessary if manipulation is required to cure the painful condition. A good rule is never to hurt the patient, although this rule cannot be applied universally, as Robert Maigne[88] advocates in *Les Manipulations Vertébrales. Le régle de la non douleur* is a good rule because it is a safe rule, but there are indications for manipulations which cause pain—for example, when adhesions are blocking the movement rather than displaced disc fragments. When the pain is slight then the patient may well be able to relax sufficiently for release of the adhesion, but if this is impossible and yet the indications are clear that manipulation should be performed then it is better to use an anaesthetic rather than to force the manipulation against the resistance of the patient.

Occasionally a patient actually resents having treatment. For example, a wife may be sent by her husband who insists on her coming, or a youth may be driven unwillingly by anxious parents so that the boy feels it is an indignity to be treated. This resistance to treatment is quite different from that engendered by fear. It is the resistance of merely being touched or handled. This can happen even if there is a clash of personalities or a clash of hormones!

Rapport between patient and doctor must be cultivated to the fullest. Not only must the patient have confidence, but she must understand what is wrong and how it is being dealt with. Explanations are not always easy, especially when trying to simplify the matter by using lay terms, but a useful method is to show the X-rays to the patient so that she can see what is wrong and see the point in manipulating. But as patients are not usually accustomed to looking at X-rays and the films are in any case in two dimensions only, it is even more helpful if they can be shown a vertebra or a vertebral column so that the condition can be visualised in three dimensions. A mental picture of what is wrong and what is being done greatly facilitates the rapport and relaxation which is half the battle of recovery. Furthermore follow-up treatment, such as correction of posture, alteration of occupation or habits, the performance of exercises, etc., will be carried out more willingly and more diligently if the patient understands why she should comply.

It will be appreciated that although manipulation is the crux of the matter, it is but part of the whole procedure in the art of osteopathy.

APPENDIX 1

CONTRA-INDICATIONS TO MANIPULATION

During the study of the preceding pages, the reader will have noticed the stress placed upon manipulative procedures. This is because manipulation is our chief modality amongst the various physical methods of treatment which can be used when dealing with structural problems. However, sometimes there are disadvantages or even dangers in manipulation. For example, manipulation is *absolutely contra-indicated* in the following diseases: malignancy, tuberculosis, osteomyelitis, active osteoporosis, fractures, ruptured ligaments, acute arthritis of any form, and large disc prolapses in which there are serious neurological changes from pressure on the spinal cord, cauda equina, and nerve-roots.

In many conditions manipulation is contra-indicated not because it may be dangerous, as in the above diseases, but *merely because manipulation is ineffective* in any case. This applies to most established diseases: the fevers, venereal disease, tropical diseases, parasitic diseases, endocrine diseases, metabolic disorders and vitamin deficiencies, blood dyscrasias, gastro-intestinal diseases other than functional disturbances, cardio-vascular diseases except some disorders of vasomotion, respiratory diseases except those due to mechanical hindrance to breathing, genito-urinary diseases, neurological diseases except cervical myelopathy, organic dementias and psychoses, and skin diseases.

Then there are some conditions in which great care must be taken in manipulation—these are not absolute but *relative contra-indications*—not necessarily contra-indications for the experienced practitioner but certainly contra-indications for the tiro: cervical disc prolapse, osteoarthritis, lumbar disc herniations, lumbar disc prolapses with abnormal central nervous system signs, bilateral root signs, or sciatica with a straight-leg raising test of less than 30°, hypermobility, and scolioses.

Manipulation is best avoided when the general health is depleted and when attempted manipulation provokes too much resistance on the part of the patient either from fear or pain.

One must remember that manipulation does not always imply

specific techniques and while specific procedures are sometimes in-appropriate other manual methods, like articulatory techniques and soft-tissue techniques, might be quite safe and eminently beneficial. The reader will have gleaned this from the main body of the book. Some types of manipulation are more effective or less effective according to which stage the condition has developed in its natural history.

When in doubt we should not manipulate, but play for time and be content with soft-tissue and articulatory methods.

Although any effective treatment has its attendent dangers—and this applies to every surgical operation—the rare adverse effects from such procedures must not lead to the wholesale condemnation of the method.

If the occasional death under anaesthesia, or fatal haemorrhage, or surgical shock, or failure in surgical technique led to the total condemna-tion of surgery then the human race would be sadly worse off; and yet there are people who would not have an operation at any price. Similarly, it would be equally foolish to condemn all manipulation simply because on one or two occasions patients have been made worse by it. The fault lies with the technician rather than with the subject.

With proper training, and with knowledge and long experience, there is immense value in manipulation and even greater value in the wide application of osteopathic principles in the treatment of human ills.

APPENDIX 2

Osteopathic research has been directed along four main channels.

1 Clinical and radiological observations upon groups of patients.
2 Animal experiments to study the effects of artificially induced mechanical sprains in their spines.
3 Observations upon the effects of artificially induced mechanical strains on human subjects.
4 The study of spinal mechanics, spinal anatomy, and related physiology with a view to improving and rationalising manipulative procedures.

During the history of osteopathy these lines of research have not followed any pre-ordained plan but have evolved gradually.

A. T. Still, the founder of osteopathy, expounded a theory and his followers, having found that the theory worked well in practice, wanted to find out why. This question has not yet been answered fully and the search goes on.

1 Clinical research is greatly hampered by the complexity of the problem and the wide range of variables in which mechanical problems present themselves. The standard clinical procedure used in medicine for research is to take a large number of patients with a specific disease or symptom and then apply a single technique or administer a single drug, then watch the effect and compare the results with some placebo treatment. This method seeks to simplify and to reduce the number of variables, admirable in its motive, but an almost impossible task in the clinical study of mechanical problems. As has been seen in the preceding chapters there are many syndromes and the allocation of a patient to one of these is not always easy. The syndromes are varying constantly with the passage of time. Patients are of different ages, occupations and sporting activities, all of which influence their symptoms and progress. Then the techniques of manipulation are difficult to standardise. Each one is far from being applicable in every case and in order to obtain statistical results a large series of patients have to be treated on exactly the same lines by equally competent practitioners. A placebo manipulative technique is impracticable. The task of devising a clinical trial taking all these points into consideration may be possible but it has so far been beyond the scope and resources of the osteopathic profession.

A task of primary importance was undertaken by Denslow.[106] He studied the incidence of osteopathic lesions in a group of young adults to observe any correlations which may exist between the incidence and location of lesions on the one hand, and the general health of the individual, the position of the vertebral column and pelvis, and certain aspects of the vegetative nervous system activity, on the other.

Each adult was examined independently by two physicians to make sure that their clinical observations tallied. Eighty per cent of the observations did so and the observations were therefore considered valid. Denslow summarised the findings as follows:

> Two osteopathic physicians can agree on methods and interpretation of palpation to a point where they observe essentially the same tissue texture findings in a given case, even though they examine the case independently and without knowledge of the history and physical examination.
>
> Tissue texture abnormality occurs predominantly in the upper cervical, mid thoracic, and lumbosacral areas of the vertebral column and pelvis and at the angles of the upper ribs.
>
> In general, tissue texture abnormalities are associated with positional and weight-bearing disturbances of the vertebrae and pelvis. However, there are certain important exceptions which must be noted in that an exceptionally robust young adult may have a major disturbance in position without abnormality in the texture of the tissues; conversely, a patient may show a major disturbance in the texture of spinal tissues without a corresponding disturbance in the position of spinal joints.

Radiological observations on groups of patients have been recorded. One of the earliest studies was made by Schwab (1934).[107] He reported on a ten-year study of 540 low back cases. He X-rayed them in the erect position and found that 64 per cent had a 'primary anatomical short lower extremity'. This study was the first of its kind and showed, for the first time, the importance of the short leg and its influence on the spine. Pearson (1949)[108] made radiological and clinical studies of 800 school children and found that standing X-rays helped in the study of predisposing lesions and showed the indications for correction of these mechanical faults before symptoms appeared. Sixteen years of study of postural X-rays was reported on by Krause in 1948.[109] Bailey and Beckwith[67] studied 432 cases of low backache with erect X-rays.

Early osteopathic research was designed to demonstrate the close links between visceral and somatic function, at a time when medical thought kept visceral function and structural problems in water-tight compartments. Neither of these extreme standpoints have stood the test of time.

Clinical observations were made by recording changes on patients following osteopathic treatment. For example, Bandeen[110] showed that manipulation of the spine at 8–9T in unselected cases leads to an average fall in systolic blood-pressure of 10 mm and a fall of diastolic pressure of 5 mm. Northup[111] has shown a more sustained fall in blood-pressure in a small number of cases. In 100 selected cases of hypertension the average reduction of pressure immediately following treatment to the cervical spine and the mechanical faults elsewhere in the spine, was 33 mm of systolic and 9 mm of diastolic pressure.

Norris[112] studied the effect of general osteopathic treatment in both hypotension and hypertension and found that in hypotension the blood-pressure tended to rise towards normal and in hypertension the blood-pressure tended to fall towards normal. He also used control subjects and gave them a period of rest of two hours to compare them with patients having the osteopathic treatment. Twenty-six per cent of the controls had a lowered systolic pressure after two hours of rest but 40 per cent of treated patients had a lowering of systolic pressure.

Castlio and Ferris-Swift[113] showed that manual stimulation of the spleen, consisting of alternate compression and relaxation of the tissues overlying the spleen for five minutes, produced an increase in leucocyte count in 59 per cent of the cases within five minutes and 31 per cent showed a further increase at the end of thirty minutes. The average increase was nearly 2000 cells per cubic mm. They also found that the red-cell count actually fell in 76 per cent of the cases by an average of 726,000 cells per cubic mm.

McConnell[114] studied the anatomy and mechanics of viscera and stressed the importance of a mobile chest wall and an efficient diaphragm for good visceral function as well as for vascular and lymphatic drainage. He also pointed to the fascial links with the neck and abdomen through the cervical fascia, Sibson's fascia, the pericardium, and diaphragm and stressed the need for good posture to maintain the normal relationship of thoracic as well as abdominal viscera.

Sutherland made a careful study of the cranium, its contents and the mechanics of the skull. He developed a whole system of techniques for treating the cranium and claimed widespread beneficial effects. The method is described in detail by Magoun.[115]

2 *Animal experiments* have been used to provide evidence of the validity of the osteopathic theory. As early as 1898 Littlejohn[116] at Kirksville started experiments on dogs. C. P. McConnell[117] experimented for five years (1907–1912) on thirty-four dogs and six guinea pigs. He produced spinal subluxations in animals under anaesthesia and under traction. The object was to obtain a slight maladjustment of the articular surfaces. Post mortem examinations were made ranging from three to eighty days. A thorough autopsy was carried out before a more detailed examination of the lesioned area was made. The following quotation is noteworthy because of its influence on osteopathic thought between 1915 and 1930:

> In the lesion itself I fail to see where there is any perceptible partial occlusion of the spinal foramen by the encroaching bony tissues. *Slight tension of the encased fibrous tissue anchoring the structures passing through the opening is common.* This in itself in one sense will act as an occluding factor. But careful microscopic examination does not reveal any greater damage to nerves or vessels here than at several other places, and the *theory of pressure per se at this particular area is untenable. It is found that the permanent vertebral lesion is maintained by overstretched and damaged articular ligaments.* Sever either the capsules of the articular processes or the ligaments of the vertebral bodies and considerable motion is immediately obtained. The ligaments of the articular processes are the ones most damaged. The intervertebral cartilage itself· is usually only slightly damaged. The cartilages of the articular surfaces are little involved, that is, in slight and moderate degrees of lesion. One other point in lesion dissection was frequently noted, viz. hemorrhagic points along the fiber sheaths of the dorsal and ventral root bundles and within the membranes of the cord, notable between the pia and the arachnoid.

The other conclusions which McConnell came to, following artificially produced lesions on animals, were that there were degenerative changes in the neurones of the spinal cord but that these changes were not extensive or severe. The blood-vessels showed some endarteritis and the spinal cord and the ganglia were hyperaemic; diapedesis had occurred and leucocytic infiltration had developed. The paravertebral muscles showed increased connective tissue and atrophy of muscle fibres. The ligaments showed proliferation and thickening but the articular cartilage and bone structure showed no change.

Further serious and sustained research efforts were made in the early days of osteopathy by Dr. Louisa Burns. The A. T. Still Research Institute in Los Angeles was under her direction for nineteen years. In 1936 the American Osteopathic Foundation merged with the A. T. Still

Research Institute and more research work was undertaken by the individual Colleges of Osteopathy, notably by the Philadelphia College of Osteopathy and the Kirksville College of Osteopathy. A complete survey of the Osteopathic research from 1893 to 1954, can be found in the 1958 Year Book of the Academy of Applied Osteopathy—an excellent exposition by W. V. Cole.

Dr. Louisa Burns[118] continued the work of McConnell and produced mechanical lesions artificially in the spines of animals, then examined the effects of these at post mortems undertaken at varying intervals after the injury. She summarised her results in a survey in 1931 but the results of her animal experiments have been criticised not only by outside medical opinion but also within osteopathic circles, and much of the evidence is not acceptable.

However, more recent animal experiments have been performed by Hix[119] and these have been reported and accepted in the medical press. At the Kirksville College of Osteopathy in the department of physiology and pharmacology Hix, made extensive studies of renal physiology and by using exteriorised kidneys in experimental animals he demonstrated that there is a uretero-renal reflex, i.e. mechanically stimulating the ureter of the kidney leads to vaso-constriction and a reduced flow of urine. He also demonstrated that applying cold to the skin in the same dermatome linked segmentally with the kidney caused vaso-constriction of the kidney vessels on the same side. Only the ipsilateral kidney responded in this way but when the stimulus was considerable the contra-lateral kidney also reacted by vasoconstriction. This skin-to-kidney reflex (somatico-visceral) is in keeping with the osteopathic emphasis upon the close linkage between soma and viscera.

The most recent work on animals at Kirksville is directed by Korr.[120] His paper on 'Axonal Delivery of Neuroplasmic Components to Muscle Cells' has important implications regarding the trophic function of nerves as distinct from their motor or sensory function. The method adopted involved the injection of radioactive isotopes into the nuclei of the cranial nerves to observe the progress of these isotopes along the track of the nerves right into the substance of the tissues supplied by the nerve:

Our observations indicate that, when radio-active substances were selectively introduced into hypoglossal neurons, these substances, or their derivatives, were conveyed down the axons only to the muscle cells of the tongue and that they reached the muscle cells only via these axons—or very nearly so. The labelled molecules apparently crossed the neuromuscular junction into intracellular components of the muscle. We suggest that the proximo-distal conveyance and intercellular transfer of substances from the nerve cell may underline the so-called trophic and other long-term influence not based on impulses, of peripheral neurons on the metabolism, function, develop ment, differentiation, growth, and regeneration of the structures that they innervate.

Although the above animal experiments appeared to confirm osteo-pathic theory, there is one serious drawback to such research (applicable incidentally to all animal experiments), namely, that the animal's reac-tions are not directly applicable to human problems. The anatomy and physiology of animals and man differ and this is especially so from the structural point of view. Weight-bearing and postural factors are not at all comparable. It is possible that structural lesions in animals have a more serious effect than they have in human beings and although Louisa Burns showed that lesions induced in guinea pigs led to sterility it is improbable that such effects occur more than occasionally in human beings.

3 A change of emphasis, away from animal experiments and towards *human research*, commenced in 1940 when Denslow started to analyse the osteopathic lesion electromyographically. Instead of, as in the past, performing animal experiments to prove a theory, the new approach was that observations should be made on the human spine to measure, with newly developed apparatus, the altered skin, muscle, nerve, and bony changes which accompanied the spinal lesion. Instead of designing experiments to prove a theory, the new emphasis was to observe the facts and then to try to evolve a theory which could explain all these observations. Such research not only helps to elucidate the problems of spinal lesions, but contributes to the general fund of medical knowledge. The standard of osteopathic research was raised and reports began to be accepted in current scientific journals. The first of these papers by Denslow and Clough[121] was on 'Reflex Activity in the Spinal Extensors'.

Denslow demonstrated that when pressure is applied to spinous processes a contraction occurs in adjacent paravertebral muscles and that if pressure is applied to tender spinous processes, the adjacent paravertebral muscles contract with less stimulus than is required by muscles adjacent to normal spinous processes. The method used was to apply a calibrated pressure meter and record the electromyographic impulses in the erector spinae muscles adjacent to the spinous process. Less pressure was required to evoke the same reflex muscular activity in the lesioned segment compared with the normal segment.

Later experiments[122] were conducted to determine whether the tenderness itself was responsible for the lowered threshold of muscular activity or whether spinal reflexes at the same segmental level were in a facilitated state. It was shown that even when the tender spinous process was anaesthetised with procaine, the increased excitability of muscles was still demonstrable. Many experiments were performed and the results and interpretation were summarised by Korr[123] as follows:

An osteopathic lesion is associated with a segment of the spinal cord which has a low motor reflex threshold, i.e. it represents a hyperexcitable segment of the cord. At least in the lesioned segments studied by us it may be said that the balance has been shifted too far for too long toward the excitatory side.

The lowered reflex thresholds are demonstrable independently of the related spinous process. Even though changes in the palpable characteristics and in pain sensitivity of the spines are important diagnostic features, they are apparently secondary to other, more fundamental alterations in the cord.

The lesion represents an anterior root at least some of whose motoneurons are maintained in a state in which they are relatively hyper excitable to all impulses which reach them. In a severe lesion many of the motoneurons are so close to threshold, even when the subject is at rest and reclining comfortably, that it requires very few additional impulses from the neurons which synapse with them to trigger those motoneurons into overt activity. Those additional impulses may come apparently from almost any source; the spinous process is but one such source.

The lesion, therefore, is to be conceived, not as a radiating centre of irritation, spreading excitation to other segments, but rather as a segment upon which irritation is focussed. It represents a place in the cord where barriers to motoneuron excitation have been lowered and which, therefore, channelises impulses into muscles receiving motor innervation from that segment.

By 1947 research had confirmed that at the site of the vertebral lesion there was tenderness, pain, paraesthesiae and abnormal muscular tension. Further studies were then devised to record and measure changes in sympathetic activity in the region of the faulty joint.

It had been observed clinically that in the region of the spinal lesion there was increased sweating—a palpable dampness of the skin over the tender spinous processes and there was increased sensitivity of the skin to scratching, together with an increased histamine or 'red response' to such scratching, compared with other normal levels of the spine.

One way of determining the sudomotor activity of the skin is to test the resistance to the passage of an electrical current through the skin. Dry skin offers more resistance to the electrical flow compared with the moist skin. By adjusting the voltage to that which will not evoke a response on dry skin and yet will evoke a response in moist skin, areas of increased sudomotor activity can be delineated.

Repeated exploration over long periods on many subjects have shown that low resistance areas are present in all subjects; that the distribution of low resistance areas, that is, of sympathetic hyper-activity, varies from individual to individual, but that in a given individual the segmental distribution may remain constant for many months.[124]

These areas of lowered electrical skin resistance were found in subjects with visceral disease at segmental levels related to the diseased viscus. The lowered electrical skin resistance areas were increased by fatigue and by altering posture—e.g. by sitting in a tilted position for an hour, or by wearing a heel lift for a day. Injecting hypertonic saline intra-muscularly close to the spine also had a similar effect on sympathetic activity in the dermatome related to the injection site.

Another and quicker way[125] of recording the change in electrical skin resistance was evolved using a photographic method called a photo-graphic dermometer and the results of using this method tallied well with the slower hand method previously mentioned.

There is also a colorimetic method using the changes of colour of cobalt chloride from blue to red when moistened but this method is not as convenient as the photographic method. There is yet another way of evaluating the vasomotor activity in the lesioned area—i.e. by using thermocouples to measure temperature changes not only in the skin but in the subjacent muscles.

The next stage in research was to correlate the clinical palpatory findings, the lowered electrical resistance, the 'red' response to scratching the skin and the electromyographic activity in the same individual. There was a remarkable correspondence in all these changes in lesioned areas.[126]

4 The *study of spinal mechanics*, spinal anatomy and related physiology was the first preoccupation of the founder of osteopathy, A. T. Still. He was often seen with a femur under his arm—a constant reminder of his skeletal interests. Ashmore[127] made an excellent clinical study of spinal movements and scolioses which proved to be a guide to manipula-tive techniques, most of which have stood the test of time. Fryette continued these studies and in 1910 prepared an articulated mounting

of the bones of the body. Later in 1920 Halladay[128] prepared flexible spines and made observations on movements from it. His book contains the first really detailed study of spinal and rib movements.

Downing[129] in 1923 wrote about the concept of anatomical and physiological locking of the spine, both of which have helped in the development and rationalising of techniques. Beckwith[130] emphasised that manipulative forces should be directed along the plane of the facets. After forty years of applied study of spinal movements and mechanics, Fryette[131] published his book on *Principles of Osteopathic Technique* in 1954, and added to the range of techniques, but unfortunately he confused the issue by introducing the idea that flexion of the spine meant increasing the curve so that forward-bending in the thoracic area was called flexion, whereas in the cervical and lumbar areas forward-bending was called extension. This created considerable confusion and because the use of the terms was contrary to the standard medical definitions, I think he did a disservice to osteopathy in this way. In my own book on osteopathic technique I have attempted to dispel the confusion by using all terms in a standard medical sense. Bowles[132] helped to shift the emphasis from a structural static diagnosis of mechanical faults and stressed the importance of functional diagnosis. He went further than making mobility tests and described a sense of 'bind' or 'ease' in an articulation. This is most appropriate and even necessary when the ranges of movement are so small as to be impalpable or inaccessible.

My own small contribution in research is to establish *radiologically* that side-bending in the cervical spine is always accompanied by rotation to the same side whether there is any forward or backward-bending combined with the side-bending, whereas in the thoracic and lumbar areas of the spine, side-bending is accompanied by rotation to the opposite side if the commencing position is an erect one of extension. If, however, the starting position is full flexion, side-bending is then accompanied by rotation to the same side. This tallies with Ashmore's[127] clinical observations made in 1915.

In the context of modern medicine, research on the spine has been concentrated on the intervertebral disc especially since Beadle's[133] report on Schmorl's morbid anatomy studies (1925–1931) of the spine. Schmorl had made a close study of 7000 spines, 1000 of which were dissected in great detail. This work was continued with the help of Junghans, and their monumental studies were translated into English in 1959.[63] But it is interesting to see that early osteopathic research did not neglect the intervertebral disc even though more attention was paid to the apophyseal joints. The A. T. Still Research Institute[134] in 1931 recorded the changes in intervertebral discs of laboratory animals following artificially-produced spinal strains. The animals were examined post mortem and at intervals after the trauma:

The intervertebral discs of the lesioned area show swelling very soon after the lesion has been produced and this increases in amount for about one day, in ordinary laboratory animals. The swelling increases the size of the nucleus pulposus and increases the pressure upon the bodies of the vertebrae, and also upon the peripheral fibrous substance of the disc. The fibers of the substantia fibrosa become edematous, their extensibility is increased and their flexibility diminished. The bodies of the vertebrae are thus slightly separated, the mobility of the affected joints is slightly increased, and during this period spontaneous correction of the lesion is considerably facilitated. During the few weeks following the lesioning, the discs are subjected to persistent pressure due to the abnormal bony relations. Water is absorbed and the disc diminishes in thickness. The nucleus pulposus becomes progressively smaller and less resilient and in old cases the area originally occupied by this nucleus pulposus may show only a few thin, brittle, connective tissue fibers, enclosing only a few remnants of the original soft, elastic, resilient structure.

In 1933 Guy[135] postulated that disc protrusions into the vertebral bodies and spinal canal could be mistaken for osteopathic lesions. He says 'there is no doubt that once a disc has been affected by over-straining, there must be some change in the alignment of the vertebrae which to the uninitiated would appear as an ordinary vertebral lesion'.

Considerable confusion has occurred in the past and still occurs to this day between the syndrome of the simple spinal lesion of restricted mobility and the syndrome of the disc protrusion but *it is my earnest hope that this book will help to clarify the differences as well as to point the way to the diagnosis and treatment of all the varied conditions which affect the spine.*

REFERENCES

1 Still, A. T. *Autobiography*, p. 87. Kirksville, Missouri, 1908.
2 Downing, C. H. *Principles and Practice of Osteopathy*, p. 17. Williams, Kansas City, 1923.
3 Cole, W. V. 'Osteopathic Research', *J. Amer. Osteop. Ass.*, 1964, **63**, 821, 832.
4 Korr, I. M. 'The Emerging Concept of the Osteopathic Lesion', ibid., 1948, November issue.
5 Goldthwait, J. E., Brown, L. T., Swain, L. T., and Kuhns, J. G. *Essentials of Body Mechanics in Health and Disease*, p. 1. Lippincott, Philadelphia, 1945.
6 Korr, I. M., Wilkinson, P. N., and Cornock, F. W. 'Axonal Delivery of Neuroplasmic Components to Muscle Cells', *Science*, 1967, **155**, 342.
7 Denny-Brown, D., and Brenner, C. 'Lesions in Peripheral Nerve resulting from Compression by Spring Clip', *Arch. Neurol. Psychiat.*, 1944, **51**, 1.
8 Barlow, E. D., and Pochin, E. E. 'Slow Recovery from Ischaemia in Human Nerves', *Clin. Sci.*, 1948, **6**, 303.
9 Frykholm, R. 'Cervical Nerve Root Compression resulting from Disc Degeneration and Root Sleeve Fibrosis', *Acta chir. scand.*, 1951, **101**, 345.
10 Korr, I. M., Thomas, P. E., and Wright, H. M. 'Symposium on the Functional Implications of Segmental Facilitation', *J. Amer. osteop. Ass.*, 1955, January issue.
11 Glover, J. R. 'Back Pain and Hyperaesthesia', *Lancet*, 1960, **1**, 1165.
12 Denslow, J. S. 'Analysis of Variability of Spinal Reflex Thresholds', *J. Neurophys.*, 1944, **7**, 207.
13 Eble, J. N. 'Patterns of Responses of the Paravertebral Musculature to Visceral Stimulation', *Amer. J. Physiol.*, 1960, **198**, 429.
14 —— 'Reflex Relationships of Paravertebral Muscles', ibid., 1961, **200**, 939.
15 Spanos, N. C., and Andrew, J. C. 'Intermittent Claudication and Lateral Lumbar Disc Protrusions', *J. Neurol. Neurosurg. Psychiat.*, 1966, **29**, 273.
16 Joffe, R., Appleby, A., and Anjoua, V. 'Intermittent Ischaemia of the Cauda Equina due to Stenosis of the Lumbar Canal', ibid., 1966, **29**, 315.
17 *Samson Wright's Applied Physiology*, 10th edition, edited by C. A. Keele and E. Neil, pp. 160, 356. Oxford University Press, London, 1961.
18 Cox, A. G., and Bond, M. R. 'Bowel Habit after Vagotomy and Gastro-jejunostomy', *Brit. med. J.*, 1964, **1**, 460.
19 van Slyke, D. D., Rhoads, C. P., Hiller, A., and Alving, A. S. 'Relation-

ships between Urea Excretion, Renal Blood Flow, Renal Oxygen Consumption and Diuresis', *Amer. J. Physiol.*, 1934, **109**, 336.

20 Hix, E. L. 'The Influence of the Autonomic Innervation on Renal Function', *J. Osteop.*, 1956, **63**, 15.

21 Herlin, L. *Sciatica and Pelvic Pain due to Lumbo-sacral Nerve Root Compression*, p. 15. Thomas, Springfield, Ill., 1966.

22 Roberts, R. A. *Chronic Structural Low Backache*, p. 66, Lewis, London, 1947.

23 Love, J. G., and Emmett, J. Z. 'Asymptomatic Protruded Lumbar Disc as a Cause of Urinary Retention', *Mayo Clin. Proc.*, 1967, **42**, 249.

24 Lewis, T., and Kellgren, J. H. 'Observations Relating to Referred Pain, Viscero-motor Reflexes and other Associated Phenomena'', *Clin. Sci.*, 1939, **4**, 47.

25 Freude, E., and Ruhmann, W. *Z. ges. exp. Med.*, 1926, **52**, 338.

26 Hansen, K., and von Staa, *Reflektorische und Algetische Krankheitszeichen der Inneren Organe*, p. 166. Thierne, Leipzig, 1938.

27 Dittmar, E. 'Cutaneo-Visceral Neural Pathways', *Brit. J. phys. Med.*, 1952, **15**, 208.

28 Farkas, A. 'Low Back Syndrome and Osteoporosis of the Spine', *Rheumatism*, 1950, **6**, 157.

29 Charnley, J. 'The Lubrication of Animal Joints in Relation to Reconstruction by Arthroplasty', *Ann. rheum. Dis.*, 1960, **19**, 10.

30 Eckholm, R., and Norbäch, B. 'On the Relationship between Articular Changes and Function', *Acta. orthop. scand.*, 1951, **21**, 81.

31 De Puky, P. 'The Physiological Oscillation of the Length of the Body', ibid., 1935, **6**, 338.

32 Davis, P. R. 'Posture of the Trunk During the Lifting of Weights', *Brit. med. J.*, 1959, **1**, 87.

33 Wyke, B. 'The Neurology of Joints', *Ann. roy. coll. Surg. Engl.*, 1967, **41**, 10.

34 Ibid., p. 5.

35 Ibid., p. 6.

36 Elliott, F. A. 'Tender Muscles in Sciatica', *Lancet*, 1944, **1**, 47.

37 Strange, F. G. St. C. 'Debunking the Disc', *Proc. roy. Soc. Med.*, 1966, **59**, 955.

38 Strong, R., Thomas, P. E., and Earl, W. D. 'Patterns of Muscle Activity in Leg, Hip and Torso during Quiet Standing', *J. Amer. osteop. Ass.*, 1967, **66**, 1035, 125.

39 Stoddard, A. 'The Short Leg and Low Backache Syndrome', a paper read to the International Congress of Physical Medicine, London, 1952.

40 *Epidemiology of Chronic Rheumatism*, edited by J. H. Kellgren, M. R. Jeffrey, and J. Ball, vol. I, p. 106. Blackwell, Oxford, 1963.

41 Lewis, T. *Pain*, p. 99. Macmillan, London, 1942.

42 See reference No. 5, p. 25.

43 Lewis, T. 'Suggestions Relating to the Study of Somatic Pain', *Brit. med J.*, 1938, **1**, 321.

44 Keele, K. D. 'Pain Sensitivity and the Pain Pattern of Cardiac Infarction', *Proc. roy. Soc. Med.*, 1967, **60**, 418.
45 See reference No. 41, p. 99.
46 Herlin, L. *Sciatic and Pelvic Pain due to Lumbo-sacral Nerve Root Compression*. Thomas, Springfield, Ill., 1966.
47 See reference No. 17, p. 322.
48 Gough, J. G., and Koepke, G. H. 'Electromyographic Determination of Motor Root Levels in Erector Spinae Muscles', *Arch. phys. Med.*, 1966, **47**, 9.
49 See reference No. 17, p. 323.
50 Mennell, J. B. *Physical Treatment by Movement, Manipulation and Massage*. Churchill, London, 1945.
51 Mennell, J. McM. *Joint Pain*. Churchill, London, 1964.
52 Roston, J. B., and Wheeler Haines, R. 'Cracking in the Metacarpo-phalangeal Joint', *J. Anat.*, 1947, **81**, 165.
53 See reference No. 17, p. 274.
54 Ibid., p. 277.
55 Ibid., p. 233.
56 *Joint Motion: A Method of Measuring and Recording*, published by the American Academy of Orthopedic Surgeons, 1965.
57 Crisp, E. J. *Disc Lesions*, p. 27. Livingstone, London, 1960.
58 Charnley, J. 'Orthopaedic Signs in the Diagnosis of Disc Protrusions', *Lancet*, 1951, **1**, 189.
59 Cyriax, J. *Textbook of Orthopaedic Medicine*. Cassell, London, 1957.
60 Hackett, J. S. *Joint Ligament Relaxation*. Thomas, Springfield, Ill., 1957.
61 Williams, P. C. *The Lumbosacral Spine*. McGraw-Hill, New York, 1965.
62 Mennell, J. McM. *Back Pain*, Churchill. London, 1960.
63 Schmorl, G., and Junghans, H. *The Human Spine in Health and Disease*. American edition, Grune and Stratton, New York, 1959.
64 Robson, P. N. 'Hyperextension and Haematomyelia', *Brit. med. J.*, 1956, **2**, 848.
65 Hettinger, T., and Müller, E. A. 'Muskalleistung und Muskeltraining', *Arbeitsphysiologie*, 1953, **15**, 126.
66 Gillespie, H. W. 'The Significance of Congenital Lumbo-sacral Anomalies', *Brit. J. Radiol.*, 1949, **22**, 270.
67 Bailey, H. W., and Beckwith, C. G. 'Short Leg and Spinal Anomalies', *J. Amer. osteop. Ass.*, 1937, **36**, 7.
68 Brain, W. R. 'Spondylosis, the Known and the Unknown', *Ann. rheum. Dis.*, 1954, **13**, 2.
69 Frykholm, R. 'The Lower Cervical Vertebrae and Intervertebral Discs', *Acta chir. scand.*, 1951, **101**, 345.
70 *Any Questions?*, vol. II, p. 875, published by the British Medical Association, London, 1966.
71 See reference No. 63, p. 195.
72 Brain, R. 'Some Unsolved Problems of Cervical Spondylosis', *Brit. med. J.*, 1963, **1**, 772.

73 Collins, D. H. *The Pathology of Articular and Spinal Disease*, p. 302. Arnold, London, 1949.

74 See reference No. 40, p. 100.

75 Ferguson, A. B. *Roentgen Diagnosis of the Extremities and Spine*, p. 382. Hoeber, New York, 1941.

76 Henderson, E. D. 'Results of the Surgical Treatment of Spondylolisthesis', *J. Bone Jt Surg.*, 1966, **48A**, 619.

77 Newman, P. H. 'The Etiology of Spondylolisthesis', Ibid., 1963, **45B**, 39,

78 Barlow, E. D., and Pochin, E. E. 'Slow Recovery from Ischaemia in Human Nerves', *Clin. Sci.*, 1948, **6**, 303.

79 Masturzo, A. 'Vertebral Traction for Treatment of Sciatica', *Rheumatism*, 1955, **11**, 62.

80 Christie, B. G. B. *Proc. roy. Soc. Med.*, 1955, **48**, 814.

81 Armstrong, J. R. *Lumbar Disc Lesions*, p. 60. Livingstone, Edinburgh, 1952.

82 Shepherd, R. H. 'Diagnosis and Prognosis of Cauda Equina Syndrome produced by Protrusion of Lumbar Disc', *Brit. med. J.*, 1959, **2**, 1434.

83 Young, J. 'Relation of the Pelvic Joints in Pregnancy', *J. Obstet. Gynaec. Brit. Emp.*, 1940, **47**, 493.

84 Sashin, D. 'A Critical Analysis of the Anatomy and the Pathologic Changes of the Sacro-Iliac Joint', *J. Bone Jt Surg.*, 1930, **12A**, 895.

85 Payne, E. E., and Spillane, J. D. 'The Cervical Spine: An Anatomico-pathological Study', *Brain*, 1957, **80**, 571.

86 Cook, J. B. 'Relationship of Spinal Cord Damage to Cervical Spinal Injury', *Proc. roy. Soc. Med.*, 1959, **52**, 799.

87 Bowden, R. E. M., Abdullah, S., and Gooding, M. R. in *Cervical Spondylosis*, edited by Lord Brain and M. Wilkinson, p. 68. Heinemann, London, 1966.

88 Maigne, R. *Les Manipulations Vertébrales*, p. 63, Expansion Scientifique Française, Paris, 1960.

89 Donald, H. R. 'The Carpal Tunnel Syndrome', *Lancet*, 1965, **2**, 740.

90 See reference No. 17, p. 281.

91 Bickerstaff, E. R. 'Headaches', *Proc. roy. Soc. Med.*, 1967, **60**, 600.

92 See reference No. 1, p. 32.

93 Ryan, G. M. S. and Cope, S. 'Cervical Vertigo', *Lancet*, 1955, **2**, 1357.

94 Campbell, A. M. G., and Lloyd, J. K. 'Atypical Facial Pain', ibid., 1954, **2**, 1034.

95 Trevor Hughes, J. *Pathology of the Spinal Cord*, p. 118. Lloyd-Luke, London, 1966.

96 Kremer, M. 'Sitting, Standing and Walking', *Brit. med. J.*, 1958, **2**, 63.

97 Roberts, A. H. 'Myelopathy due to Cervical Spondylosis treated by Collar Immobilisation', *Neurology (Minneap.)*, 1966, **16**, 951.

98 James, J. L., and Miles, D. W. 'Neuralgic Amyotrophy: A Clinical and Electromyographic Study', *Brit. med. J.*, 1966, **2**, 1042.

99 Scheuermann, H. 'Kyphosis Dorsalis Juvenalis', *Z. orthop. Chir.*, 1921, **41**, 305.

100 Beadle, O. A. *Spec. Rep. Ser. med. Res. Coun.* (*Lond.*), 1931, no. 161, H.M. Stationery Office.

101 Roaf, R. *Scoliosis*, p. 73. Williams and Wilkins, London, 1966.

102 See reference No. 61, p. 129.

103 Bloom, H. J. G., Ellis, H., and Jennett, W. B. 'The Early Diagnosis of Spinal Tumours', *Brit. med. J.*, 1955, **1**, 10.

104 Gautier-Smith, P. C. 'Physical Factors in the Production of the Myelopathy of Cervical Spondylosis', *Brain*, 1967, **90**, 359.

105 Mackenzie, J. *Symptoms and their Interpretation*, p. 74. Shaw & Sons, London, 1920.

106 Denslow, J. S. 'An Approach to Skeletal Components in Health and Disease.' Paper presented to the 45th Annual Convention of the American Osteopathic Association, Chicago, July, 1950. Reprinted in 1963 *Year Book, Academy of Applied Osteopathy*.

107 Schwab, W. A. 'Principles of Manipulative Treatment. The Low Back Problem', *J. Amer. Osteop. Assn.*, March, 1934.

108 Pearson. 'Research of Ten Years of Progress', *J. Osteop.*, February 1949.

109 Kraus, E. R. 'Postural Roentgen Study', 1966 *Year Book, Academy of Applied Osteopathy*, p. 106.

110 Bandeen, S. G. 1948 *Year Book, Academy of Applied Osteopathy*.

111 Northup, T. L. 'Manipulative Management of Hypertension', 1957 *Year Book, Academy of Applied Osteopathy*, p. 43.

112 Norris, T. 'A Study of the Effect of Manipulation on Blood Pressure', 1964 *Year Book, Academy of Applied Osteopathy*, p. 184.

113 Castlio, Y., and Ferris-Swift, L. 'Effects of Splenic Stimulation in Normal Individuals in the Actual and Differential Blood Cell Count and the Opsonic Index', College Journal of the Kansas City College of Osteopathy and Surgery, 1932, **16**, 10. Reprinted in the *Year Book, Academy of Applied Osteopathy*, 1955, p. 111.

114 McConnell, C. P. 'Ventral Technique', 1951 *Year Book, Academy of Applied Osteopathy*, p. 1.

115 Magoun, H. J. *Osteopathy in the Cranial Field*, 1951. Published by the Journal Printing Co., Kirksville, Missouri.

116 Littlejohn, J. M. 'The Beginnings of the Research Movement', *The Osteopathic Physician*, 1908, Dec., p. 11.

117 McConnell, C. P. 1951 *Year Book, Academy of Applied Osteopathy*, p. 48.

118 Burns, L. 'The Laboratory Proofs of the Osteopathic Lesion'. Presented at the American Osteopathic Association Convention, Seattle.

119 Hix, E. L. 'Uretero-Renal Reflex Facilitating Renal Vasoconstriction Responses to Emotional Stress', *Amer. J. Physiol.*, 1958, **192**, 1, 191.

120 Korr, I. M., Wilkinson, P. M., and Chornock, F. W. 'Axonal Delivery of Neuroplasmic Components to Muscle Cells', *Science*, 1967, **155**, 342.

121 Denslow, J. S., and Clough, H. G. 'Reflex Activity in the Spinal Extensors', *J. Neurophysiol*, 1941, **4**, 430.

122 Denslow, J. S., Korr, I. M., and Krems, A. D. 'Quantitative Studies of

Chronic Facilitation in Human Motoneuron Pools', *Amer. J. Physiol.*, 1947, **105**, 229.

123 Korr, I. M. 'The Neural Basis of the Osteopathic Lesion', 1947. Reprinted in 1963 *Year Book, Academy of Applied Osteopathy*, p. 49.

124 Korr, I. M. 'The Three Fundamental Problems in Osteopathic Research', 1950. Reprinted in 1963 *Year Book, Academy of Applied Osteopathy*, p. 83.

125 Thomas, P. E., and Korr, I. M. 'The Automatic Recording of Electrical Skin Resistance Patterns on the Human Trunk', *Electroenceph. clin. Neurophysiol.*, 1951, **3**, 361.

126 Korr, I. M., Thomas, B. S., and Wright, H. M. 'Symposium on the Functional Implications of Segmental Facilitation', J. Amer. Osteop. Ass. Jan. 1955. Reprinted in the 1963 *Year Book, Academy of Applied Osteopathy*, p. 121.

127 Ashmore. *Osteopathic Mechanics*, 1915. Journal Printing Co., Kirksville.

128 Halladay, H. V. 'Applied Anatomy of the Spine.' Reprinted in 1957 *Year Book, Academy of Applied Osteopathy*, p. 119.

129 Downing, C. H. *Principles and Practice of Osteopathy*, p. 202, Williams Publishing Co., Kansas, Missouri, 1923.

130 Beckwith, C. G. *Vertebral Mechanics*, reproduced in 1957 *Year Book, Academy of Applied Osteopathy*.

131 Fryette, H. H. *Principles of Osteopathic Technique*, 1954. Academy of Applied Osteopathy, Carmel, California.

132 Bowles, C. H. 'Functional Orientation for Technique', 1957 *Year Book, Academy of Applied Osteopathy*.

133 Beadle, O. A. 'The Intervertebral Discs. Observations on their Normal and Morbid Anatomy in Relation to Certain Spinal Deformities', 1931.

134 A. T. Still Research Institute, Bulletin No. 7, Chicago, Illinois, 1931, p. 12.

135 Guy, A. E. *J. Amer. Osteop. Ass.*, 1933, **32**, 7, Reprinted in 1949 *Year Book, Academy of Applied Osteopathy*.

The above *Year Books of the Academy of Applied Osteopathy* are obtainable from M. W. Barnes, P.O. Box 1050, Carmel, California, U.S.A.

INDEX

Adhesions, 37, 43, 81, 117, 120, 170, 193, 210
Alkaptonuria, 265
Amyotrophic neuropathy, 235
Anaesthesia: local, 16, 106; epidural and extradural, 142, 179; general, 174
Ankylosing spondylitis, 190, 242
Anomalies, 111, 132
Apophyseal joints: cervical, 221, 226; effusions in, 91; inflammation in, 208; nerve supply, 31; osteo-arthritis of, 150, 163; synovial fringes in, 29
Articular processes, 86, 204
Articulatory treatment, 20

Bed design, 130, 148
Blood pressure, 283
Body types, 57
Bone, mechanical effects on, 23

Calvé's disease 261
Carpal tunnel, 3, 10, 218
Cartilage, mechanical effects on, 25
Cauda equina lesions, 3, 16, 182
Cervical myelopathy, 18, 234
Clicks, 45, 82
Clinical examination, 92
Coccydynia, 193
Collagen diseases, 89, 239
Collar, 209, 212, 227
Congenital faults, 132, 207, 214
Contra-indications for manipulation, 179, 279
Corsets, 34, 126, 180
Cranial technique, 283

Deltoid palsy, 217
Dercum's disease, 90
Disc lesions, xxi, 26, 44, 102, 130 acute episodic, 137; affecting 3L nerve root, 180; central type, 182; cervical, 210; herniation, 140, 143; in lordosis, 159; in spondylolisthesis, 166; in young adults, 141, 181; paralytic type, 182; prevention of attacks, 149; prolapse, 140, 172; thoracic, 199
Dowager's Hump, 239
Drop attacks, 234
Dura mater, 71

Erythromelalgia, 171
Exercises, 128, 149, 165

Facial neuralgia, 232
Facial palsy, 232
Facial spasm, 233
Facilitated segment, 8, 11, 32
Fibrositis, 32, 54, 91, 203, 210, 226, 237
Foramen (intervertebral), 10, 168, 205, 206, 213
Fractures of the spine, 251, 263
Functional disorders, 56

Ganglion (posterior root), 10, 11, 204
Gout, 136, 255
Gynaecological backache, 266

Haemangioma, 263
Hands, xix, 273
Headaches, 227, 230
Heel lifts, 134, 253
Height (diurnal variation), 27
Herpes zoster, 72, 136
History taking, 92
Hypermobility, 42, 43, 59, 80, 116,
   119, 131; etiology, 123; of
   cervical spine, 209; treatment of,
   126
Hypomobility, 37, 43, 60

Inhibition (and stimulation), 238
Intermittent claudication, 14, 105

Joint Bind, 45, 81, 114, 208
Joint Play, 75

Kissing spines, 159
Kyphosis, 206, 240, 244

Lifting, 27
Ligaments, 24, 60, 120, 127;
   dentate, 10; flavum, 25
Locking, 81
Lordosis, 65, 102, 156, 163, 206
Luschka (joints of), 204, 206
Lymphatics, 21

Malignant disease of the spine, 261
Ménière's syndrome, 231
Meralgia paraesthetica, 171, 183
Metatarsalgia, 183
Migraine, 229
Morquio's disease, 265
Multiple myelomatosis, 263
Muscles: acute episodes, 136;
   contracture, 88; exercises of, 128;
   guarding of, 54, 88, 95;
   mechanical effects, 32; occipitalis
   m., 225; pain in, 52, 67, 105,

225; scalene m., 205, 214;
   semispinatis capitis m., 225, 226;
   spinal m., 51; sustained
   contraction in muscle syndromes,
   54, 87, 237; tone, 87

Neoplasms: intraspinal, 263;
   vertebral, 261
Nerves: compression of, 7, 8;
   irritation of, 9, 10; ischaemia of,
   9; oedema of, 8; severance of, 6;
   traction of, 7
Nerve roots: anatomy, 168, 204;
   cervical level, 211; lumbar level,
   141; paralysis, 182
Nervous tension, 62, 222
Neuralgic amyotrophy, 236
Nodules, 90

Oedema, 19, 91
Osteitis condensans ilii, 186, 188
Osteoarthritis of spinal joints, 150,
   154, 163, 226
Osteochondrosis, 200, 240, 253, 261
Osteomalacia, 250
Osteomyelitis, 261
Osteopathic spinal lesion: definition
   of, 36; features of, 39; locking in,
   82
Osteopathy: art of, 270; definition
   of, xvi, 1; principles of, xx, 1
Osteophytes, 259
Osteoporosis, 95, 245, 261

Paget's disease, 252, 264
Pain (lower extremity), 170
Pain (upper extremity), 171
Pain (spinal): activity pain, 104;
   autonomic pain, 71; causes of,
   110; compression pain, 52, 68,
   101; positional pain, 101;
   referred pain, 66, 71; stretch
   pain, 52, 68, 101; visceral disease
   pain, 266

Palpation, 72, 94, 97
Panniculitis, 67, 90, 239
Paraesthesiae, 73
Partes interarticulares, 162
Position (cf. mobility), 2, 83
Position (of a vertebra), 44
Posture, 4, 20, 61, 129, 150,
    220, 243
Proctalgia fugax, 194

Rami communicantes, 11, 221
Rapport, 118, 276
Reaction (to treatment), 117
Red response, 92, 287
Research, xvii, 11, 12, 110, 281
Rib lesions, 196; cervical, 214

Sacro-iliac joints: diseases of, 186;
    lesion characteristics, 184;
    mobility of, 184; sacral springing
    test, 185; tuberculosis of, 261
Saturday night paralysis, 217
Schmorl's nodes, 24, 28, 242
Sclerosants, 126, 166, 188
Scoliosis, 34, 65, 83, 252
Short leg, 35, 106, 131, 132, 253
Skin resistance (electrical), 92, 288
Spinal cord: blood supply, 18, 21,
    169, 220; compression of, 104
Spinous processes, 46, 85, 204;
    kissing spines, 159
Spondylolisthesis, 162
Spondylolysis, 162
Spondylosis, 18, 150, 154, 203, 245
Spondylosis deformans, 191
Still, A. T.. xiii, 228, 281
Strapping, 146
Structure (and Function), xiii, 2, 4
Subluxations, 3, 208, 222
Sudomotor disturbances, 55, 97,
    287
Surgery: in disc prolapse, 172;
    in spondylolisthesis, 167
Sympathectomy, 14
Syndromes: acute episodic, 136;

adhesions, 114; anterior tibial,
    171; brachial, 203; carpal tunnel,
    218; chronic degenerative, 150;
    coccygeal, 193; costo-clavicular,
    215; costo-scalene, 214; ear, 230;
    eye, 233; facial, 232; foraminal
    compression, 213; headache, 227;
    inflammatory apophyseal, 208;
    Klippel-Feil, 233; Ligamentous
    strain, 119; lordosis, 156;
    neoplastic, 261; nerve root, 168;
    nervous tension, 222; occipital
    and upper cervical, 219;
    prolapsed lumbar disc, 173;
    psychogenic, 267; rib, 196, 201;
    sacro-iliac, 184; scoliosis, 252;
    short leg, 131; soft tissue, 236;
    stiff back, 192; tarsal tunnel,
    183; thoracic, 194; thoracic
    outlet, 214; Tietze's, 202;
    visceral backache, 265
Synovial fluid, 26
Synovial membrane, 29, 82

Temporal arteritis, 229
Tenderness, 50, 72, 287
Tests: active and passive mobility,
    94; cervical lateral mobility, 96;
    costo-clavicular compression, 216;
    costo-vertebral, 196; Ely's, 104,
    180; foraminal compression, 104,
    210; isometric muscle
    contraction, 55; mobility, 74;
    muscle palpation, 98; neck
    flexion, 103; sacral springing,
    185; skin puckering, 89;
    skin rolling, 90; spinal traction,
    115, 210; springing, 53, 95;
    straight leg raising, 103, 178, 181
Tinnitus, 230
Torticollis, 208
Traction, 25; for osteoarthritis, 154;
    adjustive manual, 144, 200, 245;
    intermittent sustained, 212, 227;
    prone, 46; rhythmic adjustive,
    116; sustained, 172, 212; test,

115, 210; types of, 143; vertical,
212
Transverse processes, 46, 85, 97, 204
Trauma, 63, 136, 207
Tuberculosis: sacro-iliac, 187;
spinal, 54, 242, 260

Ulnar neuritis, 217

Vasomotor disturbances, 3, 14, 18,
19, 55
Venous congestion, 9, 21, 22
Vertigo, 231

Visceromotor disturbances, 3, 15,
16, 55, 239

Whiplash injury, 122
Winged scapula, 217
Wolff's law, 24

X-rays: cupid's bow effect, 24;
erect, 86, 100, 134;
functional, 80, 100, 122;
in disc protrusions, 142; in
lordosis, 162; in osteoporosis,
247; in practice, 273; mobility
100, 207; of cervical spine,
207, 227; radiological research, 228